Whole Person Care

Tom A. Hutchinson
Editor

Whole Person Care

A New Paradigm for the 21st Century

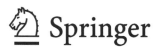 Springer

Editor
Tom A. Hutchinson
McGill University, McGill Programs
in Whole Person Care
Pine Ave W. 546
H2W 1S6 Montreal Québec
Canada
tom.hutchinson@mcgill.ca

ISBN 978-1-4419-9439-4   e-ISBN 978-1-4419-9440-0
DOI 10.1007/978-1-4419-9440-0
Springer New York Dordrecht Heidelberg London

Library of Congress Control Number: 2011926588

Springer is part of Springer Science+Business Media (www.springer.com)

Introductory

"The practice of medicine is an art, not a trade; a calling, not a business; a calling in which your heart will be exercised equally with your head."

William Osler, 1903

"The computer cannot participate in the true art of medicine. It has none of the subtle sensory perception, intellectual imagination, and emotional sensitivity necessary for communicating with people and giving clinical care."

Alvan R. Feinstein, 1967

"To be not the servants of science, nature, nations, personal beliefs or even our desire to preserve life. Understanding the reality of our own mortality, we endeavour, instead, to heal our fellow human beings and free them from constraint, so that they may flourish."

McGill Medical Class of 2012,
Pledge at White Coat Ceremony, 2009

Foreword

"Not everything that can be counted counts and not everything that counts can be counted."

Albert Einstein[1]

Why a book on "Whole Person Care"?

This book addresses issues that are profoundly relevant to each of us – both as caregivers and in our daily lives. It suggests that we have the opportunity to participate in the birth of a new paradigm, one that entails a radical reframing of both diagnosis and therapeutics; how we see those we are caring for; how we see others; how we see ourselves.

Science historian and philosopher Thomas Kuhn suggested that instead of advancing in a linear fashion, scientific progress is marked by intermittent crossroads at which the accepted conceptual world view is replaced by a new one, a perspective that scientists previously would not have considered valid. The former paradigm (the "old" way of seeing) now is considered "thinking inside the box," while the new is the product of "thinking outside the box." The new does not necessarily negate the old. For example, Newtonian mechanics still offered a good model for understanding speeds below the speed of light, even after it had given way to the new paradigm represented by Einstein's theory of relativity and quantum physics[2] [1–3].

From Hippocrates (460–377 B.C.E.) until the early years of the nineteenth century C.E., the dominant paradigm of western medicine was "humorism," a system which appeared to provide a useful framework for understanding the human body and its ills. The four humors of Hippocratic medicine were black bile (melankholia), yellow bile (cholera), phlegm (phlegma), and blood (sanguis). Each humor had its own ascribed associations and properties: health required that the four humors be "in balance" [4, 5]. As its influence waned over the early decades of the nineteenth century, humorism was folkloric in tone and passed on through brief, loosely structured preceptorship programs, many of dubious quality.

A growing array of observations during the latter half of the nineteenth century led to a new norm, that of science-based healthcare. For example, the observations, in France, of microbiologist and chemist Louis Pasteur (1822–1895) resulted in the germ theory of disease.[3]In 1864, the English surgeon Joseph Lister (1827–1912), Professor of Surgery in Glasgow, was told of Pasteur's work and correctly suspected its relevance to surgical wound infections.[4] This insight resulted in the development of antisepsis and a dramatic decrease in surgical risks. Before Lister, a two to three hundred bed hospital might record 400 operations a year, 25% of them being amputations. After Lister, the same hospital might undertake 4,000–5,000 operations a year, with less than 1% amputations! [6]. A giant step toward a science-based understanding of disease had been taken. The work of Marie Curie[5] and Florence Nightingale,[6] the development of laboratory medicine and radiology, and the founding of the Rockefeller Institute for Medical Research in 1901[7] were among the many advancements that assured the continuing growth of medical science and the increasing use of its celebrated tools, the randomized double blind clinical trial and evidence-based therapeutics. The academic seal of approval for this emerging paradigm with its inductive approach to logical thinking, took the form of a detailed review of North American medical education by the nonmedical educator Abraham Flexner, a study sponsored by the Carnegie Foundation for the Advancement of Teaching. The result, known as the Flexner Report [7], triggered sweeping reforms in medical education standards, organization and curriculum, through the adoption of a science-based model of disease coupled with obligatory hands-on clinical experience. As a result, many existing preceptorship training programs were closed and the remaining schools were reformed to conform to Flexner's recommendations. Over the ensuing years, statistically-significant data, generated by rigorous quantitative studies became the only portal to acceptability in medical research, practice, and teaching. Some voiced concern that in the process something had been lost; that the objectifying, depersonalizing, and quantifying had perhaps carried with it an element of reductionism. But the results spoke for themselves!

And yet, and yet … ! Something was missing. The science-based paradigm often failed to reflect lived experience. Why?

When, over a quiet lunch, I asked one eminent quality of life (QOL) theorist why he had casually dropped "spirituality" from the list of QOL determinants cited by respondents in his study, he commented, "It didn't correlate statistically with the other variables, and besides, they don't give research grants to study spirituality"[8] [8, 9]. That was understandable. The accepted paradigm drives the research agenda, and after all, "spirituality" seemed an unlikely source of cutting-edge scientific insight.

The lack of precision in defining some elements of subjective experience remains problematic. Concepts such as "spirit," "spiritual," "soul," "existential," "love," "suffering," "dignity," "healing," … are vague, at best. Often, such terms mean simply what the user wants them to mean; nothing more, nothing less. Furthermore, the domains in question seem to concern fantasy rather than tangible fact. The waters negotiated as one passes from considerations physical, to social, to psychological, to spiritual become mirky indeed. Why, French paleontologist, biologist, and philosopher Teilhard de Chardin (1881–1955), who spent his life trying to integrate religious experience with natural science, went so far as to say, "We are not human beings having a spiritual experience, but spiritual beings having a human experience." How can one put a p-value on such things? The social sciences have used qualitative research techniques to investigate such issues, but those strategies were deemed unreliable by quantitative science purists.

Meanwhile, daily experience has suggested that transcendence, meaning, hope, and "healing connections," may lift one beyond despair and reduce, even eliminate, suffering; conversely, uncertainty, fear, and an experience of loss of control, may amplify suffering even in the absence of physical distress. If, as suggested by the ancient metaphorical schema, we are "body, mind and spirit," (however understood), those elements are inseparable and interdependent, and, that mix of influences consistently modifies our experience of health and illness. Nevertheless, this is largely ignored in the diagnoses and therapy embodied in the science-based paradigm.

Variables that fall peripheral to the accepted science-based view of disease, appear to directly influence human suffering, sense of well-being, and even length of life. The evidence surfaces on a daily basis.

- In the midst of the unimaginable hell of a Nazi concentration camp, Viktor Frankl experienced transcendence. He described the moment. "In a last violent protest against the hopelessness of imminent death, I sensed my spirit piercing through the enveloping gloom. I felt it transcend that hopeless, meaningless world, and from somewhere I heard a victorious "Yes" in answer to my question of the existence of an ultimate purpose" [10]. Why and how did that occur?

- Amid the torrent of feelings pouring from his pen, the dying 31-year-old poet Ted Rosenthal commented, "I'm changed; I'll always be changed. I'll always be happier for what I have been through, only because it has enabled me to have the courage to open myself up to anything that happens and I am no longer afraid of death. At least I am not afraid of death the way I might have been had I not become sick" [11]. "Happier?" As a poet, Rosenthal chose the word with care. If QOL is relevant in all health care (not simply in end-of-life care) our scientific curiosity must surely be broadened to include the why and how of Rosenthal's improbable statement.

- A dying patient commented to Dr. Cicely Saunders on admission to St. Christopher's Hospice, "I never would have dreamed that it would be safe to die here." Safe to die? What factors fostered the utterance of that apparent oxymoron?

- In a study of 50 cancer patients, Kagawa-Singer and colleagues found that subjective well-being did not correlate with physical status. Surprisingly, one-third of their sample assessed themselves to be "fairly well" and two-thirds rated themselves "very well," including 12 who died during the study. The coping objective common across subjects was "to maintain self-integrity" [12]. Should a medical paradigm that furthers the best interests of our patients not ask what determines a sense of "self-integrity" both in far advanced illness and in health. Should it not ask how that end is fostered?

- Cohen et al documented the significant contributions to QOL made by the existential-spiritual domain (Ex'l/Sp) using the McGill QOL Instrument (MQOL): With cancer patients: Ex'l/Sp was a significant QOL contributor for people at various stages of the disease; it was as important as any other domain measured by MQOL subscales [13, 14]; With HIV patients: Ex/Sp was only significant when CD4 count was <100 (i.e., with AIDS), but then it was the most important contributor to QOL [15].

- A woman with breast cancer observed, "I may have significant pain but no anguish, no suffering. Conversely, I may be symptom free and suffer terribly." Similarly, Eric Cassell observed, "Our intactness as persons, our coherence and integrity, come not only from intactness of the body but from the wholeness of the web of relationships with self and others." He then noted ruefully, "the profession of medicine appears to ignore the human spirit" [16]. If that is the case, based on the evidence at hand, must not our paradigm change?

- In a qualitative study with dying patients at our center, common themes at the QOL extremes ("anguish" versus "equanimity and peace") were identified. The common themes identified at the "anguish" end of the QOL continuum included: a sense of isolation, an absence of meaning, preoccupation with future and past, a sense of victimization, and a high need for control. In contrast, common themes at the "peace" end were: a sense of connectedness to something larger and more enduring than the self, meaning discovered, presence to the moment, a sympathetic connection to suffering, and a capacity to open to a present potential that is greater than the need for control [17]. Such themes are irrelevant to the existing medical paradigm with its singular preoccupation with the biology of disease.

- The quality of caregiver presence has been identified as a critical therapeutic variable – one that is ignored by the current medical paradigm. Dame Cicely reminded us, "The *way* care is given can reach the most hidden places and give space for unexpected development," [18] thus echoing Michael Balint's comment, "By far the most frequently used drug in general practice is the doctor himself, … it is … the <u>way</u> that 'drug' is given - in fact, the whole atmosphere in which the drug is given and taken (that matters most)" (quote with tense changed from past to present and underlining added) [19]. If the quality of personal presence is to be our students' "most frequently used drug," is it not curious that the science-based paradigm does not consider the issue essential in the undergraduate medical curriculum?

- Four potent existential challenges haunt us throughout life: death (existential obliteration), isolation (the unbridgeable gap between self and others), freedom (the unnerving absence of external structure), and meaning (in a world of uncertain meaning) [20]. These threats are intensified in illness, but they lie beyond the clearly drawn limits of the current medical paradigm and so are generally ignored in diagnostic and therapeutic deliberations.

- Philips and King found that meaning perceived may lead to death delayed. They documented decreased death rates in the week preceding Passover, a warmly anticipated holiday for the sample examined, and a compensatory increase in death rates following the celebration, especially among persons with unambiguous Jewish names ($p=0.045$), though not among black, oriental, or Jewish-infant control groups. The decline was particularly marked in years when the holiday fell on a long weekend, thus enabling loved ones to gather from greater distances ($p=0.001$) [21]. Yet, "meaning" is largely forgotten, both in our diagnostic considerations and as we plan our therapeutic interventions.

• The impact of meaning on immune response and an associated delay of death were reported by Bower et al. In their study, bereaved HIV-seropositive men were more likely to find meaning if they engaged in sustained cognitive processing of their loss. When greater meaning was experienced, subjects had a less rapid decline in CD4 T cell levels and lower AIDS-related mortality over 4–9 years. (all ps <0.05) [22]. The apparent association of meaning, immune response, and longevity might bring to mind the Philips and King study as we sit at the bedside asking ourselves how to best accompany this suffering individual.

Palliative Care offers a model of whole person care that includes consideration of psychosocial and spiritual factors in addition to the physical domain [23]. In a randomized study to assess the efficacy of palliative care, Temel et al. compared traditional oncology care plus palliative care (TOC+PC) to traditional oncology care alone (TOC). One hundred and fifty one patients with metastatic non-small cell lung cancer were randomized at diagnosis into one of these two treatment groups and followed for 3 years or until death. Assessments of QOL (FACT-L) and mood (MGH Anxiety and Depression Scales) were made at baseline and 12 weeks. The patients randomized to the palliative care group (TOC+PC) had: better QOL (p, 0.03), less depression (p, 0.01), greater mobility, less pain, and longer life (p, 0.02). The longer life noted in the palliative care group is of particular interest since participants in that group had requested, and received, less aggressive end-of-life care (p, 0.05) [24]. In another study, Cohen has shown that palliative care results in significant improvement in total QOL and all QOL subscale scores (MQOL) within the first week following admission to a palliative care unit [25]. The efficacy of whole person care and its counterintuitive capacity to support an increase in QOL even when introduced only days prior to dying, should be kept in mind as we consider the need for a new medical paradigm.

Tom Hutchinson asked each of the authors in this book to consider their field of personal interest from a "whole person care" vantage point to more directly address the full range of modifiers of subjective experience, suffering and "total pain," the course of disease, and optimum care. With the adoption of a whole person care paradigm, the research agenda will broaden. Among the many phenomena that may be seen as relevant to examine are the issues raised in the above bulleted list. There will be many others: such variables as the dissociated right brain functioning experienced by poststroke Jill Bolte Taylor who suggests that "we can at will choose to step into the consciousness of our right hemisphere, to be one with all that is," [26] and the possible significance of mirror neurons and their clinical relevance to empathy in health and illness [27–29].

A paradigm shift is needed. The decision, professional and personal, is up to each of us. The choice is ours.

Balfour M. Mount

End Notes

[1] While this observation is generally attributed to Einstein, the sociologist William Bruce Cameron made the same cogent comment in his 1963 text "Informal Sociology: a casual introduction to sociological thinking" (New York: Random House) and this is thought to be its first appearance in print. Some claim that Einstein wrote this quote on his blackboard at the Institute for Advanced Studies at Princeton, citing Sir George Pickering as the author. The phrases are in reverse order in some versions of this pithy aphorism. http://quoteinvestigator.com/2010/05/26/everything-counts-einstein/

[2] An example of a paradigm shift in which the new negated the old would be the assertion by Copernicus (1473–1543) that the earth rotates around the sun, thus negating the geocentric view of earlier thinkers such as Ptolemy and Aristotle.

[3] Pasteur's many contributions included vaccines for rabies and anthrax, a process for halting bacterial contamination of milk (pasteurization) and early development of the field of microbiology. www.zephyrus.co.uk/louispasteur.html.

[4] Thomas Anderson (1819–1874), Professor of Chemistry at the same University, drew Lister's attention to Pasteur's findings and to the antimicrobial effects of carbolic acid (phenol) in sewage treatment. http://www.universitystory.gla.ac.uk/biography/?id=WH2173&type=P.

[5] Marie Curie (1867–1934) was the first person to win two Nobel Prizes (Physics, 1903; Chemistry, 1911). Her contributions included: the theory of radioactivity; techniques for isolating radioactive isotopes; the discovery of two new elements – polonium and radium; the first use of radioactive isotopes in cancer treatment; the founding of research Institutes in Paris and Warsaw. http://nobelprize.org/nobel_prizes/physics/laureates/1903/marie-curie-bio.html.

[6] Florence Nightingale (1820–1910): superintendent, the Hospital for Invalid Gentlewomen, London (1853); volunteer for nursing duty in the Scutari hospital in Istanbul with the outbreak of the Crimean War (1854); founder of the Nightingale School for Nurses at Saint Thomas's Hospital, London (1860). A pioneer in the use of statistics, she collected mortality rate data for soldiers in the British army, both at home and in battle; invented polar-area (pie) charts to clarify and dramatize her findings; showed that improved sanitary conditions lead to a lowering of death rates; noted that crude death rates could be misleading and that mortality data considerations should be age-specific; introduced a system for recording sickness and mortality data in military hospitals; demonstrated that many hospital deaths were unnecessary; showed the value of maintaining accurate hospital statistics as an instrument for reform in hospital sanitation; demonstrated that "the connection between the health and dwellings of the population is one of the most important that exists." http://www.morris.umn.edu/~sungurea/introstat/history/w98/Nightengale.html

[7] The funding by John D. Rockefeller for the Institute, now the Rockefeller University, had been inspired by the vision of William Osler. It established an outstanding record for biomedical research that has led to more than 20 Nobel Prizes, beginning with Alexis Carrel in 1912. http://himetop.wikidot.com/the-rockefeller-institute-for-medical-research.

[8] Later, when the evidence supporting the significance of the spiritual domain increased, an add-on module to the FACT addressing spirituality was created. It has, in turn, further increased the evidence of its significance.

References

1. Kuhn TS. The structure of scientific revolutions. 2nd ed., enlarged. The University of Chicago Press, Chicago; 1970 (1962).
2. http://en.wikipedia.org/wiki/Paradigm.
3. http://webcache.googleusercontent.com/search?q=cache:nBLE2ZFY6qMJ:www.blupete.com/Literature/Biographies/Science/Copernicus.htm+copernicus&cd=2&hl=en&ct=clnk&gl=ca.

4. http://www.medterms.com/script/main/art.asp?articlekey=7120.
5. http://en.wikipedia.org/wiki/Humorism.
6. Clapesattle H. The Doctors Mayo. Minneapolis: The University of Minnesota Press; 1941. p. 268.
7. Flexner A. Medical education in the United States and Canada: a Carnegie Foundation for the Advancement of Teaching. New York: Carnegie Foundation for the Advancement of Teaching; 1910.
8. Cella DF, Tulsky DS, Gray G, et al. The Functional Assessment of Cancer Therapy Scale: development and validation of the general measure. J Clin Oncol. 1993;11:570–9.
9. Peterman AH, Fitchett G, Brady MJ, Hernandez L, Cella D. Measuring spiritual well-being in people with cancer: the Functional Assessment of Chronic Illness Therapy-Spiritual Well-Being Scale (FACIT-Sp). Ann Behav Med. 2002;24(1):49–58.
10. Frankl VE. Man's search for meaning. New York: Simon & Schuster; 1984 (1959). p. 51–2.
11. Rosenthal T. How could I not be among you? New York: Avon Books; 1971. p. 69.
12. Kagawa-Singer M. Redefining health: living with cancer. Soc Sci Med. 1993;37: 295–304.
13. Cohen SR, Mount BM. Living with cancer: "good" days and "bad" days what produces them? Can the McGill Quality of life Questionnaire distinguish between them? Cancer. 2000;89: 1854–65.
14. Cohen SR, Mount BM, Bruera E, Provost M, Rowe J, Tong K. Validity of the McGill Quality of Life Questionnaire in the palliative care setting: a multi-center Canadian study demonstrating the importance of the existential domain. Palliat Med. 1997;11:3–20.
15. Cohen SR, Hassan SA, Lapointe BJ, Mount BM. Quality of life in HIV disease as measured by the McGill quality of life questionnaire AIDS. 1996;10:1421–7.
16. Cassell EJ. The nature of suffering and the goals of medicine. New York: Oxford University Press; 1991. p. 40, 43.
17. Mount BM, Boston PH, Cohen SR. Healing connections: on moving from suffering to a sense of well-being. J Pain Symptom Manage. 2007;33:372–88.
18. Kearney M. Mortally wounded: stories of soul pain, death and healing. New York: Scribner; 1996. p. 14.
19. Balint M. The doctor, his patient and the illness. London: Churchill Livingstone; (1957) 2000. p. 1.
20. Yalom ID. Existential psychotherapy. New York: Basic Books; 1980.
21. Philips DP, King EW. Death takes a holiday: mortality surrounding major social occasions. Lancet. 1988;332:728–32.
22. Bower JE, Kemeny ME, Taylor SE, Fahey JL. Cognitive processing, discovery of meaning, CD4 decline, and AIDS-related mortality among bereaved HIV-seropositive men. J Consult Clin Psych. 1998;66:979–86.
23. Doyle D, Hanks G, Cherny N, Calman K. Oxford textbook of palliative medicine. 3rd ed. New York: Oxford University Press; 2004.
24. Temel JS, Greer JA, Muzikansky A, Gallagher ER, Admane S, Jackson VA, et al. Early palliative care for patients with metastatic non-small-cell lung cancer. N Engl J Med. 2010;363:733–42.
25. Cohen SR, Boston P, Mount BM, Porterfield P. Changes in quality of life following admission to palliative care units. Pall Med. 2001;15(5):363–37.
26. Taylor JB. My stroke of insight: a brain scientist's personal journey. New York: Viking; 2008.
27. Preston SD, de Waal FBM. Empathy: its ultimate and proximate bases. Behav Brain Sci. 2002;25:1–20.
28. de Waal FBM. Putting the altruism back into altruism: the evolution of empathy. Ann Rev Psychol. 2008;59:279–300.
29. Rifkin J. The empathic civilization: the race to global consciousness in a world in crisis. New York: Tarcher/Penguin; 2010.

Preface

This is a book primarily by physicians, for physicians and medical students. For this reason, we have used the terms physician and doctor frequently throughout the book and have looked at medicine mainly from the perspective of the physician rather than from other perspectives that would be equally valid. We have done this not to emphasize or promote the inevitable hierarchy in medical practice, but to speak authentically from a perspective of which we have intimate personal experience. Nevertheless we realize that most of what we are espousing is equally relevant to other healthcare workers who are essential partners in the implementation of whole person care. We also believe that this book will be of interest to patients and members of the general public. It is the internal resources of the individual persons who become patients that constitute the major untapped resource that whole person care and medicine needs to harness effectively in the twenty-first century*. To change medical practice in the direction of whole person care will require the participation of caregivers, receivers of care, and the general public. We have therefore attempted to make the book readable by all three concerned groups.

December 6, 2010   Tom A. Hutchinson

---

*It is largely to illustrate this point that we have included many stories of patients in our book. In all cases we have changed names and details to protect identity, except in one story at the end of the book where the patient's own name is used at his specific request.

Acknowledgements

They say it takes a small village to raise a child and perhaps the same applies to a book. The headman of this village is Balfour Mount whose leadership in Palliative Care and research on Quality of Life paved the way for the foundation of McGill Programs in Whole Person Care in 1999. He subsequently formed the McGill Faculty Working Group on Healing that began to explore most of the ideas that appear in this book. Michael Kearney was the coleader of the Working Group and both he and Balfour Mount have played pivotal roles in the development of ideas about healing in medicine and in the development of whole person care at McGill, including the preparatory work that lead directly to this book. The members of the Faculty Working Group on Healing were: Barbara Bodmer (Obstetrics and Gynecology); Donald Boudreau (Respirology); Marie-Jose Caron (Palliative Medicine); Gordon Crelinsten (Cardiology); Richard Cruess (Orthopedic Surgery); Sylvia Cruess (Endocrinology); Ina Cummings (Palliative Medicine); David Dawson (Internal Medicine); Michael Dworkind (Family Medicine and Palliative Care); Allan Fielding (Psychiatry); Vania Jimenez (Family Medicine); Michael Kearney (Internal Medicine and Palliative Care); Marc Laporta (Psychiatry); Krista Lawlor (Palliative Care); Stephen Liben (Pediatrics); Balfour Mount (Surgical Oncology and Palliative Care); Mark Smilovitch (Cardiology); Yvonne Steinert (Medical Education); Mark Yaffe (Family Medicine); and Jean Zigby (Family Medicine).

The larger community in which these developments took place was the McGill Faculty of Medicine and we would like to thank the leadership of the Faculty of Medicine, particularly former Deans of Medicine, Richard Cruess and Abraham Fuks, who created and nurtured the environment in which such developments were feasible, and current Dean Richard Levin who has continued active support of these developments. We would also particularly like to thank Sylvia and Richard Cruess whose pioneering work on Professionalism in Medicine fitted so well with our work on healing to create the McGill concept of Physicianship. We thank Donald Boudreau who, as Associate Dean, with the support of Dean Fuks, initiated many important changes in the undergraduate medical curriculum, including the Physicianship Curriculum which incorporates the teaching of healing and professionalism as an integral and mandatory part of the education of medical students at McGill, and continues to provide leadership in this area. Joyce Pickering, his successor, has continued to support this development as well as adding her own innovative perspective.

Within the medical faculty our main support has come from the Department of Medicine, the Department of Oncology and the Gerald Bronfman Centre for Clinical Research in Oncology, where our offices are located. We would like to express our sincere gratitude to Dr. Gerald Batist, Head of Oncology at McGill, whose open-minded leadership has helped and supported us at so many points along the way, and to his very able Administrative Officer, Frances Ezzy-Jorgensen. Within Oncology the members of the Palliative Care Division, in particular leaders Anna Towers, Krista Lawlor, Manny Borod, and Bernard Lapointe, have been a strong source of support.

A book, like a child, needs a family and the family in this case consisted of the in-house members of McGill Programs in Whole Person Care (past and present) whose passion for this work has overcome all obstacles: Balfour Mount, Helen McNamara, Patricia Dobkin, Dawn Allen, Angelica Todireanu, Eileen Lavery, Nancy Gair, Patricia Boston, and Robin Cohen. We would also like to thank Stephen Liben who is housed in Pediatrics, Gordon Crelinsten from Cardiology, Steve Jordan from Education, Mark Smilovitch from Cardiology, Antonia Arnaert from Nursing and Gail McEachern who have played an important role in the development of our Programs. We also thank, although we cannot name all of them, the hundreds of people, including members of the Faculty of Medicine, patients, and members of the general public, who have participated in our working groups, workshops, courses, seminars, film series, and other activities over the past 6 years.

Nothing happens without funding and we would like to express our thanks to the Donner Canadian Foundation who have been our most important and consistent source of support and the McGill Max Bell Fund and Foundation who provided funding at a crucial point in our development. We also thank the following organizations and individuals for their generous support: Kidney Foundation of Canada; Webster Foundation; Jewish General Hospital Weekend to End Breast Cancer; Purdue Pharma; Open Society; Cummings Foundation; KC Dhawan Foundation; William H. Donner Foundation; Abe & Ruth Feigelson Foundation; George H. Stedman Estate; Phyllis and Robert Burns.

Of course the main work that made this book possible was carried out by the authors of the individual chapters who responded so wonderfully to my request to contribute to a book on whole person care and were so flexible in accepting editorial advice. The book would not have been conceived in the first place without Richard Lansing from Springer who suggested the possibility following a 1-day session on whole person care at the 2008 Palliative Care Congress in Montreal. The manuscript would never have been completed without the meticulous work of Angelica Todireanu who managed the process so efficiently from beginning to end.

On a more personal note I would like to thank my mentors and role models: John Seely, Alvan Feinstein, Janet Christie-Seely, and Balfour Mount. I would like to thank all of my patients who have so profoundly affected my life, including those who have contributed their stories to this book. Last but not least, I would like to thank my own family: my wife June who is such a wonderful model of competence, integrity, practical sense, and support; and my three fantastic daughters, Kate, Clare, and Nora who represent the long future to which I hope this book may make a contribution.

Montreal, December 6, 2010   Tom A. Hutchinson

Contents

1 Whole Person Care 1
Tom A. Hutchinson

2 Suffering, Whole Person Care, and the Goals of Medicine 9
Eric J. Cassell

3 The Healing Journey 23
Tom A. Hutchinson, Balfour M. Mount, and Michael Kearney

**4 The Challenge of Medical Dichotomies
and the Congruent Physician–Patient Relationship
in Medicine** 31
Tom A. Hutchinson and James R. Brawer

**5 Separation–Attachment Theory in Illness and the Role
of the Healthcare Practitioner** 45
Gregory Fricchione

6 Empathy, Compassion, and the Goals of Medicine 59
Stephen Liben

7 Mindfulness and Whole Person Care 69
Patricia L. Dobkin

8 Healing, Wounding, and the Language of Medicine 83
Abraham Fuks

**9 Death Anxiety: The Challenge and the Promise
of Whole Person Care** 97
Sheldon Solomon and Krista Lawlor

10 Whole Person Self-Care: Self-Care from the Inside Out 109
Michael Kearney and Radhule Weininger

11 Prevention and Whole Person Care 127
Tom A. Hutchinson

**12 Whole Person Care and Complementary
and Alternative Therapies** 133
Mary Grossman

13 Spiritual Dimensions of Whole Person Care 149
Abdu'l-Missagh Ghadirian

14 Whole Person Care and the Revolution in Genetics 161
David S. Rosenblatt and Jennifer Fitzpatrick

15 Whole Person Care on a Busy Medical Ward 173
Gordon L. Crelinsten

16 Teaching Whole Person Care in Medical School 183
Helen Mc Namara and J. Donald Boudreau

**17 Whole Person Care, Professionalism,
and the Medical Mandate** 201
Richard L. Cruess and Sylvia R. Cruess

18 Whole Person Care: Conclusions 209
Tom A. Hutchinson

Appendix: The Nature of Persons and Clinical Medicine 219

Index 229

Contributors

James R. Brawer
Department of Anatomy and Cell Biology, Centre for Medical Education,
McGill University, Montreal, QC, Canada

J. Donald Boudreau
Core faculty, Centre for Medical Education, Arnold P. Gold Associate
Professor of Medicine, Director, Office of Physicianship and Curriculum
Development, Department of Medicine, Faculty of Medicine,
McGill University, Montreal, QC, Canada

Eric J. Cassell
Emeritus Professor of Public Health, Weill Medical College
of Cornell University, Adjunct Professor of Medicine,
Faculty of Medicine, McGill University, Montreal, QC, USA

Gordon L. Crelinsten
Associate Physician-in-Chief, McGill University Health Centre,
Associate Professor, Department of Medicine,
McGill University, Montreal, QC, Canada

Richard L. Cruess
Professor of Surgery and Member, Centre for Medical Education,
McGill University, Montreal, QC, Canada

Sylvia R. Cruess
Professor of Medicine and Member, Centre for Medical Education,
McGill University, Montreal, QC, Canada

Patricia L. Dobkin
Associate Professor, Department of Medicine, Programs in Whole Person Care,
McGill University, Montreal, QC, Canada

Jennifer Fitzpatrick
Director, MSc in Genetic Counselling Program,
McGill University, Montreal, QC, Canada

Gregory Fricchione
Associate Chief of Psychiatry, Director, Division of Psychiatry and Medicine,
Massachusetts General Hospital, Professor of Psychiatry,
Harvard Medical School, Boston, MA, USA

Abraham Fuks
Professor of Medicine, McGill University, Montreal, QC, Canada

Abdu'l-Missagh Ghadirian
Professor, Department of Psychiatry, McGill University, Montreal, QC, Canada

Mary Grossman
Director, Lung Cancer Brojde Centre, Segal Cancer Centre,
Jewish General Hospital, Montreal, QC, Canada

Tom A. Hutchinson
Professor, Faculty of Medicine, Director, Programs in Whole Person Care,
McGill University, Montreal, QC, Canada

Michael Kearney
Santa Barbara Cottage Hospital, Visiting Nurse and Hospice Care,
Santa Barbara, CA, USA

Krista Lawlor
Assistant Professor, Department of Oncology, Division of Palliative Care,
McGill University, Montreal, QC, Canada

Stephen Liben
Director, Pediatric Palliative Care Program, The Montreal Children's Hospital,
Associate Professor of Pediatrics, McGill University, Montreal, QC, Canada

Helen Mc Namara
Unit Chair, Physicianship 3, McGill Medical School, McGill Programs in Whole
Person Care, Centre for Medical Education, Faculty of Medicine,
McGill University, Montreal, QC, Canada

Balfour M. Mount
Eric M. Flanders Emeritus Professor of Palliative Care,
McGill University, Montreal, QC, Canada

David S. Rosenblatt
Professor and Chair, Department of Human Genetics,
Professor, Departments of Medicine, Pediatrics and Biology,
McGill University, Montreal, QC, Canada

Sheldon Solomon
Department of Psychology, Skidmore College, Saratoga Springs, NY, USA

Radhule Weininger
La Casa de Maria Retreat and Conference Center, Montecito, CA, USA

Chapter 1
Whole Person Care

Tom A. Hutchinson

Keywords Palliative care • Healing • Suffering • Healthcare mandate • Transition • Stress • Growth • Presence • Self-monitoring • Whole person • Congruently • Survival • Wounded-healer • Skeleton key • Death anxiety

Pioneering Palliative Care physicians Balfour Mount and Michael Kearney noticed an interesting phenomenon in their practice. The improvement they often saw in dying patients' quality of life did not appear to depend on control of disease, improvement in function, or even control of symptoms [1]. Here is how Balfour Mount describes the paradigmatic case [2] "CD was 30-years-old when he presented with a widely disseminated germinal testicular cancer. Radical surgery and chemotherapy initially resulted in his tumor markers reverting to negative and the hope of cure, but within months his disease progressed with ensuing extreme cachexia. He died slowly over a 12-month period. CD had always stood out from his peers. He had always been a winner. Strong. Outgoing. Gracious. A world-class athlete, he was a member of the national ski team. He was successful in business and engaged to be married. A champion from a family of competitive champions, he was now melting before the raging forces of the embryonal cell. Then, just days before he died he married his fiancée and said goodbye to those he loved, observing, 'This last year has been the best year of my life'". The key change according to CD was a shift from an external focus in his life to an internal focus. That made all the difference to him.

It turns out that CD's experience was not unique, and Mount and Kearney saw this phenomenon many times in their practice. They gave the title healing to this ability of people to move from suffering to a sense of integrity and wholeness often independently of objective improvement [3]. And while this was an innate capacity of people, the palliative care that these dying patients were receiving appeared to promote this process [4]. They realized that the facilitation of healing was not a

T.A. Hutchinson (✉)
Professor, Faculty of Medicine, Director, Programs in Whole Person Care, McGill University, 546 Pine Avenue West, Montreal, QC H2W 1S6, Canada
e-mail: tom.hutchinson@mcgill.ca

T.A. Hutchinson (ed.), *Whole Person Care: A New Paradigm for the 21st Century*, DOI 10.1007/978-1-4419-9440-0_1, © Springer Science+Business Media, LLC 2011

specific characteristic of palliative care but that they were practicing an ancient part of the healthcare mandate that is relevant at all stages of illness. They suggested that this increasingly forgotten aspect of medicine needs to be reintegrated with the powerful curative aspects of modern medicine to provide the best care possible to people seeking a doctor's help [5]. This combination of curing and healing is whole person care, the subject of this book. Of course, it does not look the same in every case.

Judy Walsh was exactly the kind of patient I loved to see because she had a serious problem and she was clearly in transition. The question was to where? When I was first asked to see her she was 47 years old, had suffered from systemic lupus erythematosus since age 15, developed kidney failure and had been on dialysis for 7 years. She had left the dialysis unit the previous day saying that she was not coming back. She would probably die in a week or two if she stuck with that decision. My job was to help her with the dying process if that was what she wanted and to explore other options with her.

We began by talking about her life. She talked about the relationship with her daughter who was a teenager, lived with her father, and did not want to see her. She spoke with bitterness about how her former partner abandoned her when her daughter was born but then later obtained custody because he convinced the court that Judy was too ill to be a good mother. She had never gotten on well with her own mother. She expressed her extreme frustration that she was too highly sensitized to receive a kidney transplant. Nothing was working, life was not worth living, and she had decided to stop dialysis and die. Everyone would be happier.

We explored her decision and its implications. I said that I would need to see her in a few days as she would probably develop symptoms that would need to be controlled. She might die suddenly, but more likely she would not and would need to be admitted to hospital as she lost strength and ability to function. She would probably go into a coma before she died. This was not said to frighten her but for both of us, me as much as her, to take a look at what we were facing. I was very conscious of being very clear to myself that this might be the best course for her, and if that proved to be the case, I could accept it fully. I would attempt to make it as good an experience as I could. Like an obstetrician when the patient is due, I would attempt to support her in the suffering of labor and bring the "birthing" process to a successful and satisfactory conclusion.

Facing her imminent death got both of our full attention. In her case, it made her reflect more on her relationships. An interesting perspective came up when we discussed her mother. She felt that her mother did not love her and would be happy to see her gone. Her mother had told her on quite a few occasions in the past when Judy was critically ill that she should "let herself go". She was very mad at her mother, and I wondered to myself if part of her decision to stop dialysis was anger at the world and at her mother in particular.

I pointed out to her that a lot of people appeared to be rejecting her: her daughter; her mother, and possibly others. I asked her if, as she said, her dying would make her mother happy, did she want to make her mother happy in that particular way. This all happened very slowly, in half phrases, in an open and exploratory way. When I asked the last question, her demeanor changed. She stopped crying, she thought for a few moments, she gave me a sideways look, and said in a quiet and unemotional whisper "No". It felt almost disrespectful, but a part of me wanted to jump for joy. It was a turning point, and I sensed that she would not look back. I met her in the corridor the next day on her way to dialysis. She smiled sweetly and gently at me as if I had helped with something important – as I think I had. I will return to her story toward the end of the chapter.

What worked in my interview with Judy? To begin with, I took some time – about 40 min for this interview. And perhaps time is important. In a study of patients with irritable bowel syndrome [6], patients were randomized to a waiting list, sham acupuncture, or sham acupuncture plus a 45-min friendly interview. The patients who had the interview had a markedly better symptom severity and quality of life than the other two groups that lasted for at least 6 weeks (the last follow-up in the study) after the intervention. So, simply spending "friendly" time with patients makes a marked difference. But in whole person care, we are trying to do more than that. We are trying to make each moment count. Why? Because like Judy, patients are always to a greater or lesser extent under stress when seeing a doctor, they are virtually always in a transition of some kind, and they are hoping for something. Those three characteristics can be both problems (sometimes serious problems) if we fail to pay attention and/or opportunities for healing and growth if we use the clinical encounter to its full potential.

What does it mean to regularly practice nonroutine medicine? As in the example given, it begins with an open-minded presence to this patient and her context on that particular day. This means I was not fixed on any *past* (she is this kind of person) or any specific *future* (this is what should happen here). I believe that if I had been fixated on either of the two (or both), Judy would have picked it up right away and would not have joined me in exploring her situation. She would have known that it was not an honest exploration focused in the *present*. This open-minded exploratory presence was maintained throughout the interview as it had to be to deal with each new issue as it arose – neither taking too long elaborating or explaining the issue at hand nor rushing on to the next issue before she was ready. This process takes continual self-monitoring. We all tend to rush ahead or lag behind at different times in a clinical interaction, and the only answer is to be aware enough to catch ourselves and bring our attention back to where the patient is now. This kind of mindful presence is increasingly recognized as an important part of good whole person care [7] that we will discuss further in the book.

So, what does the "whole person" in whole person care really mean? It is perhaps easiest to start with what it does not mean. Whole person care is not knowing all about the patient in all dimensions (biological, psychological, social, spiritual, and many others that could probably be listed) and taking responsibility for taking care of all of them. Such an undertaking is doomed to failure and would probably be perceived by patients as overstepping the bounds of the medical mandate and even as invasive. When a patient comes to see a doctor he does not expect a combination biological scientist, psychologist, social worker and spiritual guidance counselor, all of them working full out at the same time. Within the context of the clinical interaction, he/she wants someone who will provide competent medical care and treat him/her seriously as a person [8], usually no more and no less. It sounds simple, and yet, there is more to it than is at first apparent. While not everything needs to be dealt with at the same time, nothing that comes up can necessarily be ruled out of bounds as a potential avenue for addressing the problem.

This is why whole person care is a challenging proposition. Because people have all of the dimensions listed above, we never can be sure what may come up in the interaction, and so, our instinct is often to narrow down the possibilities to avoid being overwhelmed. Family therapist Virginia Satir points out that at its most basic every interaction between two people has at least three elements: self, other person, and context [9]. When we are stressed and fear being overwhelmed, we automatically omit awareness of one or more of these elements [10]. For instance, if someone is blaming us for something that we have done or omitted to do, it may be easier to accept the blame rather than stand up for ourselves. Of course, it may be the right thing to do depending on the context, but we often do it automatically and unconsciously, thereby unnecessarily giving up some of our power to play our full role in the relationship. On the contrary, if the other person appears to be acting unreasonably, we may discount them as a person. Frequently in medicine, we discount both ourselves and the other person and act like we are simply trying to solve a medical puzzle. Part of our job may be solving puzzles, but there is always more going on in a clinical interaction. Satir would say that we should learn to relate congruently (staying aware of ourselves, the other person, and the context) in our clinical interactions, and this is an important component of whole person care that we discuss at more length later in the book.

There is a second challenge and opportunity in the medical encounter. As previously mentioned, the doctor practicing whole person care has two jobs that need to be carried out simultaneously: curing is an activity carried out by a healthcare practitioner to eradicate disease or fix a problem; healing is a process leading to a greater sense of integrity and wholeness in response to an injury or disease that occurs within the patient, which can be facilitated by the healthcare practitioner [5]. And the difficulty is that the roles of both the patient and the healthcare practitioner in curing versus healing are not just different, they are diametrically opposed [11].

For instance, the goal of the patient in the curing mode is survival. This is not limited to physical survival but also extends to survival of all that the patient has learned to identify as himself including physical appearance, life style, relationships, and everything else that makes up a life. In other words, the goal is to avoid change. Healing comes from the acceptance of change. This acceptance allows the patient to grow to a new sense of himself as a person (perhaps with disease) with a new experience of integrity and wholeness that is different than the old status quo. In curing, the patient depends on the expertise of the practitioner to control disease; in healing, the patient begins to realize that it is his/her own resources that will finally lead to growth and that he/she is responsible for managing those resources.

The contrast in the healthcare worker's roles in curing and healing are equally striking. In the curing mode, the physician through his knowledge and expertise concerning disease clearly has more power. That is why the patient consulted him in the first place. In the healing mode, the power shifts toward the patient. It is within the patient that healing will occur, and it is the patient who will make the healing journey. The physician's role is accompaniment. To do this effectively, the physician needs to be able to put part of himself in the patient's shoes and adopt the wounded healer role [12] – a topic for further discussion.

The epistemologies in the curing and healing roles are also very different. In the curing mode, the basis of knowledge is scientific, and this is expressed in the current requirement of evidence-base practice. In the healing mode, this approach is not helpful. Since the essence of the facilitation of healing is the relationship of one person to another, the physician's role in healing has to depend on his particular gifts and characteristics as a person and on the particular gifts and characteristics of the patient. Art rather than science is required to enable the physician to make the best intuitive use of himself in the healing relationship with the patient. The dynamics of the interaction would be different with every physician–patient pair, a complete contrast to the standardized requirements of science [11].

Given the contrasts outlined, it is not surprising that physicians and other health-care workers have had a hard time encompassing both roles in their practice. The solution is often to restrict care to one of the two poles, curing or healing, but not both [13]. To be both an effective curer and facilitate healing at the same time is a challenging task: this patient may be dying and I must remain emotionally present to that possibility and behave and communicate with the patient accordingly; at the same time, I must concentrate on clarifying the medical issues and exploring other factors that may be affecting the decision so that this patient can make the best choice possible for him/her at this transition point in his/her life. As may be apparent from this example, the enlargement of awareness required is significant but can actually result in a decrease in the psychological tension that comes from identifying exclusively with curing or healing. However, as mentioned our tendency is to restrict awareness when we are faced with stressful situations [14].

So, in my interaction with Judy where was the curing and where was the healing? And that is the point. The two are so inextricably intertwined that it is impossible to separate them completely. Before the interview even began, Judy would probably not have agreed to meet me or would not have engaged with me when we did meet if she lacked confidence that I knew what I was talking about. She knew that I had practiced nephrology for many years. My "curing" credentials were good. There was also the fact that I was now doing palliative care and that the social worker who referred her trusted me. The clinical interaction itself went back and forth between such things as the medical consequences of possible actions and her conflicted intimate relationships, with the reality of possible imminent death hovering, sometimes in the background and sometimes in the foreground.

Judy's case raises some other interesting issues about whole person care. One common objection is that it takes too long and physicians simply do not have time to be anything other than efficient technicians. There are probably situations in which this is the only feasible approach. But I wonder does our desire to get through things quickly increase our real efficiency (results achieved for time and effort spent) or does it more often leave issues unresolved in a way that uses up more time in the long run. I spent a total of just over 1 h with Judy over a 2-year-period: the 40-min interview mentioned above, a brief encounter in the corridor, and a further 20-min interview 2 years later. Would a series of shorter but more superficial interviews have worked just as well or better? I doubt it and believe that whole person care actually takes less time in the long run.

Did it require special skill and attunement to Judy's specific issues and requirements to produce the results achieved? In a way yes and in a way no. As mentioned, my previous experience as a nephrologist helped as did my relationship with her social worker. The fact that I was also a palliative care physician meant that I could discuss realistically her possible impending death and how it might be managed to minimize her suffering. But after that, it was primarily a question of taking time, being willing to face confronting issues, staying in the moment, and being watchful for realistic opportunities to move the action forward in a way that fitted the patient. We are now beginning to teach these skills to medical students at McGill under a new physicianship curriculum [15]. We are convinced that students can learn these skills given the right coaching, although everyone will perform them in their own way. It is perhaps important to state that I did not feel perfectly attuned to Judy in my interview with her and was often unsure how to proceed. How well can a 59-year-old relatively healthy male put himself in the shoes of a 47-year-old woman with lupus and renal failure? But it is not necessary to have the specific and perfect key that is unique to each person's problem. Open-minded presence in the context of medical expertise is more like a skeleton key [16] that opens many locks. We explore some of the elements of this skeleton key later in the book. We do not need to be perfectly attuned, only "well enough" attuned. We explain our attempts to make our students "good enough" whole person physicians later in the book.

An important issue already touched on is how Judy's possible imminent death affected the interview and how this relates to whole person care. I believe that the presence of possible death played a crucial role in the interview. As discussed later in the book, death anxiety is an ever-present reality in the unconscious mind that can be easily triggered to consciousness [17] as it almost certainly was in this case. We discuss later the usual responses to death anxiety that involve suppression and self-esteem bolstering by attachment to a particular world view. I have observed an additional effect in clinical interactions. An awareness of death gets people's full attention. As has been observed in Buddhist literature, it is the shortcut to being mindfully present [18]. I doubt that the same change would have occurred in Judy if the possibility of death had not been on the table. Does that mean that this is a special, even unique case? I believe not. Given the pervasiveness of death anxiety in the unconscious and how easily mortality salience can be triggered, I suspect it is an ever-present reality in any degree of illness. The physician's job is not to run from death anxiety himself and not necessarily to collude in the patient's frequent desire to suppress thoughts of possible death or serious loss. Part of whole person care is the willingness to help the patient face what may be realistic possibilities and fears in order that the person may be able to move forward out of suffering to a new sense of peace with a possibly new reality.

But what of cases where death is clearly not an issue and the illness is mild or nonexistent? Surely here, medicine can be a primarily technical encounter and the need for treating the patient as a whole person is limited on nonexistent. Nothing could be further from the truth because even when the situation is "routine" for the doctor, it is usually emotionally highly charged for the patient. A colleague was in labor. Her obstetrician was called. Everything was going well, and the labor was quite far advanced but it looked like it would take more than the 30 min the obstetrician had before a teaching session with some medical students. To my colleague's horror, the obstetrician announced he was going to use forceps to expedite matters. She was still furious when she recounted the story to a medical class *40 years later*. I asked her how her son was, had there been a complication. Her son was fine and now a successful lawyer. There had been no problem or complication. Except that there had been a huge human complication that compromised her sense of trust and relationship with the obstetrician. That wound was still incompletely healed. My own experience as a patient provides a contrasting example. I was calling up a gastroenterologist I knew to set up a routine colonoscopy. During the telephone call, he asked me how I was and I reported that I had experienced a little heartburn but not a big deal and nothing to worry about. Except, of course, I had been worried particularly as a colleague of mine had recently been diagnosed with esophageal cancer. The gastroenterologist asked me a simple question "Are you worried about it?" Somewhat embarrassed, I admitted that I was a little and he continued the exploration that led to me having a gastroscopy within a few weeks. I had the distinct impression that we were doing the gastroscopy not because he was very concerned (heartburn is a very common symptom) but because he picked up the fact that I was worried. The gastroscopy showed a small hiatus hernia with reflux. I am still grateful to that perceptive doctor who picked up my concern over the telephone. Relating to the patient as a whole person is relevant at all phases of medicine from the management of mild disease to presence at the patient's deathbed.

This brings me back to my final interview with Judy. It was 2 years later and she had asked to see me. She had been in hospital for 4 days during which time she had refused dialysis and had been seen by psychiatry who declared her competent to make that decision. The nephrologist caring for her accepted that she would die, her mother was at her bedside, and I was called to help with the dying process. Judy was very pleased to see me. She was totally clear that she was now ready to die, wanted her mother by her bedside when it happened, and asked me whether she could order pizza that afternoon. We did not discuss how this change had come about or any other details of the intervening 2 years. I had the clear sense that exploring these issues at that point would only have increased her suffering unnecessarily. It was not why she had called me but to say good-bye and to ensure that she died comfortably. I wrote the appropriate orders for potential symptoms such as shortness of breath, and when I returned to say good-bye, she waved to me. She was busy on the phone ordering a pizza, all-dressed. She died peacefully that night (quicker than expected) with her mother holding her hand.

I recently attended a meeting about admission criteria to medical school in which the speaker asked the audience to choose between a student who was academically brilliant (as evidenced by scores) but had only adequate people skills and a student who was academically adequate but had excellent people skills. The audience made various suggestions. The speaker then turned the table on us by pointing out that it is a false choice. Academic brilliance and excellent people skills are not mutually exclusive and may even be highly correlated. We can have it both ways. Whole person care is very much the same way. For too long, we have assumed that because we see science as the basis of modern medicine, we have to let go of a much older part of the medical mandate that has to do with deep relating to people and the facilitation of healing. We do not and we cannot give up this part of our job without losing our way, and our ability to help our patients. Whole person care means refocusing on our main objective in medicine – the relief of suffering in ill patients [19] – and using everything at our disposal including scientific knowledge, clinical skill, and practical wisdom in the pursuit of that laudable goal.

References

1. Kearney M. Beyond the medical model. In: A place of healing: working with suffering in living and dying. Oxford, UK: Oxford University Press; 2000. p. 3–14.
2. Cohen SR, Mount BM. Quality of life in terminal illness: defining and measuring subjective well-being in the dying. J Palliat Care. 1992;8:40–5.
3. Faculty Working Group on Healing, McGill University. Report to the Dean: a commentary on healing and the undergraduate medical curriculum.
4. Cohen SR, Boston P, Mount BM, Porterfield P. Changes in quality of life following admission to palliative care units. Palliat Med. 2001;15:363–71.
5. Mount B, Kearney M. Healing and palliative care: charting our way forward. Palliat Med. 2003;17:657–8.
6. Kaptchuk TJ, Kelley JM, Conboy LA, Davis RB, Kerr CE, Jacobson EE, et al. Components of the placebo effect: a randomized controlled trial in irritable bowel syndrome. BMJ. 2008;336(7651):999–1003.
7. Epstein RM. Mindful practice. JAMA. 1999;282:833–9.
8. Boudreau DJ, Jagosh J, Slee R, Macdonald M-E, Steinert Y. Patients' perspectives on physicians' roles: implications for curricular reform. Acad Med. 2008;83(8):744–53.
9. Satir V, Banmen J, Gerber J, Gomori M. Chapter 2, The primary triad. In: The Satir model. Family therapy and beyond. Palo Alto, CA: Science and Behaviour Books, Inc; 1991. p. 19–30.
10. Satir V, Banmen J, Gerber J, Gomori M. Chapter 3, The survival stances. In: The Satir model. Family therapy and beyond. Palo Alto, CA: Science and Behaviour Books, Inc; 1991. p. 31–64.
11. Hutchinson TA, Hutchinson N, Arnaert A. Whole person care: encompassing the two faces of medicine. CMAJ. 2009;180(8):845–6.
12. Guggenbühl-Craig A. Power in the helping professions. Dallas, TX: Spring Publications; 1971.
13. Cassell E. Prologue: a time for healing. In: The healer's art. Cambridge, MA: The MIT Press; 1976.
14. Driskell JE, Salas E, Johnston J. Does stress lead to a loss of team perspective? Group Dyn Theory Res Pract. 1999;3:291–302.
15. Boudreau JD, Cassell EJ, Fuks A. A healing curriculum. Med Educ. 2007;41:1193–201.
16. De Shazer S. Chapter 8, Skeleton keys. In: Keys to solution in brief therapy. New York: W.W. Norton & Company, Inc.; 1985. p. 119–36.
17. Pysczynski T, Solomon S, Greenberg J. In the wake of 911: the psychology of terror. Washington, DC: American Psychological Association; 2003.
18. Rinpoche S. Chapter 3, Reflection and change. In: The Tibetan book of living and dying. New York: HarperSanFrancisco; 1993. p. 28–40.
19. Cassell EJ. The nature of suffering and the goals of medicine. N Engl J Med. 1982;306(11):639–45.

Chapter 2
Suffering, Whole Person Care, and the Goals of Medicine

Eric J. Cassell

Keywords Adaptiveness • Cognition • Emotion • Function • Suffering • Person • Whole person • Meanings • Sickness • Symptoms • Pain • Intactness • Integrity • Personal • Self-conflict • Purpose • Individual • Lonely • Coherent • Empirical self • Existential • Goals • Disorder • Disease • Functioning • Communication • Functional complex • Dailiness • Sociology • Anthropology

Bodies do not suffer, only persons do [1]. This fundamental fact of suffering is revealed because in all the situations in which suffering comes about the meaning of the occurrence to the person and the person's perception of the future are crucial. Whether the stimulus is, for example, pain or other physical symptoms, or perhaps bereavement, or even hopelessness, the meaning of what is happening and its perceived future are crucial in determining whether suffering will follow. Bodies have nociception and bodies may have neuroendocrine responses to emotional stimuli, but bodies do not have a sense of the future and bodies do not know meanings, only persons do. If you reflect, as a clinician,[1] on what you know of pain or even sickness itself you will see that what is true for suffering is true for all sickness and pain, in fact all symptoms. You cannot understand this particular sick person without thinking about the person him or herself, even if you do not know that is what you are doing. This is because, as we will see in greater detail later on, *all* persons individualize their

---

[1] I use the term clinician, as noted above, to refer to those who take care of patients sick or well. There are professionals in medicine who are devoted solely to disease or its manifestation, others are historians of medicine, and still others are administrators, and so on. These (nonclinicians) can think about sick people and disease in the abstract, but clinicians (whether they are physicians or not) *must* ultimately think about the sick person even if they are most interested in diseases because it is the sick person diseased or otherwise who confronts them.

E.J. Cassell (✉)
Emeritus Professor of Public Health, Weill Medical College of Cornell University,
New York, NY 10021
and
Adjunct Professor of Medicine, Faculty of Medicine, McGill University,
PO Box 96, Shawnee on Delaware, PA 18356, USA
e-mail: eric@ericcassell.com

sickness and its manifestations – make it *their* sickness or *their* symptom. Why do we not all know this? Because we are used to thinking about sickness and symptoms as things that come from diseases – rather than as processes that inevitably unfold over time. It is as temporal processes that sickness and its manifestations pick up the individual character of the person who has them. The science of pathophysiology for processes occurring over time in sick persons provides inadequate explanations.

Suffering has most commonly been associated with pain or other physical symptoms. It is now generally accepted, however, that pain (or other symptoms) and suffering are distinct. Several facts point in this direction. For example, the magnitude of the pain is only one factor in the distress it causes; people will tolerate even very severe pain if they know what it is (its significance) and if they know that it will end. On the contrary, even pain of lesser degree may be poorly tolerated if it appears to be endless, if it is considered to have dire meaning (such as malignancy), or if it resists relief. People with no symptoms may suffer. For example, at the pain of a loved one – especially when helpless, from helplessness itself, or hopelessness. Suffering, as we said, is an affliction of persons not bodies. *Suffering is the specific distress that occurs when persons feel their intactness or integrity as persons threatened or disintegrating, and it continues until the threat is gone or intactness or integrity is restored.*

Suffering can occur in relationship to any part of a person, but it is always because the stimulus to suffering threatens the integrity of the person. Small breaches in the integrity of the person occur all the time, just as small breaches in the integrity of the skin are common (such as cuts or small burns). But when large enough, as in the following examples, loss of intactness leads to suffering. Suffering, however, is its own specific distress. When pain leads to suffering, the suffering is *suffering*, not pain, when existential issues are the stimulus to suffering it is *suffering* not the unbearable existence, and when emotional problems are the stimulus to suffering, it is *suffering*, not (e.g.,) grief. Thus, *when patients suffer it is suffering not pain, suffering not fear, and suffering not loneliness.* Suffering is suffering; it is suffering – it is what it is and not another thing. Thus, when you read discussions where suffering from physical sources is distinguished from existential suffering you will realize that the distinction is false. Whatever happens to one part of a person happens to the whole person and whatever happens to the person happens to every part, that is, what it means to speak of whole persons and whole person care. I have put together three scenarios so that you see how suffering is personalized.

(a) What if you have always been proud, of your appearance, really proud, and a careful dresser even from childhood? And then lately you start having diarrhea – all the time, for days on end. And they will not give you anything to stop it because, you are not sure why. And when you finally come into the hospital and the nurse undresses you standing up, there is feces running down your legs and on your clothes and everywhere. And everybody just goes in and out of your room.

(b) What if you have always been a good patient and tried hard to do everything they asked you to do – because you have always been good, and did the right thing even as a kid. And everybody always said that you were special. And you came to the emergency room because this time you are really sick. And you have been lying on a gurney for 11 h waiting for a bed. And you are not sure what is happening. And you are so thirsty and cold, for hours, but nobody helps. When people do stop, they tell you how busy they are and to be patient. When you try to find out what is happening, nobody listens. And some are just mean and short-tempered. And you are so cold.

(c) What if you have always been really social and have a million friends because you love that stuff. And what if you just found out last week that you had cancer in your colon and they could not operate because it is in your liver too. And you are sure that you are going to die soon. And you are afraid to tell anyone because they will stop talking to you. Like they did when your mother was dying when everybody ran away from her…and you, and left you to take care of her alone. And that was awful. And you do not even tell your daughters because – you know – they have their own lives. And you are scared, really terrified about dying.

These are abbreviated stories but the people are recognizable. The suffering that results from the threat to their integrity and intactness is because of who each one is, the specific persons they are. What is happening to each one is recognizably unpleasant, but it causes their individual suffering because of their particular natures. This is what it means when we say that suffering is always personal. The cases also demonstrate why suffering is always unique and individual. Even if two people are suffering from identical sources – say, ruptured aortic aneurysms – they will suffer the way they do not because of the pain, but because of the singular nature of each of the persons. In relieving suffering, it is a not person in general that needs to be known, but *this particular person.* Suffering can be present in varying intensity and duration with the differences again dependent on the particular person.

Here is another example:

> Jan, a 40-year-old single woman, whose sudden development of widespread metastatic breast cancer caused her to be hospitalized and near death, is suffering. But it is not the weakness, profound anorexia, and generalized edema, as distressing as they are that are the source of her suffering, but the loss of control and inability to prevent the evaporation of her career whose brilliant promise had finally been realized a few months earlier.

Suffering always involves *self-conflict* because, as with Jan, part of the person wants to resume her career, while another part of her knows her disease has made that impossible. She actually caused herself to be discharged from the hospital. Within a few days, she sustained a pathological fracture and was readmitted, aware that she should not have attempted to resume her life. Sometimes, the conflict is wanting to be alive but not wanting to live the only life offered, or wanting to be alive but not wanting to be a burden to loved ones. Suffering also always involves a loss or profound *change in central purpose*. Our central purpose when we are well is to continue the pursuit of being oneself, of being in the world of others. In suffering, purpose shifts to the removal of the source of suffering. Finally, suffering is *always lonely* – lonely because the suffering is not understood by others, lonely because of the individuality of suffering, and lonely because of the withdrawal of purpose from social engagement. Thus, suffering is *always personal, individual, marked by self-conflict, and lonely.*

While suffering, sickness, and symptoms tell us why care should be directed at persons, it does not tell us what persons are, or better, what whole persons are, it does not reveal what their care, as whole persons, should entail, and it does not point to new goals for medicine. (The relief of suffering is perhaps the reason the various forms of medicine found in the world have come into existence – it may be, therefore, the oldest goal of the helping professions.) Medicine in its clinical (patient-directed) endeavors is a field of action. Clinicians do things to and for their patients. As a consequence, they require specific goals based on what they perceive as threatening their patients or making them sick. They also require a metric that tells of success or failure in making patients better. In recent decades, we have come to understand that it is persons themselves who know whether they are better or not. Better or worse is ultimately defined by the patients themselves. When we come to define what sickness is, therefore, our definition should entail – or allow us to deduce what it means to be well *in the patient's terms*.

Perhaps we should start with the idea of the whole person. It has been believed since antiquity that it is impossible to know a person. This is obviously because persons are complex. But there are other reasons as well. For one thing, persons are constantly changing so what you knew of me yesterday has already changed. But it is also true that persons appear differently in different situations. The person in a work environment is different in many ways from the same person at home and different still from persons when they are sick, injured, or hospitalized. As we shall see presently, all persons have a secret life and in that context they may be very different than the person in his or her everyday world. Which of these presentations is *the person*? They are all aspects of the person and as such are truly the person. This complexity led philosophers in the seventeenth century a merry chase – especially John Locke – when they tried to decide whether they could consider the person they see today as the same person as the person they saw yesterday, or last year. They ended up deciding that identity was durable. By now, this is universally accepted because despite all the complexity, all these manifestations of person share so much in common that they are just different manifestations of the same person. We should leave this section, however, realizing that persons can appear and behave differently in different situations and that it does not take much imagination to realize that these differences may have an impact on sickness and the care of the sick.

A person is an embodied, purposeful, thinking, feeling, emotional, reflective, relational very complex human individual of a certain personality and temperament, existing through time in a narrative sense, whose life in all spheres points both outward and inward and who does things. Each of these terms is a dynamic function, constantly changing, and requiring action on the part of the person to be maintained – although generally the maintenance is habitual and unmediated by thought. Each of these functions that make up the person can be altered by sickness.

Persons are always in action and never quiescent. Persons can support contradictory thoughts and actions simultaneously, which, however, produce new thoughts and actions. Although basically stable in personality and overall psychological and social being, persons are always changing perceptions, thoughts, and actions in a continuous manner. If these changes are thought of as individually very small in scope and very short in time, then a picture emerges of persons as dynamically and interactively responsive to their inner and outer environment.

Virtually all of a person's actions – volitional, habitual, instinctual, or automatic – are in response to meanings. The actions and behavior are primarily reactions to ideas and beliefs about things rather than to the brute facts of the things themselves. In fact, things in themselves hardly ever exist apart from ideas about them. This should not be surprising since perception itself is an *act of thought*, not merely the registration of sensation.

A human being in all its facets interacts simultaneously outwardly into the world and with others, as well as inwardly in emotions, thoughts, and the body, and these are generally consistent and harmoniously accordant. By contrast, suffering variously destroys the coherence, cohesiveness, and consistency of the whole. The person's experience of this is of no longer being in accord and "whole," but rather of "being in pieces," of not being able to "hold themselves together." It is in this sense that suffering threatens or destroys the integrity or intactness of the person.

Persons live at all times in a context of ever-present relationships. Some relationships are as close as glue, while others are formal. Close or formal, we are all separate beings (except in intense love where two people may feel like one.) On the contrary, in every thought, feeling, and action, all ideas and beliefs about oneself and others and in every dream, fantasy, and fear, the presence of others is reflected. In normal life, physical appearance, dress, walking and other bodily movements and actions, language, speech, and gesture, everything is tuned to others in everyday life (even facial expression is a social construction). Part of the molding of individuals to each other must necessarily be physiological, although the extent of such conforming is unknown.

People want to be accepted, valued, and admired by others (and themselves) and be like those that they admire. Vanity to a greater or lesser extent is present in all and is a part of the relationship of persons to others and to themselves. They want to be seen as they would like others to see them, not necessarily as they are (or believe themselves to be). Imagine, if you can, a person in an environment in which he or she was absolutely and completely unnoticed. No one turned around or turned aside, no one looked up, no one spoke (or answered), all acted as if we were nonexistent beings no matter what we tried. What if we were lying for hours on our back, covered with a sheet except for our face, on a gurney in an emergency ward or in the hallway outside an operating room. No one looked at us; no one answered a question or responded to our speech. No one recognized our existence except occasionally to bump into the gurney without a word. Or suppose we were in a hospital bed and no one seemed to see us *as us.* Suppose when we were spoken to we felt like the person on the gurney outside the operating room or, worse, the unrecognized person. No one spoke personally to us and did only coldly or impersonally or used only our first name and perhaps the wrong name at that. Then, when things were done to our body even if they were unexplained, uncomfortable, or painful, we might even be grateful for the attention. If you can bring these painful scenes to mind, you will understand the almost animal gratitude such persons would have for personal voices, little pleasantries, answered questions, and reassuring touch from even total strangers. You will also know why medical care itself can initiate suffering.

As fundamentally true as the communal nature of human life is the fact that *all persons are different in virtually every feature of their existence – biological, physical, psychological, and spiritual.* As a result of, sometimes, differences or even conflict between the life someone must live in a family, group, or community and that person's individual inborn nature and behaviors, all persons have one or more public, private, and sometimes secret selves that are different and distinct to a greater or lesser degree. These different selves are characterized by consistent, cohesive, and coherent traits and have a disposition to behave in certain relatively distinct ways. They are sometimes marked by differences in appearance, stance, gait, and speech from other selves of the same person. Even though selves are different from one another, no one would confuse them with being a different person; executive control remains with the dominant self. (This distinguishes the phenomenon of different selves from the pathologic entity multiple personality disorder.) There are usually only a few such selves each emerging in situations similar to those that originally evoked them, usually occurring in childhood. This implies, correctly, I believe, that whatever other selves a person has, if any, all persons have an original self – an inborn and lifetime enduring constellation of personality and physical characteristics – whether it ever reveals itself fully or not. Despite the occurrence of different selves, the general belief that personality is enduring over a lifetime is supported by good evidence.

Although *there may be more than one self,* the empirical self – the self I experience now, that I experienced a few minutes and more time ago, and that I expect (without awareness of the expectation) to experience as time unrolls in front of me is what I call me. I will not be aware, usually, that I am behaving like a different self than I was (say) in the doctor's office that I just left. This me has a frame of mind and a bodily state of feelings, both of which I am more or less aware, is involved in some purposeful activity with some goal in mind. For example, I am more or less aware and involved in what I am wearing and largely influenced by my surrounding environment physically as well as cognitively, socially, and morally. Where all around me people are talking from a specific frame of reference – for example, the oncology care environment where patient survival and response to chemotherapy is the dominant frame of reference – that is the reference set that will also frame my response to the actions and words of others as well as my own. If I am in such a context, then I may experience myself in such terms. Doing so may be against my interests as I know them, but I will probably be unaware of the impact of the frame of reference or even, perhaps, of its presence. In some circumstances, we call this peer pressure and recognize its power. The point is that the self that I experience, the me of a particular circumstance is not necessarily generated solely from within me. Usually, I will not know this; I will probably not be aware of the impact of the ideas, meanings, and behaviors of others on my ideas, meanings, and behaviors. Usually (but not always), I will think these things came from within me – that they are me. This is the explanation for the participation of a person in group behaviors that may be difficult to square with the person as you know them.

How do we know ourselves? Persons know themselves as themselves by their thoughts, the sound of their own voice, and what they look like in the mirror. They know themselves by beliefs they hold about themselves and the world they live in. I am a man, a doctor, a husband, a father, a friend, an American, a liberal Democrat, and every one of those features of my identity – of me – has an influence on every aspect of my ideas, thoughts, and behaviors. A large library of ideas and behaviors past and present emerge from this identity and may easily be brought to mind. But me is not just what you see as you behold me in this minute. These other features just mentioned, which may come from the past or an anticipated future, even though you cannot see them, are also me.

Persons also know themselves to be truly themselves by their aptitudes, skills, and accomplishments, by their ability to make things, do things, and write things. Persons re-create themselves every day. What they did yesterday or last week is not sufficient; it is what they can do today that is also important – sometimes most important. This means that *persons are partially existential creatures*; it is today that matters much more than most people realize. Children are probably wholly existential; the big picture does not concern them as it does adults. But that allows them to tolerate the distress of today without dragging into it what happened yesterday or what is anticipated for tomorrow.

The empirical self includes an awareness of the body and many of its functions. The function of the special senses and the somatic senses are generally within the awareness of the individual so that if they develop abnormalities, the functional loss reaches awareness. Muscle strength, walking speed, pulmonary capacity, bowel and bladder function, and others are part of what persons know of themselves. This is true of healthy as well as sick persons, although persons will adapt to slow loss of function and sometimes be unaware of significant impairment until it is pointed out to them. This same adaptiveness allows persons to change the way they carry out tasks or the manner in which certain actions are performed so that they can do things despite major losses in function in virtually every system from cognition to the motions of the hand and other extremities. For a more complete discussion of the nature of persons and clinical medicine, see the appendix.

What should doctors do? Where should clinicians direct their attention? Since the early nineteenth century, physicians have been focused on disease (as we know it) and its symptoms, but it is apparent from what I have described that such an approach is only partway to the goal of whole person care. All the vast disease-related medical science, pathophysiology, and recorded clinical experience are of inestimable value – as far as they go. Clinicians who really want to focus on the person find themselves talking about the person and reverting back to disease-oriented medicine. How could it not be so; all the, valid, reliable, and reproducible information clinicians get is about the disease, *not the sick person.* Look at definitions of person-oriented medicine. My experience of teaching programs dedicated to whole person care, such as at the University of Rochester, is that they act as though there are two kinds of knowledge, medical science about the body and the disease, and knowledge of persons that are to be joined together at the bedside. The existence of two kinds of knowledge is not what creates the problem. Architects, for example, do not join two kinds of knowledge – aesthetics and engineering – at the end of their design. These different understandings are an entwined part of their thinking all the time from the inception of the idea to the finished design. That is how architects think. The problem is not two kinds of knowledge in medicine, the problem is that the goals of practice are almost universally divided – treat the disease and care for the patient focusing on the personal aspects of the illness – as though these were two separate elements to be brought together. That is not correct. There is only one goal; the *well-being of the whole person* who is the patient. We can think the patient is better – disease indices say things are good, but the patient does not have a sense of well-being. The patient had angina and a successful angioplasty or bypass produced a return of good coronary blood flow, but the patient is not better – has not returned to work, or the previous place in the family, or has not resumed sexual function – and the patient has not returned to a state of well-being. The patient had a malignancy and was successfully treated into remission. Unfortunately, the person fears and waits only for the recurrence. The person has not had a return of well-being.

In the last few years, person-centered medicine has come to denote medicine that is focused on the patient being in control and the patient's goals, expectations, and needs as determined by the patient. In the words of the Institute of Medicine of the National Academy of Science, it is a medicine "that is respectful of and responsive to individual patient preferences, needs, and values." This defines an accommodating and benevolent medicine, but it is not a medicine focused on the whole person that arises from consideration of both the nature of persons and of sickness. Consideration of sickness demonstrates that it has an influence on virtually every aspect of persons and vice versa. A medicine of persons seeks the origins of sickness wherever they may lie in the person recognizing that physical phenomenon may be known disproportionally because of the availability of previous knowledge and technology. This is also not a medicine whose goal is the return of the person's sense of well-being. *The key to relief of suffering is a focus on function.* What do patients have when they have a sense of well-being? They believe they can accomplish their purposes and goals. Put another way, they can do the things they need and want to do to live their lives the way they want to. Most persons are realistic, if they were sick and now better, they know they are not the same as before the stroke – but at least they can do the things that are important to them. What is important to each person is individual, personal, and important to their lives and the way they want to live and be in the world – or to put it another way, what is important is whole person being centered. In clinician's terms, what do you need to have a sense of well-being, you *need to able to function well enough to pursue your purposes and goals*. This brings us to a definition of sickness that will permit us to move forward, to begin to specify what clinicians must actually do who are treating the whole person. *Persons are sick when because of impairments of function they cannot pursue their purposes and goals*, which they attribute to something in the realm of medicine. What has happened to patients who are suffering? They have lost their intactness and integrity as the persons they believe themselves to be. They can no longer function well enough to maintain their purposes. This is individual and personal loss and at its heart is disordered, absent, or severely impaired function. Or functions at war with themselves such that the person experiences the self-conflict always present in suffering. The same belief may be at the bottom of the experience of seemingly endless or never-to-be-relieved pain – that the person's purposes and goals and the functions in their service are, at least in part, contributing to the continued pain. Not only is function disordered in suffering but also a meaning has entered the process such that the person may no longer believe that function will ever return or pain be relieved. Thus, the amelioration of sickness and the relief of suffering both require a focus on the restoration or reenabling of function.

Let us return to a better understanding of sickness itself. *What these patients actually have, independent of any assigned meaning is a disorder – "a derangement or abnormality of function"* (Dorland 1988). The disorder is the out-there-in-nature actual thing (or process) that the patient has. The response of physicians is to make a diagnosis and decide on treatment. The diagnosis "represents an attribute, not of the patient, but, rather, of the diagnostician or the diagnostic process in response to the patient. In many cases the diagnosis expresses a physician's subjective belief that the patient has the [disease], a belief that may or may not be warranted" [2]. There are, therefore, three different "entities" that describe what is wrong with the patient.

The *disorder*: A characteristic of the patient that is made up of the experience of the disturbances or derangements of function that actually exist.

The *sickness*: The patient's subjective attribution or imputation of a name for, a description of, or a belief about the manifestations of the disorder as the patient experiences them.

The *disease*: The name or pathologic process to which the physician or the diagnostic process is attributing the patient's disorder. *Disorder, sickness, and disease?* Is this just dividing up the person the way, for example, mind and body, person and body – the famous dichotomies – divide up the person? No. There is only the person who has the disorder of function that actually exists in that person. It is as if the disorder is a text about which the patient makes one reading and the physician another. To return well-being to the person requires attention to the impairments of function that make up the disorder because the patient's well-being rests on the ability to do things important to the achievement of the person's purposes and goals.

Function. Everything I have just described depends on the idea of function. Human function is the overriding, all encompassing activity that includes the entire range from the cellular to the spiritual. It is the role of something in bringing about an activity or capacity of a system of which that something is a part [3]. In physiology, it is often contrasted to structure. Things function when they perform, move from one state to another, exercise their properties, or achieve a goal or purpose. Functioning can be a simple act or a complex set of operations that require multiple subsidiary functions for its enactment. Persons must function in order to achieve their goals or realize their purposes. This dimension of functioning goes beyond the usual biological understanding of functioning, yet it is extremely important for the actions of clinicians.

These various definitions emphasize certain characteristics of functioning. The function of something in human systems is always part of, or somewhere within an increasingly complex hierarchy. One function is part of the next level which goes on to the next level and so on. For example, the function of the contractile motor unit leads in the aggregate to the contraction of a muscle fiber, which leads in the aggregate to the contraction of the muscle, which leads in aggregate (and joined to other functions involved in the motion of the part) to the motion of the part (e.g., a limb), which leads in aggregate (when joined to other functions) to the function of a part of the body, which when joined to the functioning of other parts leads to a function of a person (e.g. walking), which when joined to other functions leads to the accomplishment of a purpose or goal. Goals and purposes are often parts of further goals and so on. Writing something (requiring among many other things, the functioning of the shoulder–hand complex) that will be spoken publicly (requiring voice and speech functions) leads to recognition of skills (or not), which leads to a social act and a place in a community (or not), and so on.

It is artificial to stop considering functioning which extend past the boundaries of the body. On the contrary, all functionings up to and including the pursuit of purposes and goals involve the body. When a person is sick because they believe themselves unable to accomplish their purposes, that failure can usually be traced from the goal all the way down to a physiologic (or pathophysiologic) mechanism. Understanding function always involves at least four levels – the function(s) itself, the body structures involved, the activities that will be participated in, and the context and environment in which the activities will take place. The activity of, e.g., communication, involves (at the least) consciousness functions, intellectual functions, attention functions, psychosocial functions, memory functions, psycho-motor functions, perceptual functions, thought functions, mental functions of language, seeing functions, hearing functions, voice functions, and articulation and fluency of speech functions. Communication involves body structures as well as body functions. Structure of the nervous system, eye, ear, and related structures, structures involved in speech, and structures related to movement. Also involved are learning and applying knowledge, conversation, perhaps using communication devices and techniques, changing and maintaining body position and moving, and interpersonal interactions. The context and the environment and perhaps assistive devices are involved. The solution to the problem, however, may occur at any level if it returns the person to the pursuit of goals or purposes.

As an example, difficulties in communication between a dying patient and the family – often so important to the patient – may take place at any level in the func-tion of communication from a mouth so dry the tongue cleaves to the palate to the inability to initiate the conversation if the clinician is not there to help. In those terms, understanding human speech and communication at the level of body func-tion, structure, activities, participation, and environmental factors *is* understanding communication function. In understanding function in the terms necessary to whole person care, the distinction between the function of organ systems and their structure remains important. For example, the troubles a person is having in com-municating with others may originate in impairments of speech arising from trouble with the production of voice, articulation of speech, fluency and rhythm, and other vocalization functions. The reason(s) why the person is having difficulty being understood may originate in abnormalities of the tongue, soft or hard palate, other structures of the mouth. Or the problem may be in the activities involving communication in general such as originating or sustaining a conversation. On the contrary, the functional difficulty may come from environmental or personal problems such as inability to speak the language of the listener, the effect of drugs or other impairments on communication, or the lack of assistive devices [4].

I have started with a relatively uncomplicated example, but if well-being requires the return to a personally acceptable level of participation in sports by someone previously active in sports who has sustained an amputation of a leg above the knee, the number of levels from function to structure to activity and participation and to environmental support that must be part of the therapeutic effort is considerable. Clearly beyond the capability of a single clinician, here is where medicine as a team activity is essential. But teams require knowledgeable leaders, and patients need clinicians who understand the impact of illness and with whom a relationship has been established that continues to motivate the person.

What is the advantage of the focus on functioning as compared to the usual concentration on the disease process? Focusing on functioning and its impairments or improvements focuses on what the sick person experiences. Impact on the life of the sick person depends on *these specific particular* persons, the lives they lead, their ages, occupations, values, social existence – virtually everything that makes them who they are. Understanding the effect of a particular functional alteration in a patient brings together knowledge of physiology, pathophysiology, society, culture, and almost every facet of a person. It is difficult to think of a complex human function in its totality that does not involve and require knowledge of the whole person. A medicine that is focused on functioning is inescapably patient centered. It could not be otherwise. The sick who require crutches to walk do not despair only of the incompetence of a contractile unit or neuronal stimulation of the muscle bundle or even the weakness of an individual muscle. They will, at least initially, consider *themselves* diminished or lack confidence. For example, they may consider themselves sick in part because they have difficulty walking in public, are acutely aware of how slowly they move, and despair that they will ever not be stared at by others. On the contrary, they may feel themselves to have conquered the impairment that made them sedentary in their new-found ability to walk with crutches. Physicians are able to see that from the incompetent neuromuscular or contractile unit to stares of others or (conversely) the sense of achievement is *one functional complex*, a mosaic of elements that make up the whole. They are able also to understand the achievement that through using crutches returned the person to increased functioning and back into the world of others.

Physicians do not merely have empathy for the embarrassment of the crutch walker, they have knowledge of the functional whole that starts at the pathophysiology of the neuromuscular or contractile unit and finishes at the patient's difficulty walking with crutches and the attendant social distress. They may not understand the psychological dynamics involved in the distress of the slow crutch walker, but acquiring that knowledge does not require leaving the accepted domain of knowledge and action in clinical medicine. Clinicians, conversely, may concentrate on the disease and not see it as their basic responsibility to follow the patient through all the ramifications involved in the loss of functions that underlie the inability to fulfill goals. The great advantage physicians have, however, is that they have the ability and knowledge to understand impairments from (say) the contractile or neuromuscular unit to the fulfillment of purpose because that gives them the potential ability to intervene at any place in that process. The focus on functioning addresses the lived life of the patient that stretches from sickness to the patient's experience (definition) of health. *The role of healer extends from the fundamentals of disease to what is necessary for patients to achieve their goals and know themselves as healthy* [5]. The relief of suffering is in the same domain, but it requires acknowledging suffering for the specific distress that it is and the extra effort it demands.

Knowledge of function in a diagnostic or therapeutic sense requires not only knowledge of the structure and function of the body but also knowledge of how persons live their lives – what they do, their activities, and their participation alone and with others in the world around them. The invisible world of dailiness; how life is lived and participated in on a daily basis by everyone. Why invisible? Because it is so ordinary and flows by so steadily and constantly that it is no longer seen by the people living it. That will not do for clinicians who must know in detail (depending on the specific problem) what people do, need, and think to function in everyday life. Further, clinicians must learn how to help their patients return to function in a manner that will constitute well-being. While most people within a clinician's ken may live in a similar daily world, dailiness is highly individual and thus returning persons to function is a highly individual matter. It requires particularized knowledge about the person.

Return to the ideas above and in the appendix about the nature of persons and you will see that sickness is personal; many aspects of persons – for example, formation and maintenance of relationships, doing and making, thinking, emotiveness, the formation and use of meaning, fear and anxiety, love, sexuality, and virtually everything else – are functions open to the impact of sickness and the actions of clinicians. They all involve participation in their individual processes; they are activities involving one or many body structures and body functions.

Sickness changes patients, and the changes may occur without the patient's awareness. Sickness alters function. These changes also, in turn, alter the illness; it is a circular process. The actions of clinicians must also be personal to be true to illness. They are directed toward sick persons, the dysfunctions making them sick, and the dimensions of their altered function. As a consequence, clinicians must learn as much about persons and their functions as they do about illness itself. Their knowledge should equip them to understand this particular sick person. When someone is seriously ill, that person's being includes the illness. As these functions can sometimes, perhaps often, be improved with therapeutic support, they can be made worse by ignorance and misdirected or lack of effort.

Physicians may rightly complain that when it comes to persons their knowledge doe not come close to their scientific knowledge of disease. That ignorance, however, is not systemic. As a profession and even as individual clinicians, we have acquired an enormous amount of information and knowledge about persons. Often, clinicians do not know what they know and do not have the skills and the confidence to apply their knowledge. Even within the last 50–75 years, knowledge of persons has grown almost exponentially. Mostly, it has been considered outside the domain of medical practice in the care of the sick because of bias about things psychological or the human sciences as a whole. The investigation of human life and function in a systematic fashion has marked psychology, the social sciences (including sociology and anthropology) over the last century using well-honed and verifiable methodologies as well as impartial observation. The observation of human activities and the life of persons during the last 75 years by both objective and subjective means have hewed to standards of science that are far higher than the not uncommon biases of natural and medical scientists would admit.

All of this means that the clinicians have available a wide body of knowledge that, while far from complete, will provide them with a basis for being be able to see whole persons as a group as well as *this particular* patient. On the contrary, requiring that clinicians learn this body of knowledge and the requisite skills by their own effort and initiative will never lead to a widespread medicine of whole persons. They must be trained. If you want a doctor to do certain things, he or she must be taught. In contemporary medicine, we rarely merely teach skills. Rather, we teach the theoretical basis for the skill and then the skill itself. Communication with sick persons is an example. A body of literature on the importance of communicating with patients has developed in the last 30 or 40 years. By now, based on that theory, many, perhaps most, medical schools teach communication skills in one form or another. Once the focus is on the person, the clinical skills embodied in the clinical method become crucial. The basic skill is observation, what Sir William Osler called "that most difficult skill of all." Learning to really see the patient in all the many dimensions of appearance and presentation to the world is difficult and takes a long time.

Many have commented on the loss of expertise of history taking and physical examination, of the clinical method in general as technological methods have grown in sophistication. The inquiry into function once again is dependent on the expertise of clinicians. There are no technologies – no MRI or CAT scan or their equivalent – to discover suffering and functional loss as I have described it. The clinician and the patient and their relationship are once again the center of medicine. We do not have to start again from scratch; good work has already been done about how clinicians can adapt their histories to the discovery of functional impairment [6]. The relief of suffering is the fundamental goal of medicine. The inquiry into the impact of sickness on the person and the person's inability to pursue purposes and goals are crucial in the discovery and relief of suffering, no less so in the relief of the burdens of sickness in general whether in mild disease or the dying patient.

References

1. Cassell EJ. The nature of suffering. 2nd ed. New York: Oxford University Press; 2004.
2. Kraemer HC. Evaluating medical tests: objective and quantitative guidelines. Newbury Park, CA: Sage Publications; 1992.
3. Wouters A. The function debate in philosophy [review]. Acta Biotheor. 2005;53:123–51.
4. WHO. International Classification of Functioning, Disability and Health. Geneva: WHO; 2001.
5. Drum CE, Horner-Jonson W, Krahn GL. Self-rated health and healthy days: examining the "disability paradox". Disab Health. 2008;1(2):71–8.
6. Stewart AL, Ware JE, editors. Measuring functioning and well-being: the medical outcomes study approach. Durham, NC: Duke University Press; 1992.

Chapter 3
The Healing Journey *

Tom A. Hutchinson, Balfour M. Mount, and Michael Kearney

Keywords Alcoholic • Journey • Healing journey • Psychosocial transition • Heroe's journey • Buddhism • Inner resources • Power differential • Archetype • Function • Giving up • Giving in

If the relief of suffering is the fundamental goal of medicine, there are at least three ways that this can occur. The most obvious approach, and usually our first instinct, is to attempt to fix the problem that appears to be causing the suffering. A second approach, proposed by Dr Cassell in the previous chapter, is to widen the focus to the function, purpose, and goals of the whole person. This is an important future direction for the development of whole person care that will involve doctors and other healthcare professionals solving a different kind of medical puzzle by learning new knowledge and doing different things in their medical practice. There is a third possibility that does not primarily concern problem solving, knowing, or doing. This way of resolving suffering is a natural potential of whole persons, which we call healing. CD's experience at the start of the book is an example of this phenomenon. Let me give you an example from my own life.

My dad was an alcoholic. He did not drink all of the time and was never late home from work or missed an appointment, but his drinking was seriously interfering with his life and our lives. For many years, our bills had been mounting, necessitating frequent changes in housing and location because of unpaid rent and mortgages. He had been demoted in his job. My mother lived in constant fear of creditor's letters and sheriff's visits to repossess unpaid-for furniture and appliances. When he arrived home from work, he was often quietly drunk, which drove my mother to distraction. He was never violent or abusive, but the effects of this

---

* Although all three authors contributed to this chapter, the personal and clinical stories relate to the first author and are, therefore, told in the first person.

T.A. Hutchinson (✉)
Professor, Faculty of Medicine, Director, Programs in Whole Person Care, McGill University, 546 Pine Avenue West, Montreal, QC H2W 1S6, Canada
e-mail: tom.hutchinson@mcgill.ca

T.A. Hutchinson (ed.), *Whole Person Care: A New Paradigm for the 21st Century*,
DOI 10.1007/978-1-4419-9440-0_3, © Springer Science+Business Media, LLC 2011

disease were devastating to the whole family: my mother, my younger brother and me, and of course my dad. He had a serious problem that could not be fixed in any of the usual ways: pills, therapy, willpower, religion, advice, pleading. All of which had been tried to no effect.

He needed healing, and I remember the night it began. I was going with him into Dublin on the bus one evening. I was bound for a school debating society meeting, and he was headed to his first meeting of Alcoholics Anonymous (AA). He was 47 at the time, and I was 17. I remember thinking that he looked nervous and unsure of himself. I loved him and was touched at his courage. That night changed our lives. When my father returned from the meeting, he reported that the alcoholics that he had met at the meeting were a complete surprise to him. For a start, many of them were successful and they were very well dressed. That seemed important to him. He liked them, and they had a sense of self-respect that he wanted for himself. There was a sense of peace at the meeting. No one preached at him to stop

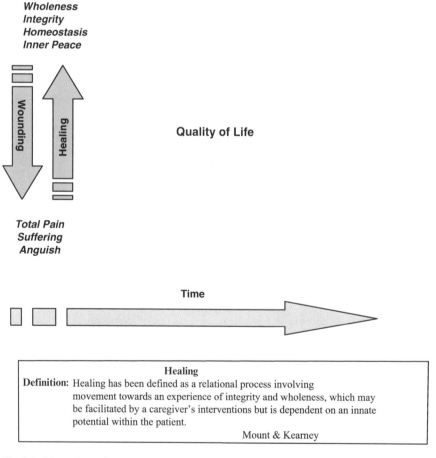

Fig. 3.1 Dimensions of the healing journey

drinking, but he did stop there and then and became a regular and proud attendee at AA meetings for years to come. He became a different man. Not just different from what he had been before, but different from other kids' fathers and other acquaintances. His alcoholism was not cured, as became evident many years later, after my mother died, but his life started to heal and he seemed happy and content. He had, I believe, found new hope in the presence of a devastating problem.

Figure 3.1 shows a diagram of quality of life, with a movement toward total pain, suffering, and anguish designated as wounding and a movement toward wholeness, integrity, homeostasis, and inner peace designated as healing [1, 2]. We all move up and down on this quality of life dimension as we live our lives through the second dimension shown on the diagram – time. It is the time dimension that makes the process a journey.

Figure 3.2 depicts the changes in well-being in a woman leaving an abusive relationship [3]. Her journey starts with the decision to leave the wounding relationship. Following her decision, her sense of well-being improves quite dramatically but is rapidly followed by a further fall when the reality of her new situation begins to sink in. At this point, many people would wonder if their decision was a wise one. Are they really better off? There follows a long period in what White calls the "betwixt and between phase" that finally leads to a return to a sense of well-being as the woman begins to come to terms with and see possibilities in her new reality. We would say that, like my dad, she was on a healing journey.

Others would have different words for this process: Colin Murray Parkes would call it negotiating a psychosocial transition [4]; Virginia Satir would see the change

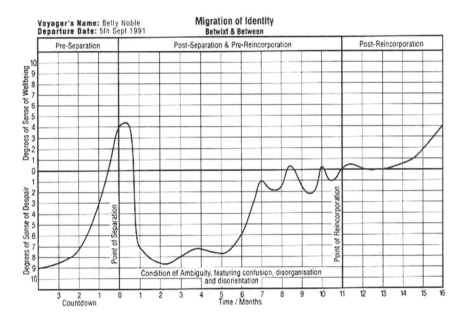

Fig. 3.2 The healing journey in a woman leaving an abusive relationship

process [5], and Joseph Campbell would recognize The Hero's Journey [6]. James Joyce would write Ulysses in an attempt to give his readers a moment-to-moment experience of the process [7]. It does not occur instantaneously and involves further wounding and suffering as well as healing. What most people want is to back away from the journey and the suffering involved and return to the integrity and wholeness that they knew before the wounding occurred. For most serious problems, like this woman's and my dad's, that is simply not an option. There is no turning back. At this point, to paraphrase Robert Frost, the best, and only, way out is through. And yet, it is sometimes startling to see the lengths that people will go to rather than face the suffering that needs to be faced to move forward.

Brian Ditty was a patient that I knew while he was on dialysis treatment for kidney failure [8]. Here is how he describes his response when he was told he would have to start regular dialysis treatment for his kidney failure: "I was 19 when my doctor called me and said it was time to start dialysis. I told him, 'No, I don't think so, it's not for me.' He said 'What do you mean, what are you talking about?' I told him again 'It's not for me, it's not my lifestyle.' He then told me if I did not start I would die in a few weeks. I told him that was fine. I'd had a good life." Brian thought that he was willing to die at 19 rather than face the suffering of life on dialysis.

As Buddhism has long taught [9], suffering is part of life and can, therefore, not be avoided. We and our patients will suffer. That is not a choice. The choice is whether we will suffer to avoid life or in the service of something that is of deeper importance to us – a something that often cannot easily be articulated by the person. The example of my father makes it clear for me. He was suffering terribly when he was a drinking alcoholic. He would do anything to avoid that suffering except stop drinking because the potential suffering of facing life without a drink was more frightening than the suffering with which he was familiar. I see the same phenomenon in people with terminal disease. They are suffering, struggling terribly to overcome a cancer or other disease that they know in their hearts cannot be cured. But to admit that the disease cannot be fixed would mean facing uncertainty and loss of the illusion of control – more terrifying than their current suffering. And so, they continue to suffer in a way that is familiar to them until the day arrives when they begin to come to terms with the fact that they are dying. When that happens a new process opens up, which involves different suffering, and possibilities for a new sense of integrity and wholeness.

Perhaps the aim of medicine is not just to eradicate the suffering that can be eradicated but also to support patients in facing the suffering that cannot be eradicated, and which they have been avoiding, with the hope that they can experience a greater sense of integrity and wholeness. Perhaps the real goal of medicine should be to support patients in their healing journey, to help patients move toward a life with a greater sense of connection and meaning and a new relationship to wounding and suffering. I think that for my father what initiated the change was the deep connection he felt with fellow (wounded) alcoholics. This enabled a change in his experience of himself and his alcoholism, which had been transformed from a source of shame to an opening for a new life. To Brian Ditty, it may have been the love he felt from his parents that made it possible for him to move forward. For each person, the catalyst will be different.

How can we help as healthcare workers? Our first instinct might be to attempt to speed up the process or to short-circuit it. But that is rarely (we would say virtually never) possible. And now, we are caught in a bind. As caregivers, we may believe that in the absence of a shortcut there are only two remaining options: (1) Go on the whole journey with the patient or (2) Withdraw from or deny the whole process. Often, the first seems so overwhelming that we opt for the second choice to the detriment of patients and ourselves.

Here is my experience of the dilemma. For most of my career (24 years), I practiced as a nephrologist. I followed patients with various kinds of chronic kidney disease. On a regular basis, one or other of my patients would have a decrease in their kidney function to the point that they needed to go on regular dialysis treatment. I dreaded this milestone. I think that it was partly my sense of having failed. I should have prevented this outcome. But the dread was even more related, I think, to facing this new phase in the patient's illness and what it meant for them. I had seen many patients start dialysis and did not like what I saw. They did usually survive, but their expected life span was shortened (average 5 years, similar to some common cancers). Their daily life would now be very difficult, requiring visits to the hospital 3 times per week for hemodialysis, a very restricted diet, and multiple medications. For peritoneal dialysis, the requirements would be different but also very intrusive. They developed recurrent complications. Just as they were adjusting to one set of problems, they seemed to be faced with another transition [10]. I simply could not face it. Why? Because I felt that if I were in their shoes I would find life unbearable. I felt overwhelmed. Being willing to put part of myself in their shoes and adopt the wounded healer role would have involved faith and trust in my own and others' inner resilience and resources – a faith and trust that I did not then possess.

So I took the second option. My conversations with them became fairly short. I did not attempt to explore with them what their concerns and expectations were in this new phase of their lives. When they did raise fears or worries, I tended to be reassuring in a general way that probably did not convince them any more than it did me. I did not attempt to help them to face this new reality of their lives. I believe that in failing to do so I did not respect them as persons with untapped inner resources and (unintentionally) did not help them to marshal those resources to get the most out of their situation. I failed them. But what else could I do?

There was another choice that I hadn't realized was possible. It is to be present to another's suffering on a moment-to-moment basis and serve them as we would want to be served. Guggenbuhl-Craig [11] describes it as the wounded healer role "The image of the wounded healer symbolizes an acute and painful awareness of sickness as the counter pole to the physician's health, a lasting and hurtful certainty of the degeneration of his own body and mind. This sort of experience makes of the doctor the patient's brother rather than his master". Our suffering may not be the same, or as intense, as the suffering that the patient is now experiencing, but we may be in as bad or worse a situation in the future and are willing to extend to them what we would like to be extended to us. And they in turn begin to find resources for healing that they may have been unaware were available.

What might that look like? After I stopped practicing nephrology, I embarked on a new career in palliative care. It taught me what I had failed to experience in my previous work – the power of emphatic presence. When people first realize that they are not going to get better and that they will die from their disease, it often initiates a period of intense suffering. It may be a chaotic process in which they oscillate between believing they will get better and a sense that all is lost. Enter the palliative care physician whose job is to join them neither in false hopes nor in hopelessness, but to be present to the real hope possible in each moment. I have done this (imperfectly) many times, and it is exactly what I would want in the same situation.

I was having a meeting with the family of a woman who was dying of metastatic breast cancer. The reason for the meeting was primarily to try to help the patient's husband, whom I had not met, but whom I had been told was "impossible". He kept asking for more tests, woke his wife up frequently at night (he spent day and night in her hospital room), and did not appear to be able to accept that she was dying. The meeting began as usual with me saying a few words about family meetings and their usefulness in helping to get everyone on the same page. I then asked for input from the family about how they saw things were going. In the course of this conversation, the patient's husband affirmed that he felt the future was uncertain. His wife might be dying, but on the contrary, she might live for years. No one could say for certain. One of the patient's sisters added that another issue of concern was that it was hard to judge how much pain the patient had because she had always been a person who thought only of other people rather than herself and rarely discussed her own needs. She was a very loving person. I interrupted the conversation at that point and asked the husband to tell me more about his wife, since I only knew her since she was sick. He did, and as he talked it was evident how much he loved her and how much he would miss her when she died. He commented "she had a better intuition for people," one that he depended on. She was a completely loving person. He did not know what he would do without her.

From that point on, the conversation went more easily. We talked for a while longer, and toward the end I said that I thought things would be easier when he (the husband) began to accept that his wife was dying and we could enter a new phase that I had often seen could be a good experience for people. But I noted this transition might take time. The husband interrupted me and said he did not think it would take more time. He would adjust to this new reality. He simply had not had a conversation about these issues with the medical team before this. He proved to be correct. From that point on, the focus of the family was the patient's comfort. The husband did not appear to struggle in the same way with the reality of his wife's dying. His hope now was that his wife could be relieved of pain and that she would die peacefully, which she did within days.

What worked in this interview? To begin with, I was open to the process and trusted that if I attended to each moment and each person that something good would open up and help the situation to begin moving in a positive direction. What came up was the sister's remark about the patient being a very loving person. That allowed me to start to ask her husband more about his wife and to begin to relate to her as a whole person (she was comatose and not in the room) while at the same time beginning to relate to the husband in the same way. I attempted to open up possibilities for her and for him rather than pushing for change. The power differential was disappearing, and we were now not just doctor and patient's husband but two caring people facing a difficult and sad life event together. With this kind of radical shift in the power relationship the healer pole of the healer–patient archetype becomes activated [12] in the patient (or relative). It is this inner healer that leads to transformation, as I believe we saw in this husband. As Guggenbuhl-Craig observes [11]: "When a patient becomes sick, the healer-patient archetype is constellated. The sick man seeks an external healer, but at the same time the intra-psychic healer is activated. We often refer to this intra-psychic healer in the ill as the 'healing factor'… The physician within the patient himself and its healing action is as great as that of the doctor who appears on the scene externally." And changing the power differential is the key step in uncovering this inner healer.

Is the healing described here encompassed by Eric Cassell's resolution of suffering through a focus on function? Yes if the idea of function is interpreted widely enough, and with an extra step that may be implied by Cassell, but often missed by patients, families and professional caregivers. The missing step is coming to terms with reality. The most frequent cause of suffering being prolonged that we see in patients and the families of patients in palliative care is that they remain focused on unachievable goals. This ranges from a hope for cure and a return to previous function to an expectation to live for months or years when the reality is closer to days or weeks. Patients suffering in this way are often working very hard to achieve their goals, but they continue to suffer intensely. This changes when they begin to accept the reality of their situation and redirect their hopes and goals. This can sound like giving up, but nothing could be further from the truth. Often, it brings with it a new focus and a new energy for the task at hand. And, as with the husband of the patient in the last story, there may be a new sense of calm. As an acquaintance of mine dealing with a difficult situation with her son said "It is not giving up, but giving in to life", which might serve as a good summary of the healing journey.

References

1. Mount B, Hanks G, McGoldrick L. The principles of palliative care. In: Fallon M, Hanks G, eds. ABC of palliative care. 2nd ed. Oxford, UK: Blackwell Publishing Ltd; 2006. p. 1–3.
2. Mount BM, Kearney M. Healing and palliative care: charting our way forward. Pall Med. 2003;17:657–58.
3. White M. Re-authoring lives: interviews & essays. Adelaide (Australia): Dulwich Centre Publications; 1995. [Chart], Migration of identity. p. 102.
4. Parkes CM. Bereavement. Studies of grief in adult life. 3rd ed. England: Penguin Books; 1996.
5. Satir V, Banmen J, Gerber J, Gomori M. Chapter 5, The process of change. In: The Satir model. Palo Alto, CA: Science and Behaviour Books, Inc.; 1991. p. 85–119.

6. Campbell J. The hero with a thousand faces. 2nd ed. Princeton, NJ: Princeton University Press; 1968.
7. Joyce J. Ulysses. 10th ed. London, Great Britain: The Bodley Head Ltd; 1964.
8. Ditty BE. Chapter 1. Phillips D, editor. Heroes. In: 100 stories of living with kidney failure. Montreal: Grosvenor House Press, Inc.; 1998. p. 7–14.
9. Wallace BA. The first point: the preliminaries. In: Buddhism with an attitude. The Tibetan seven-point mind-training. Ithaca, NY: Snow Lion Publications; 2001. p. 13–63.
10. Hutchinson TA. Transitions in the lives of patients with end stage renal disease: a cause of suffering and an opportunity for healing. Pall Med. 2005;19:270–7.
11. Guggenbühl-Craig A. Chapter 13, The closing of the split through power. In: Power in the helping professions. 2nd ed. Putnam, Connecticut: Spring Publications, Inc.; 2004. p. 87–92.
12. Kearney M. Towards a therapeutic use of self. In: A place of healing. Working with suffering in living and dying. Oxford, U.K.: Oxford University Press; 2005. p. 91–102.

Chapter 4
The Challenge of Medical Dichotomies and the Congruent Physician–Patient Relationship in Medicine

Tom A. Hutchinson and James R. Brawer

Keywords Dichotomy • Organism • Cortex • Hemisphere • Integration • Language • Prosody • Face • Perception • Right/left • Diagnosis • Externalization • Hippocrates • Asklepios • Placebo • Satir, Virginia • Communication stances • Communication • Analog • Analogic communication • Congruence

As Scott Fitzgerald remarked [1] "The test of a first-rate intelligence is the ability to hold two opposed ideas in mind at the same time and still retain the ability to function." And we would add not just function but function more effectively. It is an important ability because from the subatomic foundations of physical existence to hypercomplex patterns of human behavior and social organization, life in this world is rife with dichotomies. There always seems to be two of everything, and the two are often mutually exclusive: light/dark, knowledge/ignorance, life/death, etc. Although dichotomies are endemic to every facet of our existence, we have never gotten comfortable with them. They are perturbations in the integrated flow of life, and discordant elements disrupting our sense of harmony and unity. We feel compelled to get past them, to resolve them. The easiest way of dealing with them is to ignore them or deny their existence. Second to this is collapsing them by choosing one element over the other. The physicist can choose whether he wishes to consider the wave-like properties of light or its particulate nature. He cannot simultaneously study both. He can choose to know the position of a particle or its momentum. He cannot simultaneously know both. Moderate dichotomies may be amenable to some level of integration. Do we want a liberal or a conservative government? We cannot have both, but we can have a conservative minority government modulated by the impact of liberal coalition partners.

T.A. Hutchinson (✉)
Professor, Faculty of Medicine, Director, Programs in Whole Person Care, McGill University, 546 Pine Avenue West, Montreal, QC H2W 1S6, Canada
e-mail: tom.hutchinson@mcgill.ca

T.A. Hutchinson (ed.), *Whole Person Care: A New Paradigm for the 21st Century*, DOI 10.1007/978-1-4419-9440-0_4, © Springer Science+Business Media, LLC 2011

Medicine is not immune to the dichotomy quandary. The focus of medicine, the underlying objective unifying its diverse branches and disciplines, is the health of humanity. The problem is that the people who comprise humanity are peculiarly dichotomous creatures. The patient who walks into the doctor's office is, on the one hand, an organism, constructed of molecules and governed by natural law. His life processes can be described in physical terms and are amenable to scientific investigation. Although more complex, he is fundamentally no different than the rodent, or, for that matter, the yeast, from which he has learned so much about his own biology. As in the case of yeast, one organism is, more or less, the same as another.

On the other hand, the patient is a human, a wondrous form of life, endowed with individual identity, awareness of self, and an array of faculties, sensibilities, and behaviors that defy scientific-reductionist methods of analysis. In addition, the human is a social being whose personality is significantly shaped by the history, mores, and beliefs of the civilization to which he belongs.

We are, by and large, oblivious to the contradiction that we embody. For most of us, it is an interesting theoretical oddity of no practical import. For the healthcare professions, however, it is a defining issue that, in great measure, determines the direction in which medicine evolves.

Consider what happens when a patient visits a doctor with a new complaint. The patient has symptoms and is "dis-eased" but does not yet have a named disease. The physician takes a history, does a physical examination, perhaps orders some tests and then makes a diagnosis. The resulting effect is diagrammed in Fig. 4.1. The disease is now separated from the patient with multiple resultant beneficial effects. For the patient, this is first of all a validation. The problem is not in his head or imagination, and in an interesting way it is no longer his fault that he feels unwell [2] – he simply has a disease that both medicine and society recognize afflicts people against their will. To appreciate the power of this effect, consider those with problems that are not fully validated as bona fide diseases (Chronic Lyme disease [3], Chronic Fatigue syndromes [4], and other examples). Organizations representing people with these partially recognized diseases have gone to great lengths to obtain recognition [3, 4]. On the other side of the coin, consider the frequent relief of people who finally receive a diagnosis defining a condition as one recognized by the profession and by society as a bona fide disease, even if is very serious and even fatal. There is another effect – people appreciate a definitive diagnosis because it empowers them to focus on what they can do to mitigate the effects of this now externalized problem on their lives. This empowering externalization effect is probably as old as medicine itself and has also more recently been explicitly employed to great effect outside mainstream medicine by groups as diverse as Alcoholics Anonymous dealing with alcoholism [5] and family therapists dealing with "non-medical" problems such as bedwetting and encopresis [6].

A diagnosis also makes the doctor's job easier and facilitates the collaboration between doctor and patient. If I know that your frequent voluminous urination (polyuria) is due to diabetes mellitus rather than diabetes insipidus, it makes a radical difference in the treatment that I will prescribe and the prognosis and potential complications that I need to discuss with you. Without this diagnostic process

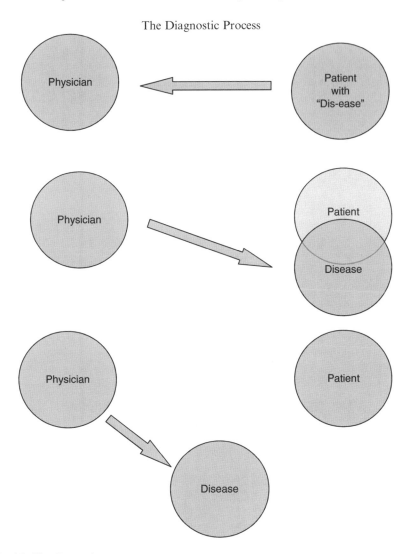

Fig. 4.1 The diagnostic process

around which almost all medical information is organized, whether in a textbook, the Internet, or the doctor's head, medicine could not function and yet it creates a major challenge for the doctor, the patient, and clinical medicine – a dichotomy that becomes more problematic, the more medicine advances.

The problem is simply this: after the diagnosis is made, the doctor has two relationships rather that one to manage at the same time (Fig. 4.2). He has the relationship with the disease where his job is to cure the problem or do everything in his power to limit its progression and effects. No patient should accept any less. At the same time, he has the relationship with person who has the disease (the patient) where his job is to facilitate healing. As Kearney [7] points out, we have realized

The Two Therapeutic Relationships

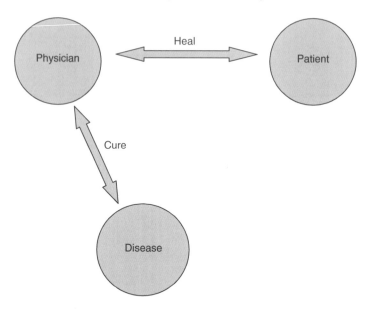

Fig. 4.2 The two therapeutic relationships

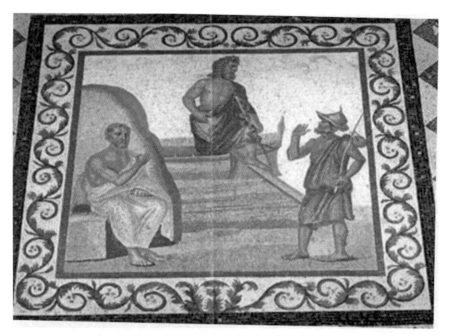

Fig. 4.3 Mosaic from the island of Kos

this at least since the classical Greeks. Figure 4.3 shows a mosaic from the Greek island of Kos in which a patient (on the right of the figure) is coming to see a doctor. But as the Greeks realized, he is actually coming to see two doctors. In the foreground is Hippocrates the physician who will attempt to cure the patient's disease. In the background on a boat and holding a staff with a snake is Asklepios, the god of healing. We believe the Greeks were right in believing that we need both and therefore we have used their titles (Hippocratic and Asklepian) to label the two sides of the medical dichotomy in Table 4.1.

The problem might be relatively straightforward except that curing and healing are a very real dichotomous pair. In Table 4.1, you notice that each characteristic on the left-hand Hippocratic (curing) side of the table is matched by an opposite characteristic on the Asklepian (healing) side. For instance, on the Hippocratic side under "ACTION" the patient is holding on, whereas on the Asklepian side he needs to learn to let go. On the Hippocratic side, his goal is to survive (meaning as mentioned in Chap. 1 not just physical survival but also survival of his current life and identity with as little change as possible), whereas on the Asklepian side the goal is growth. The contrasts in communication, epistemology, and validity are equally striking. We return to the contrasts in communication and epistemology later but want to highlight here the last line of the table referring to validity.

Scientific medicine, at least since the late nineteenth century, accentuated by the development of evidence-based medicine in the late twentieth century, has implicitly dismissed the Asklepian side of medicine as invalid. Double-blind randomized clinical trials (the gold standard of good evidence) are specifically designed to erase the placebo effect and with it healing and all of the effects in the patient that result from a healing relationship with the individual healthcare practitioner or the team responsible for care. It is as if those effects do not exist although we know from those same clinical trials that the "placebo" effect is often of apparently comparable size to the "real" effect being studied. We have dealt with this dichotomy in the way we frequently deal with other dichotomies. We focus on one side and act as if that were the whole. In doing so, we engage in a strategy that is often utilized by the brain in processing information. Our brains are designed in such a way as to simplify our perceptions and reduce ambiguity. As a consequence, however, the information that we receive is often highly selective

Table 4.1 Medical dichotomy

	Hippocratic	Asklepian
Patient		
Possibility	Being cured	Healing
Action	Holding on	Letting go
Goal	Survival	Growth
Doctor		
Communication	Content	Relationship
	Digital	Analog
	Conscious	Unconscious
Epistemology	Scientific	Artistic
Validity	Real	Placebo

and incomplete. To take a very simple example, consider for a moment how we see human faces.

A common organizational theme in the brain is the spatial distribution of functional capacities in reciprocal pairs. The complementary functions of the right and left cortical hemispheres, for example, have been so well established as to have captured the public imagination. There is no end of Web sites extolling the virtues of the musical, artistic, fun-loving right brain over its dry, colorless, mathematical/linguistic counterpart on the left. Pop science notwithstanding, the distinctions are real and consequential.

The impact of the left/right cortical dichotomy on our conscious experience can be appreciated through the picture in Fig. 4.4 below [8]. The top image is a full

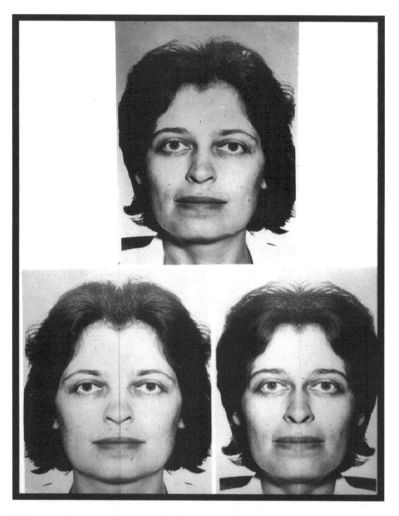

Fig. 4.4 Composite images from a single photograph of the same face

frontal facial photograph of a colleague at McGill. At the lower left is a picture constructed of the left half of face and its mirror image (i.e., two left halves fused to form a full face representation). At the lower right is a face assembled from the two right halves of the face. The lower right face clearly resembles the original (top image) far more than does the face at the lower left. The reason for this is that the human face is asymmetrical and that the two halves are notably dissimilar. When one views a person face on, the neuroanatomy of the visual system is such that the right half of the observed face ends up in the right cerebral hemisphere of the observer, whereas the left half is represented in the left hemisphere. Inasmuch as the right hemisphere outperforms the left in appreciating spatial relationships and imagery, the left "defers" to the right and what we see is pretty much what our right hemi-spheres show us [8]. However, she does not see herself the same way. Although we identify the individual with the image on the lower right she thinks she looks more like the image on the lower left constructed of the two left facial halves. The reason is that her view of herself is what she sees in a mirror, and in a mirror image, the left half of the face is represented in the right cerebral hemisphere. There are, thus, two of her; the "her" identified by herself and the "her" perceived by others [9]. Because the stakes are not very high, the choice (made by?) to consider only the right cortex to avoid confusion is not of major consequence either on the down side (direct adverse effects) or on the potential loss of an upside (a potential synergy that might result from encompassing both sides of the dichotomy in our awareness).

However, more directly relevant to the medical dichotomy, pioneering family therapist Virginia Satir would say that we habitually do the same thing when the potential losses and benefits are extremely high, in relating to whole people, and not just their faces. In a very simple diagram (Fig. 4.5), she depicted any relationship between two people as having three essential elements: self, other, and context [10].

Components of an Interaction between 2 people

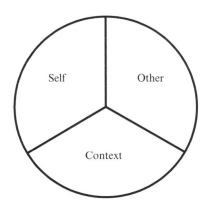

Fig. 4.5 Components of an interaction between two people

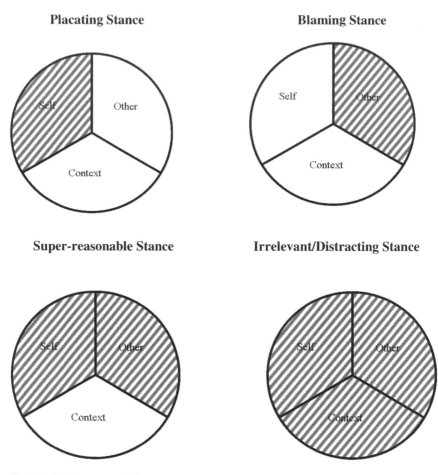

Fig. 4.6 Satir's communication stances

This is very close indeed to the relationship that set up the medical dichotomy in the first place – the relationship of the physician (self) to the patient (other) and to the disease (context). She pointed out that people regularly blot out or extinguish one or more of these elements when they interact with other people under stress. She identified four major communication stances [11] diagrammed in Fig. 4.6: placating in which the self is ignored or blotted out, blaming in which the other is ignored as a person, superreasonable in which both self and other are forgotten about as people, and irrelevant in which the person under extreme stress loses touch with all three elements – self, other, and context. The stance we adopt in a clinical interaction will determine how we handle the medical dichotomy.

And in medicine we see all four stances. Placating is a natural starting place for many young medical students and nurses. They understand that the essence of medicine is service to others. Their professional self-esteem is often not very high (they believe they have very little to offer) but are willing to do whatever they can to help the patient get better. If a patient or a supervisor indicates that they are not doing enough, their usual response is to try harder, stay later, and forget about their own needs. This is not bad in itself and perhaps a good place to start but in the long run hard to sustain. Despite our tendency to deny them, we do have needs that if not met lead to fatigue, poor functioning, emotional reactivity, and possibly in the long run burnout. Sometimes, in reaction to the risk of being consumed by the needs of patients and/or the system, students or practitioners adopt the blaming response. In this response, my own vulnerability and needs are paramount and I identify any problems or deficiencies as someone else's fault. The reason my supervisor gave me a poor evaluation is that he himself is insecure. The reason this family is angry at me is because they are dysfunctional. Both of these assessments may be true, but in the blaming stance this is not a balanced assessment but a defensive reaction aimed at bolstering by own self-esteem.

Both of these first two stances (placating and blaming) involve an element of relationship and overt emotional reactivity and can in the long run be exhausting. Perhaps for this reason, the favored stance is often for physicians to focus exclusively on the Hippocratic side of the medical dichotomy and adopt the superreasonable stance in which the personhood of the patient and the doctor are ignored in a single-minded focus on curing or fixing the disease. This may sound somewhat neutral and not too harmful but in practice can be disastrous and very wounding.[1] For doctors who are close to or beyond the point of burnout [13] (emotional exhaustion, depersonalization, low sense of personal accomplishment) the irrelevant stance may become frequent. In this stance the physician has lost contact with himself, the other person and the context. Doctors in this stance are both embarrassing and dangerous.[2]

---

[1] A colleague was admitted to an intensive care unit following esophageal surgery for cancer. He was relatively stable, although bleeding from a nasogastric tube, when visited by a group of residents who had to have known him well previously as a colleague and teacher. They completely ignored any prior relationship as they discussed his case including a vivid description of his GI bleeding. As they turned to go, one said to the other obviously within his hearing "It is a pity but I suppose he should have 6 or 7 good months left." There was no acknowledgement of him or his probable reaction to this statement. Not surprisingly he reacted strongly (internally), but the residents did not notice. They had already moved on to the next patient [12].

[2] Here is an example from one of our medical students: "We're still following surgeon A around the wards – A family friend asked him to visit her husband, who's being treated on the wards. We walk into the room, and are confronted by an elderly man in severe pain – eyes clenched, back arched, breaths coming in short bursts. Pt's med student is present. Four family members are present. Family friend, in tears is grateful surgeon A came - hugs him. Surgeon A turns away from the pt and tells us a joke. I can't listen – my attention is directly at the pt, who's in obvious distress, and the family who have anxious looks. Surgeon A examines the pt's urinary catheter, the assumed source of the pain. Uses a large syringe to pump water in and out of the bladder and comments that everything looks ok. Meanwhile the pt's eyes fly open and he shakes his head back and forth in obvious agony as the fluid is moved in and out of the catheter. Surgeon A is satisfied with the placement of the catheter and leaves the room assuring the family that nothing can be done - the prescribed pain killers are appropriate he says. Surgeon A never once addressed the patient. I'm disgusted. Before leaving, surgeon A invites us to rounds the next week. I'm tempted, since he's the first tutor to offer, but I don't think I will for fear that I'll acquire his bed side manner, which I find reprehensible."

It is easiest to see how specifically the communication stances relate to Table 4.1, and particularly to the parts on communication and epistemology, by starting with physicians in the superreasonable stance who obliterate the Asklepian side of the dichotomy. In the superreasonable stance communication is about content using digital means (each word has a specific meaning) and is conscious. This aspect of communication does not involve a relationship between people. This is why it can be done equally effectively (in terms of transfer of information) by a written document. But this entirely neglects the Asklepian side where the purpose of communication is relationship which is transmitted by analogic means and is largely unconscious. Here is description of analog communication from Watzlawick et al. [14]: "What then is analogic communication? The answer is relatively simple: it is virtually all nonverbal communication. This term however, is deceptive, because it is often restricted to body movement only, to the behavior known as kinesics. We hold that the term must comprise posture, gesture, facial expression, voice inflection, the sequence, rhythm, and cadence of the words themselves, and any other nonverbal manifestation of which the organism is capable, as well as the communicational clues unfailingly present in any context in which an interaction takes place."

Significantly, the dichotomy between the appreciation of analogic and digital communication is reflected in the way that the brain processes these two dimensions of language perception. And in this case the brain can and does encompass both sides. The capacity to understand the grammatical, syntactic, and semantic (digital) aspects of language resides primarily in the left cerebral hemisphere in most individuals. In contrast, corresponding areas of the right hemisphere are essential for the appreciation of the analogic dimensions of language referred to as prosody [15].

Speech comprehension is, therefore, the product of a synergy between disparate modes of neurological processing localized in different regions of the brain. In order for speech comprehension to be complete, each of these distinct linguistic dimensions, digital and analog, must reflect its own unique characteristics unimpeded and undiluted by the other.

And where relationship is the issue it is our analog communication that matters. According to Watzlawick et al.: "Indeed, wherever relationship is the central issue of communication, we find that digital language is almost meaningless. This is not only the case between animals and between man and animal, but in many other contingencies in human life, e.g., courtship, love, succor, combat, and of course, in all dealings with very young children or severely disturbed mental patients. Children, fools, and animals have always been credited with particular intuition regarding the sincerity or insincerity of human attitudes, for it is easy to profess something verbally, but difficult to carry a lie into the realm of the analogic."

If, as Watzlawick et al. claim [14], it is difficult to fake analog communication how do we do something about it? The answer is not to fake better but to be aware of, and if necessary change our relationship with the patient. We do this by changing our stance in our interaction with the patient. By moving from a superreasonable stance to a placating stance, or even a blaming stance, for instance, we are beginning (although incompletely) to move into relationship with the patient, and the analog communication messages will quickly follow. The objective, however, is to move past blaming and placating to include both ourselves and the patient fully in the relationship. This is what Satir calls congruence [16]. This is a learned process that cannot be standardized and will look different in every physician–patient pair – hence the use of the term artistic on the Asklepian side of the epistemology dichotomy in contrast to scientific on the Hippocratic side. Like an artist, the physician who wishes to master communication on the Asklepian side needs to learn more about himself and his inbuilt reactions so that he can get in touch with and authentically convey his presence and caring to the patient.

Congruence does not solve dichotomies, but rather transcends them. A colleague reported that he could not get through to a young psychiatric patient for whom he was caring. The specific problem was relatively straightforward. The patient was part of an inpatient group who had to stick to certain rules as part of their therapy. One of the rules was that they could not take snacks at certain times of the day. However, many of them did anyway, and our patient asked, given this reality, whether he could have a snack. He was told no. This infuriated him and led to a number of interviews with my colleague. My colleague to calm the situation took a fairly analytic and unemotional approach to the situation trying to explore with the patient why he reacted so strongly to the situation and what he could learn from it. This made the patient worse, and my colleague presented the situation to our group because he was concerned the patient was becoming increasingly psychotic. My colleague felt that he was doing the right thing in attempting to help the patient learn from the situation. The patient felt that he was right in seeing the response to his question as unreasonable and infuriating. Neither person felt (correctly) that the other was listening to him. In a role play, it became evident what needed to happen. To the observers, it was evident that both were right and one or both of them had to come to that realization. With some coaching, the psychiatrist put himself in the patient's shoes (while also staying in his own shoes), and everything began to change in the role play. There is a clear relationship here to earlier discussions (Chap. 3) of the wounded healer role. The person playing the patient felt listened to, the demeanor of the psychiatrist changed (unconscious analog communication perfectly evident to the observers), and the two became engaged with each other again in a productive therapeutic alliance. This kind of problem usually cannot be solved by convincing arguments on either side, by one or other side dominating or giving in (though we often strive for exactly that outcome) or by the manipulations that sometimes occur to us in situations of disagreement or conflict. This is a very real difference between two people both of whom *are* right, although the greater the intensity of the interaction the harder it will be to open ourselves to that realization. A difference between two people might be seen as a microcosm of all the other difficult to resolve dichotomies in our lives. The answer is to move to a different level (congruence) where we can see both points of view. Dr Ofri's relationship with her patient in Chap. 7 is an example of this process and of congruence. In that wider perspective, both sides of the medical dichotomy are encompassed, new healing possibilities become available, and a synergy is sometimes created that appears energized by the intensity of the original divergence. We explore some of this synergy further in the last chapter of the book.

It is difficult to get a full sense of congruence by reading about it, and Dr Dobkin and I [17] have begun to experiment with teaching mindful congruence to physicians in practice and to medical students using role plays and simulations that recreate real clinical encounters. It is surprising how often experienced clinicians (as above) can be caught in an unconscious communication stance, how they can change (by adding back the missing part) when it is pointed out to them, and what a difference it makes to the interaction. So, part of the way forward is to explicitly teach congruent relating to medical students and physicians. And part will consist of a change in how students are taught, supervised, observed, and evaluated when doing clinical rotations. As this skill becomes more appreciated and developed, they will also have more opportunities to see it practiced by role models. But this is not a new skill, and we suspect that master clinicians have always behaved this way. We suspect that this is what Dr Francis Peabody meant [18] when he said that"the secret of the caring of the patient is in the caring for the patient," although we would have been happier if he had added "and the awareness and caring for ourselves."

References

1. Fitzgerald FS. The crack-up. Esquire. Feb 1936.
2. Arnowitz RA. Conclusion. In: Making sense of illness: science, society and disease. Cambridge, UK: Cambridge University Press; 1998. p. 166–89.
3. Arnowitz RA. Chapter 3, Lyme disease: the social construction of a new disease and its social consequences. In: Making sense of illness: science, society and disease. Cambridge, UK: Cambridge University Press; 1998. p. 57–83.
4. Arnowitz RA. Chapter 1, From myalgic encephalitis to yuppie flu: a history of chronic fatigue syndromes. In: Making sense of illness: science, society and disease. Cambridge, UK: Cambridge University Press; 1998. p. 19–38.
5. Anonymous. Chapter 2, There is a solution. In: Alcoholics anonymous big book. 3rd ed. New York, NY: Alcoholics Anonymous World Services; 1976. p. 17–29.
6. White M, Epston D. Chapter 2, Externalizing of the problem. In: Narrative means to therapeutic ends. New York, NY: W.W. Norton and Company; 1990. p. 38–76.
7. Kearney M. A place of healing: working with suffering in living and dying. Oxford, UK: Oxford University Press; 2000.
8. Milner B. Complementary functional specializations of the human cerebral hemispheres. In: Levi-Montalcini R, editor. Nerve cells, transmitters and behaviour. Vatican City: Pontificia Academia Scientiarum Scripta Varia; 1980. p. 601–25.
9. Brawer JR. The value of a philosophical perspective in teaching the basic medical sciences. Med Teach. 2006;28:472–4.
10. Satir V, Banmen J, Gerber J, Gomori M. Chapter 2, The primary triad. In: The Satir Model: family therapy and beyond. Palo Alto, CA: Science and Behavior Books; 1991. p. 19–30.
11. Satir V, Banmen J, Gerber J, Gomori M. Chapter 3, The survival stances. In: The Satir Model: family therapy and beyond. Palo Alto, CA: Science and Behavior Books; 1991. p. 31–64.
12. Drazen RY. The choice is yours [DVD]. Drazen Productions; 2001. Distributed by the American Board of Internal Medicine Foundation.

13. Maslach C, Jackson SE, Leiter MP. MBI: The Maslach Burnout Inventory. Palo Alto, CA: Consulting Psychologists Press; 1996.
14. Watzlawick P, Bavelas JB, Jackson DD. Chapter 2, Some tentative axioms of communication. In: Pragmatics of human communication: a study of interactional patterns, pathologies, and paradoxes. New York, NY: W.W. Norton & Company; 1967. p. 48–71.
15. Pell M. Cerebral mechanisms for understanding emotional prosody in speech. Brain Lang. 2005;96:221–34.
16. Satir V, Banmen J, Gerber J, Gomori M. Chapter 4, Congruence. In: The Satir Model: family therapy and beyond. Palo Alto, CA: Science and Behavior Books; 1991. p. 65–84.
17. Hutchinson TA, Dobkin PL. Mindful medical practice: just another fad? Can Fam Physician. 2009;55:778–9.
18. Peabody FW. The care of the patient. JAMA. 1927;88:877–82.

Chapter 5
Separation–Attachment Theory in Illness and the Role of the Healthcare Practitioner

Gregory Fricchione

Keywords Attachment theory and health • Neurobiology of separation and attachment • Illness experience • Caregiving • Transitional relatedness

The Separation Challenge of Illness

In an important book titled *Health Wars: On the Global Front Lines of Modern Medicine*, Richard Horton, physician editor of the Lancet, focuses on the crisis in clinical medicine and the patient–doctor relationship today [1]. Horton makes the point that modern medicine, while continuing to push its scientific frontiers, must remain true to its roots in the relationship of trust between the patient and the doctor.

Empathy joins *trust* as the keys to maintaining the soul of clinical medicine, as Alfred Tauber [2], a Boston University Professor of Medicine and Philosophy emphasizes in his "new medical ethic": "While basic science and the conceptual network of physical terms can tell us much about phenotypic symptoms and signs and pathologic cellular damage and genetic descriptions of disease, they tell us nothing about what the disease causes in the human being who is a patient" [2].

Science is limited when faced with the most important driver for the patient's visit to the doctor in the first place. Horton states: "It is neither a wholly mechanistic nor a wholly metaphysical question, yet it remains, for many patients, a deeply important one: what is this disease doing to me? Doctors tend to recoil from these more holistic matters. In asking the question, I am not seeking an ultimate final meaning of human disease, teleology of illness so to speak, instead I am trying to find a way to make sense of what it is that disease does to us, not only as human

G. Fricchione (✉)
Associate Chief of Psychiatry, Director, Division of Psychiatry and Medicine,
Massachusetts General Hospital, Professor of Psychiatry, Harvard Medical School,
Warren 615, 55 Fruit Street, Boston, MA 02114, USA
e-mail: gfricchione@partners.org

bodies but also as human beings. It is a question of ontology as much as it is of pathology" [1].

Suffering is what brings the patient to the physician. Indeed, the word "patient" derives from the word for suffering. A physician will ask a patient what his chief complaint is, and in the word "complaint," there is the plaintive suggestion of the pain that has stimulated the visit to the doctor.

It is this "dis-ease" in Horton's view – this sorrow, regret, disappointment, grief – that motivates the patient to enter into a relationship with the doctor. Horton writes, "The patient is not merely categorized as a pathological diagnosis: there is a mental expression of whatever biological process is evolving, the expression that precipitates the need for a medical opinion" [1]. The doctor, therefore, begins the encounter with the humanistic appraisal of the person rather than a purely scientific evaluation of the case.

The seasoned physician intuitively uses a conceptual network of mental and spiritual terms as opposed to a conceptual network of physical terms in speaking with patients. At its most effective, the language of the medical encounter is a humanistic language designed to reduce fears and to convey reassurance in a process that has been called "concordancing" [3].

Medical research has a quality of objectivity or at least intersubjectivity leading to the "disembedding" of evidence from its site of origin in the unique experience of the clinical consultation. In this way, medicine has a tendency to privilege "desituated evidence over situated experience" [1]. This can persuade doctors, enamored with evidence-based medicine and clinical guidelines, to avoid the complicated psychosocial concerns of the patient and ignore the fears of separation that the patient often has when facing the overwhelming challenges of serious illness. Patients and doctors have mutually agreed upon ways of knowing only in a medical encounter where they can both come to understandings of *dis-ease* as well as disease.

In the clinical encounter, an experienced doctor is able to elicit a full, impressive, and nuanced illness narrative from the patient. This narrative, replete with details and signs and symptoms of underlying pathology, also contains deep fears and sadnesses. Once appreciated, the illness narrative can be *analogically* compared with thousands of other illness narratives the experienced physician has been privy to in other consultations at the bedside. The full repertoire of *source* narratives in the physician's mental portfolio can lead him to match one up with the *target* narrative of the patient he sees and touches before him. The patient's details emerge in the comparisons and join up with emotional intuitions, flowing up from the physician's own emotional brain center – the limbic system. These insights converge in a brain region called the paralimbic cortex, the anterior cingulate area to be specific, and surface as a diagnostic response selection.

> Narrative shapes clinical judgment. In medical practice, the vast body of knowledge about human biology is applied to the patient analogically through the narratives of the experience of comparable instances.... [4].

The ultimate situation presented by serious illness (and the separation challenge that goes with it) is an inescapable human reality. Technological medicine is increasingly "disembedded" from this reality. This becomes the disconnection, the schism in modern medical practice. It is a separation challenge to medicine itself as a profession, and Horton intuitively sees the need for an attachment solution: "The solution is to discover a way to *reconnect* doctor to patient through a *bridge* of *common* understanding and *shared* ways of knowing about disease. We need nothing less than a new philosophy of medical knowledge" [1]. The use of attachment terminology in this suggestion is telling. Attachment behavior is integral to medical knowledge and to shared meaning.

Those who practice medicine must be both competent and compassionate. As a profession, medicine must strive to integrate the scientific and the spiritual. Both methods of relating serve as potential reflections of compassionate love at the bedside where *dis-eased* patients are facing the crisis of illness. In the final analysis, this is the only option for a medicine that professes to be humanistic.

The crisis of physical illness can be understood conceptually using a model proposed by Moos and Tsu [5]. Genetic endowment and personal factors, physical and social environmental factors, and illness-related factors all impact on the illness experience of the individual. The experience itself is a composite of emotional valencing in the limbic system and cognitive appraisal in the neocortex, resulting in the perceived meaning of the illness in what has been referred to as the emotion–cognition amalgam. This amalgamation seeks to meet the adaptive tasks that test one's coping skills, which in turn help determine the outcome of the illness crisis.

The contribution of the limbic system is essential to the illness experience. This area mediates the basic drives to self and species preservation, attachment behavior, and territoriality [6]. Thus, while the cortex cognitively appraises illness and its threat, understanding is not reached without limbic-mediated fear of excessive depending or of final separation. Illness attacks territoriality. Patients are removed from their homes, have their clothes taken away, are invaded by multiple tubes, and must yield control to strangers. Attachments are strained as patients are separated from family members both literally and symbolically. The amygdala, in collaboration with the hippocampus and thalamo-cingulate areas, among other limbic regions, mediates these experiences [7].

The emotional salience of the illness condition obviously affects appraisal of the illness threat and allocation of cognitive focus. This is rooted in what I have called the *separation–attachment dialectical process* [8, 9]. A response selection would take place in the paralimbic circuit that includes the anterior cingulate cortex (ACC) [10]. This particular circuit, like several other circuits that are integrated yet segregated in the brain, contains a motor area (the basal ganglia), a sensory locus (the thalamus), and an analyzer–effector section (the cortex) [11]. It evolved in mammals to enable us to employ parent–offspring and social attachments as our survival strategies [6]. The paralimbic zones (the ventromedial prefrontal and insular cortices) are tightly connected with the prefrontal cortex, which enables us to plan and execute our attachment behaviors. As mutation provided brain area in the general pallium, it was exapted in the mammalian trajectory in the service of finding survival advantage through more enhanced and refined attachment solutions to separation challenges. An example in the primate line would be the evolution of mirror neurons, which aid us in developing our capacity for empathy.

When talking about the separation–attachment dialectic and the evolution of the brain, we come to an understanding of how the "directed selection pressure" of the separation threat biased cerebrotype evolution in the direction of enhanced and refined attachment solutions [12]. These solutions required certain underlying neuronal constructs that appeared in the segregated yet integrated forms of basal ganglia-thalamocortical loop evolution [9]. These forms proceeded from a *protolimbic circuit*, with an amygdala-centered emotional "hot" memory system balanced by an inhibitory hippocampus-centered cognitive "cold" memory system, to a *paralimbic cortical circuit*, with a medial orbital frontal/anterior cingulate cortex (MOF/ACC) adding emotional-cognitive manipulation with inhibitory output to the amygdala and stimulation of the hippocampus, and then on to a *prefrontal cortical (PFC) circuit* with working memory/memory of the future capabilities and with connections to the ACC to do response selection based on a memory of the past and an error detection network. The PFC and ACC work together to modulate down amygdalar flow stemming from fear conditioning.

Thus, the brain can be viewed as a highly complexified organ for finding attachment solutions to separation challenges [9]. Reflecting this fact, the patient's main questions revolve around the uncertainty of future attachments and fear of future separation, perhaps even final separation. This limbic-stimulated struggle accounts for much of the threat and challenge of any separation–attachment experience. The illness condition is an especially vivid example of a separation challenge in search of an attachment solution.

The Attachment Solution

Using an approach informed by ethology, biology, and control theory, as well as psychology, Bowlby [13] arrived at several main propositions about attachment behavior. First of all, emotionally significant attachment bonds between individuals serve a basic survival function and, therefore, have a primary status. Second, an understanding of these attachment behaviors can be arrived at using cybernetic theory wherein each partner's CNS contains a system designed to maintain proximity or accessibility of one to the other. Third, working models of self and other interaction patterns develop over time in each partner's mind, allowing for efficient operation of the relationship. Fourth, instead of developmental stages to which one becomes fixated or regresses, Bowlby favored a developmental psychiatry that primarily involves the study of the parent–child bond. "The key hypothesis is that variations in the way these bonds develop and become organized during the infancy and childhood of different individuals are major determinants of whether a person grows up to be mentally healthy" [14].

The emotional bonds that form between parent and child serve several functions including *careseeking* and *caregiving*. Ethology – the field that extrapolates from animal behavior to find clues to the origins of human behavior – sees the parent–child bond as an integral part of human nature present at least from the beginning of extrauterine life. Infants and children bond with their parents or adult caretakers to whom they look for protection, solace, and care. In adolescence and on into adulthood, these persistent parent–child attachments are supplemented with new attachments particularly with peers and usually of a heterosexual nature.

Bowlby [14] argues that while the drives for food and sex often play important roles in the parent–child bond, the relationship itself is primary with its survival value of protection as its core function. This human capacity to seek and secure comfort from attachment is not to be seen as regressive dependency, but rather as an important characteristic of adaptive character behavior and reflective of mental health. At times, the individual in a mature bond will be careseeking, while at other times he/she will be caregiving.

Bowlby speculated that a physiological process in the CNS was responsible for maintaining the optimal distances between child and parent within a limited spatial–temporal range. Accessibility, thus, becomes prioritized in all contexts. Bowlby entitles this "environmental homeostasis," though today we might call it environmental *allostasis* [15]. The inputs that stimulate careseeking include fear, loss, or sickness. The inputs that terminate careseeking and stimulate exploration include a sense of comfort, solace, reassurance, and mastery.

From Bowlby's [14] evolutionary perspective, "human attachment behavior is constructed so as to promote survival in the environment in which man evolved". Given the key cornerstone survival value of security and protection that a caretaker provides, the child's attachment control system will be structured to perform most efficiently and to support healthy development when bonding can take place with a person who is effective, responsive, and caring.

The other side of the careseeking coin is caregiving. Here too, ethology and evolutionary theory can provide us with some answers. Kin selection altruistic care of the infant can be understood as the promotion of offspring survival, a reflection of the "selfish gene" hypothesis if you will. Still, Bowlby cites the ethological appraisal of altruism as a far cry from Freud's pessimism about man's essential selfishness and disdain for the interests of others. If we are not all primary narcissists, then perhaps we can aim at least as high as secondary narcissism (showing care in exchange for social reward – reciprocal altruism) and sometimes even for genuine altruism wherein we do loving acts with no reward in mind.

The closest we can get to a neurobiological understanding of this process of altruistic caregiving involves the interrelationship of the thalamofrontocingulate and neofrontocerebellar pathways mediating the mammalian behavioral triad (the infant separation cry, maternal nurturance, and play behavior), which is then embellished not only by a "memory of the past" but also by a "memory of the future" [6, 16]. In addition, the essential action of specialized mirror neurons in frontal and paralimbic cortical regions that provide the human being with the magic of mapping another individual's intellectual and emotional mindset onto one's own is key to the empathy that drives altruistic behavior [17].

Bowlby [14] saw one attachment behavior pattern leading to healthy development and two others leading to dysfunction [14]. When the child becomes confident that a parent or parent figure will be responsive and caring, especially when he is challenged by fear and threat, *secure attachment* is the result. Secure attachment kindles in the child a confidence that he is competent to explore the world. Bowlby points out that healthy development leading to security in the parent–child bond requires "a parent (in the early years, especially the mother) being readily available, sensitive to her child's signals, and lovingly responsive when he or she seeks protection and/or comfort and/or assistance" [14].

In the *anxious resistant attachment* pattern, there is uncertainty on the part of the child whether the parent will be forthcoming in a responsive caring manner. The residual state is one of proneness to *separation anxiety*. These children are extremely wary about exploring their world. A clinging dependency emerges when the parent is inconsistently available – responding on one occasion but not another. Repeated separations as well as the threat of abandonment as a means of control are other factors in the development of anxious resistant attachment.

A third pattern is *anxious avoidant attachment*. In this scenario, the child actually comes to expect rebuffing at the hands of the parenting figure when they seek solace and assistance. This constant rebuffing leads the child to a strategy of avoidant withdrawal sparked by the rationale that life can be lived without the support and love of others. Children who have sustained abuse, institutionalization, and constant rejection will develop severe personality disorders characterized by dependency–independency struggles sometimes eventuating in the condition called *Borderline Personality*.

The separation–attachment dialectical process helps us to understand these behavior patterns. In meeting the challenge of disordered attachment some choose overattachment in the extreme and become what we call insecure-anxious types, while others choose a separation solution and become insecure-avoidant children.

Object Relations Theory

When one drills down into the mechanisms of attachment theory using the psychodynamic theory of object relations, certain insights become available. In a paper on the "internal world," Meissner reviewed the history of object relations theory [18]. He dates the beginnings of Freud's important thinking on *internalization* to *Mourning and Melancholia* (1917) [19]. In this treatise on depression and narcissism, Freud thought of the internalization mechanism as one of "narcissistic identification." In other words, when we psychologically internalize an object of our attention, it is assimilated into the ego's image and needs. Meissner points out that, later, any external conflict between ego and object was transformed in Freud's thinking to an internalized structural conflict between superego and ego.

The British school of object relations pursued independent lines of thought. Fairbairn [20] focused on ego relations to objects, hypothesizing the erection of an inner world dependent on processes of *splitting* into good and bad objects and *introjection* [18]. The splitting can create parallel images in both ego and object, leading to schizoid positions that foster psychopathology. Instincts to Fairbairn do not primarily seek to discharge libidinal energies, but rather are objectseeking. Drives attach to objects on the basis of an ego appraisal of which potential objects can fulfill the role of the introjected split-off object representations, which are usually of either an all-good or all-bad variety.

In the work of both Michael Balint and Donald Winnicott, there is a shift in emphasis from the internal frame of reference to the mother–child interaction. Balint's [21] "primary love" notion is a description of the infant's object relatedness as it arises from the very beginning of life. As opposed to Freudian primary narcissism, it explores "The need for harmonious fitting-in and mutual responsiveness between mother and child and the related symbiotic matrix within which this occurs – elements which are essential to the child's normal development – are better understood in the perspective of object-relatedness…." [18]. Balint, thus, more concretely examines the qualities of the real interaction occurring between child and mother and the potential for love as it arises in this formative relationship.

Balint and Winnicott emphasized the basic ego pathology that results from a dysfunctional early mother–child relationship. Balint called this early misattachment the "basic fault," while Winnicott referred to the development of the "false self" [18].

Morse [22] found a common theme in these concepts. The ego starts out in a unified state; however, fundamental pathogenetic splits emerge (reflected in insecure attachment behavior patterns) when early object relationships are disruptive [20]. *Here, again, we note that the language of the separation–attachment process is crucial to understanding what is common in object relations theory.*

In Winnicott's concept of *transitional phenomena*, a breakthrough was made in understanding how the internal psychological structure interrelates to the external world [23]. Transitional phenomena allow for the examination of that part of the human being's life that encompasses both the internal subjective and external objective (intersubjective really) worlds he inhabits. Here is Meissner's statement on Winnicott's contribution, "Basing his approach on the analysis of the transitional object, the infant's first not-me object which replaces the symbiotic mother, he describes an area of illusion which provides a transition between the child's infantile solipsistic world of self-absorption and the emerging capacity to relate to objects" [18]. In other words, the child transitions from a merged self-object to a separate self, capable of attaching to an object at a refined and enhanced level – if all goes well. This transitional paradigm helps us understand a child's developing awareness of separate objects, object-relatedness as transitional relatedness, and the ways by which transitional relatedness will affect object relations.

For Winnicott, the capacity for *illusion* as reflected in the power of transitional phenomena is an essential part of human character extending throughout the life cycle. Indeed, it is powerful enough to serve as the inspiration for, as Meissner puts it, "creative, cultural, artistic and even religious expressions and experience" [18].

> There is a no-man's land between the subjective and what is objectively perceived that is natural to infancy, and this we expect…In religion and the arts, we see the claim socialized so that the individual is not called mad and can enjoy in the exercise of religion or the

practice and appreciation of the arts the rest that human beings need from absolute and never-failing discrimination between fact and fantasy [24].

The term "illusion," which carries the connotation of unreality, is insufficient to describe transitional phenomena. Transitional objects may be viewed as symbols or representations of a reality (a secure maternal child attachment, for example) that has been experienced and will, through the power of the representation object to stimulate human brain biology, be experienced again in the coordinated space of a certain person, place, and time. Using positron emission tomography, for example, Kosslyn et al. [25] have shown that visualizing an imaginary letter "A" stimulates the same brain regions as actually seeing a real letter "A."

It is important at this juncture to question what may be the human being's primary natural state. From the point of view of the separation–attachment dialectical process, Winnicott's position can be restated in the following way. Our first felt experience is aloneness–separation, and it is only later that dependence–attachment enters the human condition. In this schema, the push to regress is in the direction of a peaceful unaliveness, which is Winnicott's version of Freud's inorganic Death Instinct. It would seem likely in this case that any attachment experience for one who regresses to aloneness is likely to have been unsatisfactory.

There is another version, of course, of conditions of initiality. This version sees the human-felt experience of attachment as primary. In discussing "maternal primary process presence" earlier, we noted its ability to provide a soothing emotional tone to the infant in its earliest experience of aliveness. As Horton [26] writes, "A partial explanation for the origin of the soothing maternal primary process presence is the following: An 'omnipotent sufficiency' characterizes the earliest months of life and is "maintained, for a time, by the close 'symbiotic relationship with the mother'" [26].

The *mother–infant symbiosis* when healthy provides a gratifying sustenance from which a sense of fusion emerges, providing a psychological infrastructure in the life process of the individual from childhood through adulthood. This concept of *fusion* is seen as a soothing illusion, which is normally conscious up to about the age of 3. Thereafter, it is an unconsciously held concept [27]. I would agree with Horton that the solace that serves as the "driving force behind transitional activities throughout life" finds its source in the connection between *maternal primary process presence* and *latent oceanic experience*. If a mother figure, in the developmental experience of the child, can approximate or embody an oceanic presence, solace will result [26]. In this context, "transitional solace is qualitatively separable from and more psychologically basic than all other pleasures and joys" [26].

It is only in the mystery of the separation–attachment dialectical process that the twin dangers of abandonment and engulfment can be understood. In the drive to *attach*, there is the goal of solace in the face of possible aloneness. In the drive to *separate*, there is the goal of the freedom to exist in the face of possible overdependence and engulfment. The starkness of these dangers is most vividly displayed in the tortured lives of those with the so-called Borderline Personality.

It should be noted that our condition of initiality is somehow informing of our condition of terminality. Are we initially ourselves in a state of separation or of attachment? Likewise, are we terminally ourselves in a state of separation or of attachment? Before life and after death, where are we? The core unrest responsible for movement comes from the separation–attachment dialectical process and the total dissatisfaction we feel with total separation or total attachment. For many reasons, some reflected in the biology and evolution of our brains, we need to more or less be separated and attached simultaneously in this life. Only in this dialectical way do we find a synthesis of our experience emerging. Only in this way do we feel restored enough to explore and in the process to mature as individuals capable of loving attachments in community.

The Spiritual Imperative in Medicine

Man's spiritual imperative originates in what can be understood as a dialectic of separation and attachment. As can be gleaned from the above discussion of parent–child attachment theory, spirituality, when defined as the feeling of connectedness to something greater than ourselves, can be seen to emerge in our contemplation of the emotion we orphans feel, separated as we are from what we yearn to feel – the presence of our "Parent."

Listening hard to those with illness may help us discover this "pining emotion" in our human predicament. When asked what the worst part of their illness experience is, most patients say in so many words that it is the fear of separation and loss of attachment. The medical psychiatrist, Richard Berlin, has written about the practical implications of this [28]. We may label this "dis-ease" as anxiety and depression, but it is perhaps more heuristically described as *the separation–attachment process* all humans share.

In one recent qualitative study, 13 subjects were intensively interviewed during their battles with life-threatening illnesses [29]. The object of this study was to uncover what the inner life responses to serious illness really are. The researchers, Mount and Boston, found that the power of meaning per se emerges from the psychodynamics of healing or more correctly, of *healing connection*, a marker for attachment. They found that patient responses reflected two poles: on the one hand, there were suffering and anguish as marked by a sense of wounding, isolation, disconnection, and a preoccupation with the past and the future tinged with a feeling of victimization and loss of control. On the other hand, there was healing defined by a sense of integrity and wholeness with connection at one level often leading to a connection at other levels. Even a sense of sympathetic connection to their own suffering is sometimes found.

Mount and colleagues, through linguistic analysis of subject interviews, found four levels of attachment accounting for the healing integrity. One level was attachment of the self as ego to a deeper center within the self, what some might call *atman*. On another level, there was the attachment of self to others in an "I-thou" loving way. On a third level, there was attachment of self to something larger in nature, appreciable through the senses. And then, finally, there was the attachment of self to the caregiver, to God, to the ultimate, to someone greater than self. It is important to realize that there are variations in their patients' sense of dis-ease and in the ability of individuals to meet illness challenges by forming attachments at these levels. This variation in ability stems somewhat from the quality of early attachments in their lives.

Bowlby's [30] internal working model, which provides for a consistency of attachment style over time, is based on particular neurological substrates that have come on line as a result of the sculpting of the first attachments between infants and primary caregivers. This model guides affects and behaviors in response to the threat of illness. In this schema, attachment type can be thought of as a disposition towards self-perception as well as the perception a patient has of others and their responsiveness. Self-perception and a bias toward certain overdetermined strategies are stimulated by the presence of the illness threat. In this regard, the emergence of attachment behavior is dependent on the context of the illness separation experience leading to the dis-ease of being ill.

Attachment behavior is mobilized in the face of illness events. In other words, the separation threat of illness causes the type of stress that will trigger attachment behavior. Attachment theory's internal working model helps us to distinguish between trait-like attachment patterns and attachment behaviors triggered by the stress state of illness.

Recently, the association of attachment style with adaptation to illness has been studied. In patients with hepatitis C infections, those with fearful attachment style reported more medically unexplained symptoms than patients with secure attachment, suggesting that greater adaptability comes with security of attachment [31]. In patients with chronic pain, fearful attachment was associated with more pain, depression, catastrophizing and physical disability. Preoccupied attachment style was correlated with pain-related healthcare utilization [32]. Researchers surmise that attachment style is an important consideration in assessing symptom appraisal and subsequent healthcare utilization. Both those with preoccupied dependent, anxious attachment and those with anxious approach-avoidance behavior stemming from a fear of rejection show higher symptom reporting. In those with preoccupied style, this insecurity leads to heightened healthcare utilization [33].

Attachment security and insecurity may be uncovered in the setting of illness stress, but attachment insecurity may contribute to the presentation of the disease itself through an association with the physiological stress response. There may be an increase in perceived stress, impaired regulation of stress physiology, and a reduction in social support modulation of stress, all potentially leading to an increase in the physiological stress response and a lowering of the threshold for disease. Much evidence has accumulated to support this hypothesis. Attachment insecurity may trigger all of these pathways. The converse may also be true – the bolstering of attachment security through compassionate love may be healthful. This will buffer against the effects of stress, reducing metabolic wear and tear (allostatic loading) and elevating the disease threshold [34].

Compassionate Caregiving and Its Implications

Physicians provide care when they step into that "intermediate area" Winnicott talks about between separation and attachment [35]. They become facilitators in the dialectical movement from restore to explore to mature that takes place in the arena of illness as it does in other epigenetic stages of development. It is here, then, that compassionate love in medicine can be examined and nurtured. Its developmental power cannot be minimized and indeed may promote healing. We can speculate that both cortical and limbic neurophysiochemical effects take place in such a compassionate, caring transitional relationship.

In the psychosomatic or "mind–body hypothesis," distress in response to a crisis (becoming pathogenetic when chronic or overwhelming) will be processed in cortical and limbic brain areas, resulting in *stress response system* (hypothalamic-pituitary-adrenal axis; locus coeruleus-sympathetic nervous system; vagal complex-visceral nervous system) and immune system changes that may predispose to or exacerbate disease states [15, 36, 37].

Recently, the concept of allostasis has been introduced into the field of stress medicine research by Sterling and Eyer [38] and refined by McEwen [15]. Allostasis, literally meaning "maintaining stability (or 'homeostasis') through change," refers to the capacity to adapt or constantly modify physiological parameters to adjust to ever-shifting environmental conditions. Hence, we can also speak alternatively about maintaining a "state of dynamic balance." Moreover, *allostatic load* refers to the wear and tear that the body experiences due to repeated cycles of allostasis, i.e., allostatic stress responses, as well as the inefficient turning-on or shutting-off of these activated responses. Human physiologic systems need to be pliant within certain ranges to adjust to varying conditions. Separation distress has a tendency to reduce pliancy and produce "allostatic loading." Picture losing your job and hearing that your son has cancer in the same month. This would cause severe allostatic loading and your brain and body would know about it.

As mentioned above, the worst part of the illness experience for most patients reflects the fear of separation and loss of attachment, which contributes to allostatic loading. Family members share in this separation challenge. Here is an exchange with the wife of a terminally ill man in the throes of his final struggle with glioblastoma multiforme: "I should stop giving John the chemo, for it is not fair to put him through it.... all 3 doctors agreed that was best.... they think John has a few weeks. My prayer has always been if the Lord takes him, John will be confused and never have to say 'good bye' to his girls. It looks as if that prayer will be answered, for he is not aware he is ill but he does feel love all around him. I pray John will go peacefully as if he was going to sleep. The girls and I are heartbroken, but we would never wish for John to suffer, and he cannot even hold his head upright. My head hurts from crying, so I will write more tomorrow, but I had to tell my friend. Love, Mary."

To the extent that spiritual and religious behavior on the part of the patient and spirituality in the patient–doctor relationship mollify separation distress in the brain, there may be "downstream" effects that promote health. This would be above and beyond the epidemiologic effects of a healthier lifestyle, diet, and improved compliance. The placid state achieved through spirituality in the patient, the family, the staff, and the doctor may rekindle the "remembered wellness" of "secure base attachment" in the midst of illness-induced separation anxiety and depression [30, 39]. A less stressed, neurobiologic equilibrium may, then, promote healing. All of these approaches allow humans to tap into an ability to reduce the specter of purposelessness and to limit reflection on the myriad contingencies that may hasten death.

When has healing occurred? Is it only when disease has been cured? Or does the concept also include the ability to assuage the "dis-ease," to use the terminology of Richard Horton, which uniformly accompanies the illness experience.

The word "heal" comes from the old English word hælen. While it does mean to restore to health by way of a cure, it also means "to set right; to amend" [40], as in the phrase "to heal a rift between us." In addition, it takes on another meaning in the 1993 third edition of the American Heritage Dictionary [41]. "To heal" can mean "to restore a person to spiritual wholeness." To be sure, this form of healing is the major goal of authentic religion. It is instructive to keep in mind that the root meaning of the word religion comes from the Latin word "religio," which can be translated as "to bind back."

Healing is a product not only of curing but also of caring, a caring that is spiritually inspired in the loving response of the caregiver, as Drs. Peabody and Churchill suggest. "The good physician knows his patients through and through, and his knowledge is bought dearly. Time, sympathy and understanding must be lavishly dispensed, but the reward is to be found in that personal bond, which forms the greatest satisfaction of the practice of medicine. One of the essential qualities of the clinician is interest in humanity, for the secret of the caring of the patient is in the caring for the patient" [42].

Visitors to the Massachusetts General Hospital see the last sentence of these famous words etched in the lobby's marble wall. Alongside this saying is another famous quote, this time from Dr. Edward Churchill speaking over 60 years ago, "Charity in its broad spiritual sense that is, a desire to relieve suffering, is the most prized possession of medicine."

Those who practice medicine must be both competent and compassionate. Indeed, as a profession, medicine must strive to unify the scientific and the spiritual, with both methods of relating serving as potential reflections of compassionate love at the bedside. This in the final analysis is the only option for a medicine that professes to be humanistic. As Weatherall [43] suggests, medicine must return to an ethic of "the love of our patients."

We come to a theme common to the concept of healing in both medicine and spirituality whether we are referring to curing or to caring. This common message is one of restoration and reattachment. This theme is also at the core of man's spiritual love – a uniquely human capacity for consolation in response to the challenge of separation and loss. Physicians and other caregivers ignore the power of the attachment solution of compassionate care only at their patient's peril and to their own detriment.

References

1. Horton R. Health wars: on the global front lines of modern medicine. New York: NY Review of Books; 2003.
2. Tauber AI. Confessions of a medicine man: an essay in popular philosophy. Cambridge: MIT Press; 2000. p. 114–6.
3. Skelton J, Hobbs FDR. Concordancing: use of language-based research in medical communication. Lancet. 1999;353:108–11.
4. Hunter KM. Doctor's stories. Princeton: Princeton University Press; 1991.
5. Moos RH, Tsu VD. The crisis of physical illness: an overview. In: Moos R, editor. Coping with physical illness. New York: Plenum; 1977. p. 3–21.
6. MacLean PD. The triune brain in evolution. New York: Plenum; 1990.
7. LeDoux J. The emotional brain. New York: Simon and Schuster; 1996.
8. Fricchione GL. Illness and the origin of caring. J Med Humanit. 1993;14:15–21.
9. Fricchione GL. Separation, attachment and altruistic love. The evolutionary basis for medical caring. In: Post SG, Underwood LG, Schloss JP, Hurlbut WP, editors. Altruism and altruistic love. Science, philosophy and religion in dialogue. New York: Oxford University Press; 2002. p. 346–61.
10. Devinsky O, Morrell MJ, Vogt BA. Contributions of anterior cingulate cortex to behaviour. Brain. 1995;118:279–306.
11. Alexander GE, Crutcher MD, DeLong MR. Basal ganglia-thalamo-cortical circuits: parallel substrates for motor, oculomotor, "prefrontal" and "limbic" functions. Prog Brain Res. 1990;85:119–46.
12. Clark DA, Mitra PP, Wang SS. Scalable architecture in mammalian brains. Nature. 2000;411:189–93.
13. Bowlby J. Attachment and loss. Vol. 1, attachment. 2nd ed. New York: Basic Books; 1982.
14. Bowlby J. Developmental psychiatry comes of age. Am J Psychiatry. 1988;145:1–10.
15. McEwen BS. Protective and damaging effects of stress mediation. NEJM. 1998;338:171–9.
16. Ingvar DH. Memory of the future: an essay on the temporal organization of conscious awareness. Hum Neurobiol. 1985;4:127–36.
17. Rizzolatti G, Sinigaglia C. Mirrors in the brain: how our minds share actions and emotions. New York: Oxford University Press; 2008.
18. Meissner WW. The problem of internalization and structure formation. Int J Psychoanal. 1980;61:237–48.
19. Freud S. Mourning and melancholia. In: Rickman J, editor. A general selection from the works. New York: Doubleday; 1957.
20. Fairbairn WRD. Synopsis of an object-relations theory of the personality. Int J Psychoanal. 1963;44:224–5.
21. Balint M. Primary narcissism and primary love. Psychoanal Q. 1960;29:6–43.
22. Morse SJ. Structure and reconstruction: a critical comparison of Michael Balint and D.W. Winnicott. Int J Psychoanal. 1972;531:481–500.
23. Winnicott DW. Playing and reality. New York: Basic Books; 1971.
24. Winnicott DW. Human nature. New York: Schochen Books; 1988. p. 107.
25. Kosslyn SM, Thompson WL, Alpert NM. Neural systems shared by visual imagery and visual perception: a positron emission tomography study. Neuroimage. 1997;6:320–34.
26. Horton PC. Solace. The missing dimension in psychiatry. New Haven: Yale University Press; 1981. p. 47.
27. Jacobson E. The self and the object world. New York: International University Press; 1964.
28. Berlin RM. Attachment behavior in hospitalized patients. JAMA. 1986;255:3391–3.
29. Mount BM, Boston PH, Cohen SR. Healing connections: On moving from suffering to a sense of well-being. J Pain Symptom Manage. 2007;33:372–88.
30. Bowlby J. Attachment and loss. Vol. 2, separation. New York: Basic Books; 1973.

31. Ciechanowski PS, Katon WJ, Russo JE, Dwight-Johnson MM. Association of attachment style to lifetime medically unexplained symptoms in patients with hepatitis C. Psychosomatics. 2002;43:206–12.

32. Ciechanowski P, Sullivan M, Jensen M, Romano J, Summers H. The relationship of attachment style to depression, catastrophizing and health care utilization in patients with chronic pain. Pain. 2003;104:627–37.

33. Ciechanowski PS, Walker EA, Katon WJ, Russo JE. Attachment theory: a model for health care utilization and somatization. Psychosom Med. 2002;64:660–7.

34. Maunder RG, Hunter JJ. Attachment in psychosomatic medicine: developmental contributions to stress and disease. Psychosom Med. 2001;63:566–7.

35. Winnicott D. Transitional objects and transitional phenomena. Int J Psychoanal. 1953;34:89–97.

36. Chrousos GE, Gold PW. The concepts of stress and stress system disorders. Overview of physical and behavioral homeostasis. JAMA. 1992;267:1244–52.

37. Reichlen S. Neuroendocrine-immune interactions. NEJM. 1993;329:1246–53.

38. Sterling P, Eyer J. Allostasis: a new paradigm to explain arousal pathology. In: Fisher S, Reason J, editors. Handbook of life stress, cognition and health. New York: Wiley; 1988.

39. Benson H. Timeless healing: the power and biology of belief. New York: Simon and Schuster; 1996.

40. Morris W, editor. American Heritage Dictionary. Boston: Houghton Mifflin; 1978. p. 607.

41. Costello R, editor. American Heritage Dictionary. Boston: Houghton Mifflin; 1993. p. 626.

42. Peabody FW. The care of the patient. JAMA. 1927;88:877–82.

43. Weatherall D. Science and the quiet art. Oxford: Oxford University Press; 1995.

Chapter 6
Empathy, Compassion, and the Goals of Medicine

Stephen Liben

Keywords Empathy • Compassion • Mindfulness • Detached concern • Self-esteem • Intention • Attitude • Awareness

The way empathy and compassion are currently thought about and taught in medical education is the wrong answer to the right question. This chapter begins by outlining the reasons why this is so and then suggests an alternative way that is congruent with whole person care. The question of how to educate health care providers (HCPs) so that they are empathic and compassionate in the care of the sick is a good one and is synonymous with this book's focus on care of the *whole* person that includes the personal suffering that accompanies illness. If we agree that medicine's role is to reduce suffering, then educating health care professionals to understand the cognitive and emotional experiences of those they serve (i.e., being *empathic*) is, at first glance, the right goal. However, there are two problems with setting empathy as a goal in medical education; one problem is the "dark side" of empathy that is rarely addressed, and the other problem is the question what is left when empathy cannot be elicited or fails completely. Having outlined the limitations of empathy as goal for health care professionals, we focus on how mindful self-compassion is an essential and learnable starting point in the compassionate whole person care of others.

Words elicit thoughts, perceptions, and emotions, and in your reading experience certain words, such as "compassion" and "empathy" and "healing," will be specific to your own definition and prior experiences. For example, if you had a negative religious education based on the demand that you should be "compassionate and selfless," then you may find that the word "compassion" for you triggers negative thoughts and emotions. Alternatively, if you are comfortable with the language of "compassion" and "service" as ideals that you personally uphold, then

S. Liben (✉)
Director, Pediatric Palliative Care Program, The Montreal Children's Hospital, Associate Professor of Pediatrics, McGill University, 2300 Tupper Street, Montreal, QC H3H 1P3, Canada
e-mail: stephen.liben@mcgill.ca

T.A. Hutchinson (ed.), *Whole Person Care: A New Paradigm for the 21st Century*, DOI 10.1007/978-1-4419-9440-0_6, © Springer Science+Business Media, LLC 2011

your association with these words may be positive. Once you personally associate a word as having a positive or negative connotation, then it is less possible to see new possibilities for the concepts that underlie these words. To put it another way, words are pointers that direct thoughts to experience; words are not the "thing" itself. In order to allow you the greatest possible opportunity for a meaningful reading of this chapter, I define what I mean by certain often positively and negatively charged words. One definition of authentic learning is that it is "paid for out of the pocket of what you thought you already knew."

The word *health care provider* (HCP) is used as inclusive of both professionals and nonprofessionals who care for an ill person. The word *patient* is for anyone who asks for or needs assistance for physical and mental problems and thus is inclusive of the term "client" often used by psychotherapists. The terms "Other" and "the Other" are used to describe anyone other than one's self.

Empathy

Empathy was originally a term derived for a theory of art appreciation, and its definition continues to evolve. One definition of empathy is that it is the ability to identify/understand another person's thoughts or emotional state. Sympathy is closely related in that it also involves understanding another's emotional state, but it adds a positive judgment to the shared thoughts and emotional state. For example, if I understand that another person is experiencing fear, then I am empathizing. If I also agree that the person *should* be fearful and I share some of that fear myself, then I am closer to sympathy than empathy. Emotional attunement or resonance is another way of understanding clinical empathy and comes closer to supporting whole person caregiving than does the idea of "detached concern" [1].

Detached concern is the active suppression of emotional attunement or resonance and sounds more like "don't get involved." The concept of detached concern is a failed attempt to separate cognitive understanding from emotional response, as it makes the erroneous assumption that the caregiver could be in the midst of another's suffering and pain and at the same time not be emotionally affected by any of it. This detached concern stance "don't get emotionally involved" is about as useful an educational objective as telling someone with anxiety to "just relax." This artificial cognitive isolation discounts both the caregiver themselves and the other person leaving only the cognitive puzzle to be solved (see the superrational stance of Virgina Satir in Chap. 4). While there are (rare) times when a medical problem is simply a puzzle to be figured out (e.g., how to work up a low sodium in an unconscious ICU patient), the kind of clinical problems that require a whole person care approach mandate a more nuanced and complex way of being and doing (and at specific times "non-doing").

Detached concern as a clinical approach is untenable both from the caregivers' perspective (health care professionals who attempt to suppress emotions that arise from care for others become depressed burnt-out or chronically dissatisfied) and also from patients who demand more than a "body-mechanic" approach to medical problems that have no "quick fix" (i.e., the vast majority of medical problems). Even for the small percentage of medical problems that are amenable to "quick solutions," for example a broken arm from a fall in an otherwise healthy child, an approach that neglects the emotional aspects that arise will deprive the HCP, the child, and the parent of the opportunity to allay fears and perform necessary procedures (applying a cast) with warmth humility and understanding. On the contrary, an empathic approach that utilizes the health care professionals' emotional resonance with patients then sounds closer to the kind of interactive relationship that might foster whole person care.

The recent discovery in neuroscience of "mirror neurons" in specific parts of the brain has indicated that we may be "hard wired" for empathy. Mirror neurons are cells that fire both when an animal acts and when the animal observes the same action performed by another. The neuron, thus, "mirrors" the behavior of the other, as though the observer were itself acting. An example is what happens in response to watching someone else smile and laugh; you may then find yourself smiling and even laughing without even knowing exactly why. Such mirror neurons have been directly observed in primates and are believed to occur in humans and other species [2]. In humans, brain activity consistent with that of mirror neurons has been found in the premotor cortex and the inferior parietal cortex. In this developing area of neuroscience, the mechanisms of self-awareness, mental flexibility, and emotional regulation that are essential components of empathy are being correlated with specific neuronal systems [3].

However, having empathy as a goal in HCP–patient interactions has several problems that make it an unrealistic and unachievable goal at times.

There are several problems with setting empathy as a goal in medicine [4].

1. The risk of trivialization: If empathy is taught as a learnable "skill," there is the possibility of trivializing another's experience. Reciting memorized lines (e.g., "this must be so difficult for you" or "so you feel sad") and following suggested guidelines from large class lecture presentations (e.g., "touch the patient lightly on the forearm to show concern") can become empty if devoid of authentic feeling and understanding. Empathy taught as a set of rote behaviors is bound to be dissatisfying for all involved.

2. "Not my job" phenomenon: While the humanistic aspects of medicine have gained recognition over the solely technical roles, there often remains a bias to choose technical skill over relationship-based abilities. The false dichotomy set up by the question "would you rather have a surgeon that can cut well or one that will listen to how you feel?" is a setup that evades the real-world need to have a surgeon that has both the technical skills as well as the interpersonal skills to care for patients. The splitting of technical skills from interpersonal skills is codependent on a medical system that has "experts" for almost everything so that the part of the HCP's job that calls for empathic caring and human interrelating may be "delegated" to others (e.g., the social worker) to the detriment of both the HCP who when acting only as a technician is suppressing all that comes up

in patient encounters, as well as for patients who want more than technical skills when they feel threatened [5].

3. The dark side of empathy – Overidentification. By not recognizing that we can never really "know" the Other completely, there is the danger that HCPs can overestimate their ability to empathize with patients as evidenced by the statement "I know how you feel" when it would be more accurate to think "I may know some of what you are thinking and feeling." Overidentifying and oversimplifying another person's situation is especially problematic when the HCP has had a similar experience of the patient. For example, if the HCPs have been cancer patients themselves, then they may have some idea of what it might be like for someone else to be diagnosed with cancer, but they can never really know how that other person's particular life history, culture, personality, and circumstances come together to form the unique experience for that particular patient. It is both erroneous and trivializing at the same time to believe that we can empathize with another to the point of really "knowing" another's experience. We can come close to a better understanding by being open, curious, and fully present to the Other (more on this to follow), rather than by "trying to be empathic."

4. Lack of emotional attunement – There is a spectrum of empathy from cognitive and emotional resonance to a lack of empathy (no resonance) all the way to "dark" feelings of disgust and anger at another person's situation. At the extreme is schadenfreude, a term that defines the pleasure felt in the face of the Other's misfortune. Thus, the HCP may not be able to identify at all with the patient (absence of empathy) or may even think and or feel "I do not like you." In the face of such neutral or negative thoughts and feelings, when empathy "fails," what is the alternative for the HCP who, nonetheless, has a duty to care? As explored in the last part of this chapter, the response is not aimed at "forcing" empathy but rather is oriented towards self-reflection (e.g., "what is going on here? What is the storyline I am creating that is fuelling these neutral or negative thoughts and feelings") coupled with present moment (mindful) awareness as in the thought "right here, right now, can I be with things the way they are while waiting for an appropriate response to emerge?"

Compassion

Compassion is often defined as awareness of and sympathy for another's suffering, or stated another way, it is the awareness of another's suffering coupled to the desire to alleviate it. Defined as such compassion comprises empathic *attention* to the awareness of another's state of suffering coupled with the *intention* to alleviate the suffering. Compassion, unlike empathy, does not necessarily imagine a detailed knowledge of another's thoughts and feelings but rather more simply the acknowledgement that the Other is suffering together with the desire to alleviate it. Training and encouraging compassionate HCPs would, therefore, seem to be a laudable goal of medical education. But is compassion learnable and if so how to teach it? If it is so obvious that a goal of medicine is compassionate care, then why are there not evidence-based formalized teaching programs in medical education that teach the compassionate practice of medicine?

One of the possible reasons for medicine's poor track record in teaching compassionate care is the common conflation of compassion with altruism. Altruism is defined as "unselfish regard for or devotion to the welfare of others" [6]. Altruism is listed as the first fundamental principle in a recently published "Physician Charter" [7]. Setting pure altruism as a goal is a setup for failure as there are always "selfish" reasons to act or not to act. Even the most seemingly altruistic acts (e.g., in donating an organ to a stranger) have embedded within them something back to the donor (in the case of the organ donor, the act of donation is not necessarily selfless in that it results in the donor feeling good about themselves). Health care workers who realize that they cannot eradicate their own self-interest in caring for patients may simply give up and abandon attempts at altruism and compassion. Rather than seeing compassion as conflated with altruism, the opposite view is more helpful, that is, that compassion is first based on the self, in self-knowledge and in the knowing that by decreasing the suffering of others you are also decreasing your own suffering. As stated by the 14th Dalai Lama "High levels of compassion are nothing but an advanced state of self-interest" [8].

The understanding that reducing the suffering of others has the indirect benefit back to us of reducing our own suffering has several components. First, there is the necessary understanding of interconnectedness. Interconnectedness (or "interbeing" – A state of connectedness and interdependence of all phenomena, as coined by Thicht Naht Hanh [9]) is the recognition that we are all interconnected in a complex system where things are as they are because of multiple causes and conditions where even small acts may have unforeseen large consequences. This phenomenon is described in the butterfly effect metaphor from chaos theory wherein small differences in the initial conditions of a dynamic system may produce large variations in the long-term behavior of the system. Seeing Others as completely disconnected from ourselves leads to the opposite of compassion (e.g., "since it is not me that is suffering, and I am separate from everyone else, then it does not matter") in a similar way that separating the body and mind into separate entities has led to the kind of dissatisfaction with modern medicine that underlies the motivation for developing whole person care. Understanding the idea that each of us has an individual self-identity that is at the same time interconnected with Others and with the world is one way to understand the "self-interest" of compassion quoted above. Frank Ostaseski, founder of The Zen Hospice Project in 1987, the largest Buddhist hospice center in USA, makes the connection between self-interest and compassion: "I work on myself so that I can be of service to others; my service work with others is also for me" [10].

Another component to the connection between our own suffering and that of others is that the only way to truly offer help to others comes from first understanding the difference between our issues and those of others. In order to differentiate what are self-generated thoughts and feelings from those that emanate from the patient (i.e., is this empathy I am feeling or is this my own issue that is coming up?), we need to know how to separate our own reactions from those we pick up from others. For example, if fear and the desire to run away arises in the HCP when a patient brings up their fear of dying, how can the HCP know if what they are feeling is their own fear of dying versus empathic attunement with the patient? Such levels of self-knowledge may not always be attainable, but there are ways to respond to such thoughts and feelings that help the HCP reanchor themselves in the present in such a way as to maintain curiosity about what the patient is saying without getting swept up in personal emotions. For example, acting out on unexamined feelings may lead the HCP to avoid difficult situations typified by the statement "I better go now to give you some time to yourself" when what the HCP really means is "I am going to leave now to get away from this uncomfortable feeling I have, but I will put it in such a way so as to make it sound like I am doing this for your benefit and not for mine." One way to respond to the arising of difficult thoughts and emotions in the HCP is with on the spot, in the moment, reanchoring of thoughts back to the present moment. This awareness of the thought process and need to return to the present is also illustrated by Pema Chodron's suggestion to "drop the storyline and stay with the energy" [11] wherein the HCP recognizes that they are no longer listening to the patient and instead are inside their heads creating an ongoing story about what is happening that may or may not be true. Once this internal storyline (narrative) is recognized by the HCP, they can then reanchor themselves in the present by means of different kinds of practices. For example, they can momentarily shift their focus of attention from the "storyline" on to the raw sensation of their breathing for one or two breaths so that they can then return their focus of attention back on to the patient. This redirection of awareness is a core component of "mindfulness" defined as the practice of moment-to-moment openhearted awareness, focused in the present moment [12].

Understanding oneself and developing practices that promote awareness of the way things actually are (versus the ongoing "internal story of me" that is the default background) is a prescription for self-care and a prerequisite for compassionate care of others. In other words, caring for yourself is a sine qua non for giving care to others. William Osler put it so: "Dealing as we do with the poor, suffering humanity, we see the man unmasked or, so to speak, exposed to all the frailties and weaknesses. You have to keep your heart pretty soft and pretty tender not to get too great contempt for your fellow creatures. The best way to do that is to keep a looking-glass in your own hearts, and the more carefully you scan your own frailties, the more tender you are for the frailties of your fellow creatures" [13]. How exactly can we train HCPs to self-reflect ("keep a looking glass in your own hearts…scan your own frailties") without being self-indulgent and narcissistic is a question that is addressed in the next section.

Self-Esteem Versus Self-Compassion

Both self-compassion and self-esteem involve positive emotions toward the self, but there are important differences that make self-compassion a mindful practice oriented toward the emergence of compassion and whole person care. Self-esteem, on the contrary, is based on self-evaluations of the self as worthy, likable, or competent. Self-compassion does not involve self-evaluation, but rather entails positive feelings of care and connectedness [12]. Problems with self-esteem are that it is difficult to increase and maintain as it implies being above average and can lead to narcissism & self-centeredness. Unlike self-esteem, self-compassion de-emphasizes a view of self as separate from others and may be a healthier way to experience positive emotions toward the self. Self-compassion means taking responsibility for past mistakes while at the same time being less personally distressed by them (e.g., "I made a mistake, I guess I remain human and will learn from this and try better the next time"). The alternatives to self-compassion are either blaming others ("it is not *my* fault") or self-blame ("there I go again, I am such an idiot"). Self-compassion encourages kindness toward self and others as it recognizes that everyone wants to be happy and that we all experience dissatisfaction and suffering as a lived experience. The difference between pity and self-compassion is the difference between "poor me" and "it is not easy being human." Instead of greeting difficult emotions by fighting hard against them, we can bear witness to our own pain and respond with kindness and understanding – that is self compassion. In other words, self-compassion means that we take care of ourselves in the same way we would take care of someone we loved or deeply cared for.

Self-compassion teaches us to be kind to ourselves no matter what happens, even as, at the same time, we continue to shape our behavior for the better. In difficult times, this is achieved by returning to our intention. As outlined earlier, compassion is the combination of attention to the Other coupled with the intention to help. By returning to the simple (but not easy to maintain) practicable act of paying attention, on purpose and nonjudgmentally we foster the environment wherein compassion arises on its own. We cannot fall asleep by commanding ourselves, but rather by creating the conditions (physical comfort and mental letting go) that allow sleep to happen to us. In a similar way, we cannot force ourselves to be compassionate, but by mindful awareness and returning over and over again to the present moment, we create the conditions for compassion to happen to us. What follows is a side-by-side outline of the spoken words contrasted with the inner dialogue of a HCP with and without mindful self-attention.

Example of inner and outer dialogue: HCP = health care professional P = patient

Outer (spoken) dialogue	Inner (unspoken) dialogue of HCP Without mindful self-attention	Inner (unspoken) dialogue of HCP With mindful self-attention
HCP: Hello my name is Dr. MB, what brings you to see me today?	HCP: I am tired and hungry and I really hope this is something simple that this patient's problem is something I can fix real quick so that I can finally take a break and get something to eat.	HCP: I am tired and hungry and I really hope this is something simple that this patient's problem is something I can fix real quick so that I can finally take a break and get something to eat.

(continued)

(continued)

P: My life is a mess and I feel so miserable trying to live with terrible back pain. I have constant back pain and nothing makes it better. You are the fourth HCP I am seeing for the same problem and I sure hope you can help me. HCP: Can you tell me when it started and if there was something obvious that started it like a fall?	HCP: Oh no,no, no, no, not chronic back pain. I hate these cases. He probably just wants narcotics, no, from the look of him he probably just wants me to sign a whole bunch of papers so he can go off of work. This is so unfair! Why do I always get these unhelpable cases when I need a break? HCP: For sure this is going to take forever and there is no way he will be satisfied. I can see it already, he is just like my brother, always complaining and never satisfied....	HCP: Oh no,no, no, no, not chronic back pain. I hate these cases. He probably just wants narcotics, no, from the look of him he probably just wants me to sign a whole bunch of papers so he can go off of work. This is so unfair! Why do I always get these unhelpable cases when I need a break? HCP: This sounds familiar! – this is my "its not fair" broken record playing again. Alright, my intention is be present & to be helpful if I can even if it not easy. Now can I focus on one breath .... and bring my attention back to this person who is coming to me because of a problem they want help with.

In the above external and internal dialogue, the mindfulness-trained HCP has a moment of insight into what for him is a familiar thought process ("It's not fair"). In the moment of awareness that he is having familiar negative thoughts (as opposed to attention to what he is thinking it is awareness *that* he is thinking), he is able, with self-compassion, to bring his intention back to be of service to the patient before him. Without the noncognitive element of self-compassion, it would have been just as likely that he could have berated himself for his lack of attention ("here I go again with my broken record, I am always doing this, I am not that good a person, etc..."). Mindful self-compassion means bearing witness to one's own pain (mindfulness) and responding with kindness and understanding to self – in the same way we set our intention to be compassionate to others.

Mindful self-compassion helps to parse the extremes of complete disconnection from the Other at one end (Virgina Satir's superrational stance – see Chap. 4) from overidentification and secondary vicarious traumatization at the other end. Is it possible that compassion, as a human response to suffering, is always there as a baseline, ready to arise, if only the conditions that block it (too much "self-ing") could be removed? This idea of compassion as a constant underlying intention, often covered over, but always ready to be expressed if the conditions are right, is an alternative to the usual medical model of compassion that sees compassion as a finite resource, more like the contents of a container that gets filled up and emptied with use. Thus, the right answer to the question of how to educate HCPs so that they are compassionate in the care of the sick is oriented toward self-care and self-compassion skill rather than an exclusive focus on the patient. Practicing in this way has three components: intention, attitude, and awareness. The *intention* is to focus on ourselves and the patient at the same time. The *attitude* is one of compassion toward both ourselves and our patient. *Awareness* is what allows us to keep this broad focus and to catch ourselves when it narrows down or wanders. This skill of "awarenessing" can be learned by formal and informal meditation practices, group work, and writing and journaling exercises [14], and we believe in the future it will come to be seen as an essential clinical skill for all health care practitioners who wish to practice compassionate whole person care.

References

1. Halpern J. What is clinical empathy? J Gen Intern Med. 2003;18(8):670–4.
2. Dinstein I, Thomas C, Behrmann M, Heeger DJ. A mirror up to nature. Curr Biol. 2008;18(1):R13–8.
3. Decety J, Jackson PL. The functional architecture of human empathy. Behav Cogn Neurosci Rev. 2004;3(2):71–100.
4. Edwards KA. Critiquing empathy. Second Opin. 2000;4:35–47.
5. Broyard A. Intoxicated by my illness: and other writings on life and death. New York: Fawcett Columbine; 1993.
6. Merriam Webster Dictionary [Internet]. Accessed 21 Nov 2010. http://www.merriam-webster.com/dictionary/altruism.
7. ABIM Foundation, American Board of Internal Medicine, ACP-ASIM Foundation, American College of Physicians-American Society of Internal Medicine, European Federation of Internal Medicine. Medical professionalism in the new millennium: a physician charter. Ann Intern Med. 2002;136(3):243–6.
8. Davidson R, Harrington A. Visions of compassion: Western scientists and Tibetan Buddhists examine human Nature. USA: Oxford University Press; 2002.
9. Hanh T, Eppsteiner F. Interbeing: fourteen guidelines for Engaged Buddhism. Berkeley: Parallax; 1998.
10. Dimidjian V. Journeying East: conversations on aging and dying. Berkeley: Parallax; 2004.
11. Chodron P. Comfortable with uncertainty: 108 teachings on cultivating fearlessness and compassion. USA: Shambhala; 2003.
12. Germer C, Salzberg S. The mindful path to self-compassion: freeing yourself from destructive thoughts and emotions. NY: Guilford; 2009.
13. Osler W. Address to the students of the Albany Medical College. Albany Med Ann. 1899;20:307–9.
14. Neff K. Exercises to increase self compassion [Internet]. Accessed 21 Nov 2010. http://www.self-compassion.org/.

Chapter 7
Mindfulness and Whole Person Care

Patricia L. Dobkin

Keywords Mindfulness • Healing • Self-compassion • Mindfulness-Based Stress Reduction • Participatory medicine

Mindfulness

'Being mindful' implies that the mind is full. "Full of what?" one may ask. *Awareness* of what is occurring in the present moment within one's self (e.g., recalling a previous encounter with the upcoming patient; feeling tired) as well as of others (e.g., noticing that the patient enters the examination room leaning on a cane), and the setting (e.g., a waiting room full of patients). Mindfulness involves specific attitudes such as "openness" toward what is happening, curiosity, patience, perceptual clarity, and the complementary abilities of focusing and shifting attention. In the context of medical practice, mindfulness has the potential to foster healing [1]; how this may occur and its application to the twenty-first century health care paradigm described in this book are considered in this chapter. Given that mindfulness is an innate universal human capacity that allows for clear thinking and open-heartedness, it fits the overarching goal in medical practice to cure disease when possible and alleviate suffering in a compassionate manner.

Mindful Practitioners

The McGill University Medical School new curriculum was launched in 2005; it systematically teaches professionalism and healing throughout the 4-year undergraduate program [2]. When examining this 'Physicianship' program – which focuses on

P.L. Dobkin (✉)
Associate Professor, Department of Medicine, Programs in Whole Person Care,
McGill University, 546 Pine Avenue West, Montreal, QC H2W 1S6, Canada
e-mail: patricia.dobkin@mcgill.ca

clinical observation skills, attentive listening, clinical reasoning, self-reflection, bioethics, and communication that takes into consideration the "social contract" – it is evident that being mindful would further this approach to clinical practice. For example, when fully present in the moment, with an open, curious mind, one can listen attentively to patients' accounts of who they are, what brings them to a particular encounter, and why they believe they are sick. The physician will hear and see clearly the patient through spoken words, "paralanguage" (e.g., tone of voice, pitch, etc.) as well as body language. The patient is likely to feel "heard," validated, and understood. As mentioned in the first chapter, the health care practitioner's open-minded presence with the patient in the context of medical expertise is like a master key that opens many locks.

Self-Compassion: Taking Care of the Self To Take Care of Others

In order for a health care professional to possess and use this key effectively she/he must first know and accept herself/himself deeply. Research has shown that those who are self-critical tend to be so with others as well, including their patients. When one can experience the full range of human expression within oneself – including joy and sorrow, strength, and weakness – one touches on the essential human condition. From here one can relate to others with authenticity. When one includes oneself on the roster of those deserving of being cared for, stress and burnout are more likely to be prevented or dealt with. However, health care professionals often neglect to include self-care on their lengthy 'to do' lists. Acts such as taking a vacation, exercising regularly, or enjoying an evening out with friends are often viewed as sufficient. The notion of self-care is much more than these 'time out' types of activities, and it is distinct from selfishness. In the Mindfulness-Based Medical Practice course that we teach, we hear narratives describing the extent to which physicians omit themselves from the wellness equation. This is often rationalized through references to an altruistic sense of duty, severe time constraints, and the "culture of medicine," which has little tolerance for "weakness." Nonetheless, when we explore the negative consequences of not making space for themselves in their lives such as emotional exhaustion, depersonalization, early retirement, or health problems, it becomes clear that being kind to oneself is a necessity rather than luxury.

Training Health Care Professionals How to Practice Mindfully [3]

Epstein, a physician at the University of Rochester School of Medicine and Dentistry, has written eloquently and extensively [4–6] on how to teach mindfulness to medical students and physicians. A recent study by Krasner et al. [7] examined an intensive education program for 70 family physicians, which included didactic material on burnout and meaning in medicine, mindfulness, narrative, and appreciative inquiry exercises. The authors reported short-term and sustained improvements in well-being and attitudes associated with patient-centered care. Furthermore, increases in mindfulness were significantly correlated with decreases in burnout and distress, as well as enhanced empathy toward patients. These promising findings are consistent with a study conducted at Monash University in Australia with medical students, all of whom took a Health Enhancement Program as part of the required core curriculum [8]. With mindfulness training, the students were less distressed even during exam periods following the program. We have found similar improvements with medical students taking the "Mindful Medical Practice" elective at McGill University, with significant reductions in stress (despite being matched to resident programs at the time when the survey was completed), as well as increases in mindfulness and self-compassion. Other medical schools such as Jefferson Medical College [9], University of Massachusetts Medical School, the University of Arizona Medical School in USA, and Dalhousie School of Dentistry in Canada have also integrated mindfulness practices in their training programs of Medicine and Dentistry.

Mindful Patients

While the spotlight on professionalism emphasizes health care providers' characteristics, duties, and functions, there is another important factor that should not be overlooked: the patient. In the past 25 years, the roles of physicians and patients have shifted in terms of power and responsibilities. While physicians used to make decisions unilaterally, now they are less paternalistic, patients are more likely to voice their preferences, and other germane (often unacknowledged) influences (e.g., the patient's culture, information from the Internet, and advertising directed at both parties) are "in the room." Along with these changing dynamics, patients and physicians need to collaborate and negotiate treatment plans for mutually agreed upon goals to be reached.

Given what research has shown about the effects of stress on physical and mental health, as well as the critical role lifestyle plays on development and exacerbation of various chronic illnesses, patients' mindfulness matters. How? Here is an example. A 50-year-old man notices that he is out of breath when climbing stairs, fatigues easily, and has frequent heart palpitations. When he visits his family doctor, he describes what he is experiencing, when things began to change, what improves or worsens these symptoms. In other words, he must *know* (i.e., be aware of) and be able to communicate his direct experience effectively, i.e., the quality, intensity, and frequency of the symptoms. His attitude toward these symptoms may be noteworthy. Is he in denial of the potential seriousness of the problem? Or is he very worried? Equally as important, the physician needs to ask about relevant factors, such as overtime work hours or use of over-the-counter medications and/or complementary therapies. Perhaps the patient has comorbid conditions, such as hypertension or diabetes. This is all part of the complex picture that directs decisions regarding the best course to take. Medical practice in the twentieth century often missed the critical role that patients played in their own health. Rather than be passive recipients of care, they must engage in self-care activities (e.g., eat well, exercise, get enough sleep, not smoke, drink with moderation, etc.). Moreover, they need to adhere to medical recommendations especially if the disease is complex requiring multidisciplinary directives (e.g., changes in diet, exercise, as well as insulin injections, and attending regular health care visits for a diabetic patient).

Several programs that teach patients how to be mindful have been developed over the past 25 years. One well-known program, Mindfulness-Based Stress Reduction (MBSR), was developed at the University of Massachusetts Medical Center [10]. In this structured 8-week group program, patients with various illnesses (e.g., cancer, chronic pain, and autoimmune disorders) meet for 2.5 h/week to learn how to be mindful and manage stress better. Patients practice various forms of meditation together and on their own to learn to respond rather than react to illness, symptoms, and other difficulties in their lives. During the group meetings, they share how practicing meditation and taking better care of themselves influence their symptoms and their lives. This program has been adapted to meet the needs of depressed patients (Mindfulness-Based Cognitive Therapy), those suffering from alcohol and substance abuse (Mindfulness-Based Relapse Prevention) and eating disorders (Mindfulness-Based Eating Awareness Training). It is taught around the globe in more than 250 centers. Studies (cohort and randomized clinical trials) have consistently demonstrated reductions in distress, physical symptoms, and increases in patients' quality of life after participation in this program [11].

Mindful Medical Encounters

Dr. Ofri: A physician in action [12] (The bold in the quoted text are those elements of this account of one doctor's experience with a patient that illustrate mindfulness in medical action.).

"After they'd left, I saw that Mrs. Uddin was already waiting for me, and I knew I'd never get through the morning session. Whoever invented the fifteen-minute patient slot had never met Nazma Uddin. Mrs. Uddin – a heavyset woman from Bangladesh – always had a thousand complaints, endless aches and pains, never-ending misery. Today she was wearing her usual dark blue heavy polyester robe, head scarf, and veil. Only her eyes and forehead were visible. But when I closed the door, she immediately unsnapped the veil, and we smiled sympathetically at each other, gearing ourselves up for the inevitable frustrations that lay ahead. At this point in our relationship, however, a visit with her did not unnerve me. But it hadn't always been that way. She used to be my torment.

I had become Mrs. Uddin's doctor eight years before. She was only thirty-five years old, but she'd seemed so aged and infirm that **it shocked me** to see that we were the same age. Each visit was an endless litany of hiccups, headaches, shin pains, stomach pains, ear pains, coccyx pains. Despite innumerable CT scans, blood tests, specialty consultations, cardiac stress tests, lung function tests, endoscopies, and MRIs, there was nothing concrete I could find to explain her complaints. No therapy I offered seemed to help. There was **clearly a psychological**

element to her condition, but she never followed through with referrals to psychiatrists or trials of antidepressant medications. She had some amorphous blend of chronic pain syndrome, osteoarthritis, fibromyalgia, depression, dyspepsia, somatization disorder, migraines, stress- all of which I treated. But nothing ever got better. **I dreaded her visits.**

In those years, Mrs. Uddin always brought along her young daughter, Azina…

I was annoyed that Mrs. Uddin kept Azina out of school for these appointments. I was exasperated by her extravagant overuse of the medical system. **I always felt as if I were going to drown** in Mrs. Uddin's unremitting complaints, as though she were deliberately trying to torture me with her unsolvable issues. **If I didn't control my feelings**, my **mind would spin with frustration, perseverating** about how much I hated the whine in her voice, hated seeing her name on my roster, hated the fact that she'd emigrated thousands of miles from some random village in Bangladesh and somehow managed to end up in *my* clinic with her intractable and dispiriting complaints. And especially how **I hated that stultifying veil**.

The tension between us finally broke one day when Azina piped up and asked if we were done yet because she wanted to get back to school in time for recess. The shock of her own voice and her own words was like ice water. **I realized that I had slipped too far in my own irrational feelings, that my anger was flagrantly displaced, and that I had lost all sense of the humanity of my patient and her daughter.**

Azina quietly told me what it was like at home with a mother who was depressed and in pain, how the burden of caring for her mother and the family had fallen on her shoulders, how she ached to just worry about homework, like the rest of the fifth-graders. **This revelation open my eyes and helped me regain my empathy – and energy –** for Mrs. Uddin. After that, I no longer saw Mrs. Uddin as a torment; **Azina had cured me** of that.

Today Mrs. Uddin was here with her usual complaints, none of which had changed – or progressed – since we first met. Over the years, we'd acquired a familiarity with each other's quirks, and in some ways we felt like an old married couple… Our visits still ran generously over the allotted fifteen minutes, **but I no longer felt angry…**

I still had **my own personal discomfort with the concept of the veil**. The theme of finding women's bodies and sexuality threatening, something that needed to be controlled, seemed to be a commonality in so many cultures. My children were still young, but at some point they'd notice that in Orthodox Judaism, women had to sit behind a barrier in the synagogue… However, I recognized that many Muslim women chose the veil… Still **I needed to keep my political and feminist concerns out of my individual encounters with women who wore the veil…**

I didn't have any solutions for Mrs. Uddin today, but the **very act of unloading her concerns seemed to relax her. I offered my sympathy for her pains.** I suggested that we try physical therapy again. I reminded her that weight loss would help her aching knees. I recommended that she consider acupuncture – she'd always been leery about that one – and I refilled her panoply of prescriptions. I convinced her to give the antidepressants another try. She assented this time, but I knew there was only a fifty-fifty chance that she'd take them.

She snapped her veil back on and stood to go. We **gave each other a hug**, as we always did now. We had a lot of years behind us, and it was clear that we had a lot ahead of us too."

What is apparent as Dr. Ofri contends with what some may label as "a difficult patient" is the doctor's awareness of herself, the other, and the context. She is honest with herself about the strong negative emotions that arise in her. She is cognizant that the patient likely has psychosocial problems that contribute to her numerous conditions. Dr. Ofri acknowledges her own religious and cultural views and recognizes how these may impact her relationship with a woman similar in age but very distant from her own background culturally and geographically. By accepting all of her own thoughts and feelings, however unpleasant they may be, she is able to open up to this other human being, so different from her, and tap into her reserve of compassion. By giving her care when there is no cure, she invites the patient to unburden herself. In the end, these two women hug each other with warmth, knowing that they will meet again and do what patients and physicians have done together for centuries.

Do all doctors practice like this? Should they? How did Dr. Ofri learn to be like this? Is it simply a reflection of her personality, emotional intelligence, upbringing or culture? In our research with health care professionals who took our Mindfulness-Based Medical Practice program, we found that after the program there were improvements on depressive symptoms, perceived stress, mindfulness, and self-compassion [13]. Significant increases were observed on the environmental mastery subscale of the Ryff-Well-Being Scale as well as the self-kindness, common humanity, and isolation subscales of the Neff Self-Compassion scale. A formal test of moderation was conducted to explore whether mindfulness moderates the relationship between stress and wellness. Mindfulness predicted wellness positively ($R=0.35$, $p<0.01$), while stress demonstrated a negative effect on wellness ($\beta=-0.62, p<0.00$). A significant moderation effect was observed in the interaction effect; as mindfulness increased, stress had less of a negative impact upon wellness ($\beta=-0.04$, $p<0.01$). Out of the 51 participants who were in the quantitative phase of the study, a subgroup of 26 (13 each year) took part in focus group interviews after the Mindfulness-Based Medical Practice program. Preliminary results suggest that participants experience the program as enhancing their ability to observe, tolerate, and regulate emotions, particularly anger and sadness. Other recurrent themes included an increased willingness to set time aside for self-care practices. Mindfulness was frequently described as a tool to improve listening skills and presence in the face of organizational challenges associated with time pressures and heavy patient loads.

Multidisciplinary Teams

Patients in the twenty-first century often have illnesses that require the services of various health care professionals. This can pose a problem from several standpoints. It requires patients to keep track of multiple appointments, recommendations, and navigate the medical system. Since communication between health care professionals may not be optimal, patients need to inform their doctors about their procedures, results, and medications. This can be especially hard for the elderly and infirm, adding another aspect of stress to the illness experience. Some are fortunate to have family members willing to help them, but for those who are isolated or have language barriers such management can be overwhelming.

Furthermore, health care professionals work with 'others'. While not readily acknowledged, a portion of stress in the medical system can be attributed to working with colleagues from the same and other disciplines. There is a fixed hierarchy in medicine both within (e.g., attending staff, residents, medical students) and between professionals (e.g., physicians, nurses, psychologists). Exchanges between these individuals may be limited or problematic. Multidisciplinary treatment is considered essential in many areas in medicine such as chronic pain, diabetes, and heart disease. Thus, communication must be effective and respectful between those who join in the common goal of helping patients cope with interventions and live with disease.

We have found that by giving 1-day workshops to a mixed group of health care professionals they gain insight into the ways others view situations, how misunderstandings may occur, and how they may be resolved. For example, in one role play an emergency room (ER) doctor described an elderly male patient who refused a critical medical procedure and how he (the doctor) thought things began to unravel when a specialist was called in for a consultation. One workshop member played the patient, another was the ER doctor, and one was the specialist. While the specialist thought it essential to "convince" the patient to undergo an invasive test (using an authoritarian style), there was discord in the room. Unfortunately, no one had elicited from the patient why he had refused the procedure. The ER doctor expressed his anxiety about time passing and the patient's condition worsening. Employing mindful communication skills taught in the workshop, these "actors" were able to *experience* what hindered effective collaboration and "replay" it until they reached a point in which all parties felt heard and respected. Moreover, the other workshop members observed this and all entered into a discussion about the process once the role play was completed.

Mindless Medical Encounters

Dr. Gawande in his book, *Complications* [14] describes "when good doctors go bad." Just as an excerpt from Dr. Ofri's book showed how effective mindful doctors can be, the following, based on a real case, depicts how one doctor "lost his mind" with disastrous consequences for his patients. "Dr. Goodman" (a fictional name) had been a well-respected surgeon before losing his privilege to practice medicine. (The bolded text emphasizes his difficulties.)

"Mrs. D was twenty-eight years old, a mother of two, and the wife of… She had originally come to Goodman about a painless but persistent fluid swelling in her knee. He had advised surgery, and she had agreed to it. The week before, he had done an operation to remove the fluid. But now, the assistant reported, she was back; she felt feverish and ill, and her knee was red, hot, and tender. When he put a needle to the joint, foul-smelling pus came out. What should he [the assistant] do? It was clear from the description that the woman was suffering from a disastrous infection, that she had to have the knee opened and drained as soon as possible. But Goodman was **busy**, and he never considered the idea. He didn't bring her to the hospital. He didn't go to see her. He didn't even have a colleague see her. 'Send her out on oral antibiotics', he said. The assistant expressed some doubt, to which Goodman responded, 'Ah, **she's just a whiner.**'

He used to enjoy being in the operating room, **fixing people**. After a while though, it seemed that the **only thing he thought about was getting through all of his patients as quickly as possible. ...** He was far busier than any of his partners, and that fact increasingly became, in his mind, a key measure of his worth...he became fixated on his status as the No. 1 booker. His **sense of himself as a professional** also make him unwilling to turn people away...Yet, no matter what he did to keep up, unforeseen difficulties arose – a delay in getting a room ready, an unexpected problem in an operation. Over time, he **came to find the snags unbearable**."

When dismissed by his hospital, Dr. Goodman could not comprehend what went wrong. Later, he was evaluated for burnout and treated for major depression. Before this expulsion, many of his patients were injured, some permanently. From a mindful whole person care perspective, Dr. Goodman's failure to work a reasonable number of hours (he clocked 80–100 h per week in the last decade of his working life), his attitude towards patients, his sense of himself ("I am what I do"), and his orientation toward fixing rather than helping patients to heal all contributed to a mindless practice that spun out of control.

High Stakes of Not Being Fully Present: The Evidence

There is an emerging literature on medical students', residents', and physicians' burnout and depression that indicates that unwell physicians have a negative impact on patient outcomes [15]. In one cross-sectional study, residents who scored high on a burnout scale self-reported providing at least one type of suboptimal care [16]. Importantly, Halbesleben and Rathert [17] found that the depersonalization aspect of burnout was associated with patient outcomes of lower satisfaction, and longer post-discharge recovery time. Burnout in medical students gradually develops over the course of medical education, with a prevalence of a moderate to high degree of burnout in years 1, 2, 3 as 22, 37, and 41%, respectively [18]. If future physicians can learn to cope early on with the stressors inherent in the practice of their profession both the healers and those they treat may benefit [19]. For example, Jones et al. [20], in a series of studies, showed that the introduction of stress management courses in hospitals reduced medication errors and malpractice claims. While more evidence is needed linking burnout to patient outcomes, such serious implications compel us not to wait until things get worse. We at McGill Programs in whole person care believe that what is missing is a paradigm that works in the context of twenty-first century medical education and practice.

Mindful Health Care Delivery in the Twenty-First Century

"How, in the face of the constant seeming wild dance of the reality of the stimuli bombarding the system from subsystems and suprasystems, does one separate information from noise, make sense of one's world?" [21]. This may sound like an apt description of an ER, but it was written by Antonovsky, a medical sociologist. If one were the patient being rushed into hospital, what would the experience be like? If one were the nurse conducting the triage, what may she notice about her encounter with the patient near the end of her 12-h shift? While he did not use the term "mindfulness," Antonovsky wrote about the importance of maintaining a "sense of coherence" in one's life. He purported that this sense of coherence stems from viewing life as comprehensible, manageable, and meaningful. He noted that individuals with a strong a sense of coherence coped well with stress. Clearly, both patients and their health care providers need to find their way through the maze we call the health care system.

What we are proposing is a radical change in the culture of medicine, which currently is 'ailing' [22, 23]. Chronic stress coupled with social changes and considerable changes in the organization and delivery of health services have taken their toll. Burnout and distress may negatively impact career trajectories (e.g., choice of specialty, early retirement). Our society cannot afford to lose its highly trained workforce. It is in the public interest to prevent burnout in health care providers. Achieving this will require a fine balance given that an important aspect of professionalism is altruism. Solutions need to take into account the social context as professionalism exists within the dynamic interplay of system actors, system structures, and broader environmental influences [24].

When we teach mindfulness to patients and health care professionals we are, in essence, helping them find meaning, change reactive patterns, and be able to manage whatever occurs in life. In a study that included 83 patients with various chronic illnesses, we found that increases in mindfulness was significantly correlated with increases in total sense of coherence ($r=0.54$, $p<0.0001$) at the end of the 8-week MBSR program [25]. This shows that both mindfulness and sense of coherence can be cultivated and that they positively influence each other.

Participatory Medicine

Mindfulness allows for a trusting relationship to emerge between the physician, nurse, or other health care provider and the patient. This, we contend, is the 'space' in which healing can take place; the physician accompanies the patient on the journey toward wholeness, even when no cure is possible. She/he invites the patient to approach the illness experience in a deeper way, exploring its meaning and opportunities. This is accomplished through what we call an "analogic" form of communication. In addition to the words spoken, the physician's genuine concern for the patient is shown through his or her posture, gestures, facial expression, voice inflection, sequence, rhythm, and cadence in speech. Knowing when to be silent, when to allow time for integration of information, when to gently touch the person tells a patient that he/she is not abandoned to his/her fate. Being present in this way provides a safety zone in which the dark side of illness can be explored: the fears, losses and implications. When the health care professional accepts the "wounded healer" role (i.e., his/her own humanity), then it is possible to open to the patient's suffering in a way that is meaningful. To do so, she/he must be able to tolerate uncertainties, strong emotions and address existential questions. This is not about "bedside manners"; rather, it is empathy in action. Herein lies the heart of medicine.

Kabat-Zinn [26] wrote eloquently about "participatory medicine" in the context of rehabilitation. He noted that for a patient to be restored to good health and function he needs to be "reenabled" i.e., learn to live fully in one's body, being, and life – in whatever state it is now – and accept personal agency for it. He states, "This embodied attention, this consciousness *in* the body, this willingness to work at the boundaries of what makes an intentional effort to be with, accept, and work with things as they are is a condition of body and mind known as mindfulness" [26]. Yet, the patient cannot do this work alone. It requires an equal degree of mindfulness on the part of treating professional, who applies knowledge, carries out procedures, prescribes medicines while remaining sensitive to the patient's response to these interventions.

Figure 7.1 seen below shows numerous factors that need to be kept in mind when a patient seeks treatment for a disease or illness. There are three intersecting foreground elements: the health care professional, the patient/person, and the disease. These are embedded in two overlapping "contexts": the medical and social systems. In the left circle is the health care professional who arrives with her/his professional experiences and personal history. She/he meets the patient in "A," encounters the patient and disease together in "B," and the disease itself in "C." "A" is a place where healing may be promoted. "B" is the intersection of the physician, patient, and disease; this is where curing may occur. "C" contains the health care professional's "tool box" containing medical knowledge, procedures, diagnostic tests, surgery, and medications. The person, in the circle on the right, arrives with his/her genetic loading, psychosocial characteristics, personal and medical history as well as health-related behaviors. These will impact the disease in "D" (e.g., being overweight and smoking with coronary heart disease). Moreover, the patient/person approaches disease or illness with certain beliefs, expectations, and hopes. Some call this the placebo effect (with negative cognitions or emotions it would be a "nocebo" effect).

The picture would be incomplete, however, if we did not take into account the context as well. Clearly, the medical system with its structure and processes impact both the health care professional and the patient directly and indirectly. For instance, if a patient has to wait a month to see her family physician to get a referral for a rheumatologist, then wait another 5 months to meet that doctor, and then another month for laboratory results to be given to her, the window of opportunity to start medication in a timely manner may be missed. Keeping this hypothetical case in mind, suppose the patient comes from a culture that values stoicism and the patient has endured painful joints for some time before finally agreeing with her adult children that it would be a good idea to let the family doctor know that it is

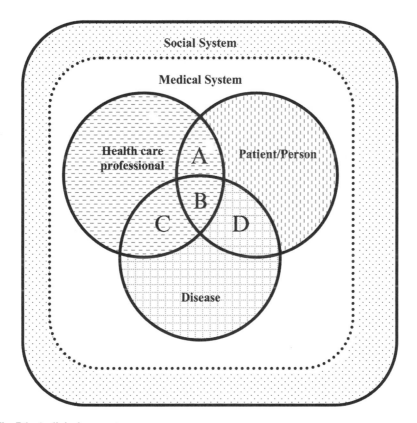

Fig. 7.1 A clinical encounter

becoming hard to open jars and sleep through the night due to pain. In this case, the delay is much more that the 6–7 months due to access issues. This may very well contribute to disability and disease progression.

To approach all this from a mindful perspective, the doctor may open a dialogue with the patient that includes both the medical aspects of arthritis care and coping strategies that the patient may find useful to live as fully as possible with the disease. The patient, in turn, needs to take responsibility by engaging in self-care behaviors (e.g., exercise, adhere to medications). While it may not be possible to change the cultures of medicine or society, one could acknowledge how they either promote health and well-being or hinder it, and work with them or around them as best as the situation allows.

Mindfulness in the Health Care Setting

To our knowledge, the concept of a "mindful health care setting" is just that: a concept (some may say a flight of fancy). Yet, the Canadian Medical Association (CMA) published a policy paper a decade ago on physician health and well-being stating "physicians need to manage professional and personal stress to maintain their own health and well-being and to maximize their ability to provide quality health care to their patients" [27]. For this idea to move from policy to practice, the setting must accommodate it. Mindful medical practice can be effective, evidence-based, and acceptable to physicians from a wide range of cultural backgrounds. It would build on rather than conflict with current practices. A successfully developed approach would commence in medical school, continue in residency training, and recur throughout the physician's career. Thus, there would not be a "disconnect" between the values and practices inherent in the care of patients.

Ruff and Mackenzie [28] wrote a policy paper concerning the role of mindfulness in health care reform. While this editorial is oriented toward the American health care system, many of its ideas can be applied to other jurisdictions, such as Canada, that offer universal health care to their citizens. The review examines what drives health care costs up, such as advances in technology, administrative practices, and the aging population. The authors note that by leveraging preventive medicine there is a humane solution. They underscore the relative neglect of low-tech strategies to promote health and prevent disease. Ruff and Mackenzie emphasize, as I do in this chapter, the importance of patients taking a proactive stance. The review highlights how mind–body interventions (e.g., meditation, use of guided imagery prior to surgery, massage for premature infants) are associated with cost savings. This is especially relevant to the growing number of patients living relatively long lives with various chronic conditions, such as renal disease, cancer, diabetes, and chronic pain. Finally, the authors also acknowledge the importance of mindful practitioners for the reasons previously summarized. Not only would acting in this way benefit the caregivers but also when they, in turn, recommend such approaches to patients they may do so in a credible and convincing manner.

Barriers to Mindfulness and Whole Person Care in the Twenty-First Century and Overcoming Them

The first potential barrier that *appears* to prohibit being mindful in medical practice is time. This idea is based on a misconception of what mindfulness entails. It is not what one *does*, but how one *is* that matters. As noted in Chap. 1, Dr. Hutchinson's time spent with his patient was less than 1 h over 2 years, but it made a significant difference in the patient's experience. Rather than be distracted, he was with her and attended to her needs fully. Notably, mindfulness is the antithesis of multitasking. This statement may lead one to conclude that it, therefore, cannot fit in a setting in which phones ring, beepers beep, monitors' alarms are activated, and personnel is burdened by paperwork. Yet, if one does one's work with full attention, it may be time-efficient in that fewer errors are made and necessary tasks get done, one after the other.

A second barrier is that training does not emphasize this aspect of clinical practice. Dr. Hutchinson and I have initiated Mindful Medical Practice workshops and more extensive programs to fill this gap. While we do not receive funding from the medical school, we are supported indirectly (e.g., office space) and our work is gaining momentum. Other medical schools have also found creative solutions to teaching mindfulness in the interest of providing integrated whole person care.

Third, the medical setting's house staff may not "buy in" to the idea that wellness in practitioners is crucial for patient care and that mindfulness helps a doctor stay well. They may fail to model the "art of medicine" in which caring is viewed as important as curing. Senior staff may inadvertently teach medical students and residents that getting the job done first and foremost as quickly as possible is what is most valued when practicing the "science of medicine." Then, even the most sincere trainee may set aside his/her views and feelings to conform to the setting demands.

A fourth barrier results from "top-down" decision making that does not involve employees directly. Studies pertaining to job stress and burnout consistently show that dictating schedules, heavy paperwork loads, imperfect computer systems, and limited autonomy contribute to job dissatisfaction. If administrators do not include those most affected by their decisions, all are likely to be negatively impacted. Thus, it is recommended that a standing "Wellness Committee" pertaining to optimizing work conditions that prevent burnout and dissatisfaction be formed and supported in medical settings. A new culture in which wellness is promoted can result in a win-win-win situation: health care providers, their patients, and the system may all reap the benefits.

References

1. Dobkin PL. Fostering healing through mindfulness in the context of medical practice. Curr Oncol. 2009;16(2):4–6.
2. Boudreau JD, Cassell EJ, Fuks A. A healing curriculum. Med Educ. 2007;41(12):1193–201.
3. Irving JA, Dobkin PL, Park J. Cultivating mindfulness in health care professionals: a review of empirical studies of mindfulness-based stress reduction (MBSR). Complement Ther Clin Pract. 2009;15(2):61–6.
4. Epstein RM. Mindful practice. JAMA. 1999;282(9):833–9.
5. Epstein RM. Mindful practice in action (I): technical competence, evidence-based medicine, and relationship-centered care. Fam Syst Health. 2003;21:1–9.
6. Epstein RM. Mindful practice in action (II): cultivating habits of mind. Fam Syst Health. 2003;21:11–7.
7. Krasner MS, Epstein RM, Beckman H, et al. Association of an educational program in mindful communication with burnout, empathy, and attitudes among primary care physicians. JAMA. 2009;302(12):1284–93.
8. Hassed C, de Lisle S, Sullivan G, Pier C. Enhancing the health of medical students: outcomes of an integrated mindfulness and lifestyle program. Adv Health Sci Educ Theory Pract. 2009;14(3):387–98.

9. Rosenzweig S, Reibel DK, Greeson JM, Brainard GC, Hojat M. Mindfulness-based stress reduction lowers psychological distress in medical students. Teach Learn Med. 2003;15(2): 88–92.

10. Kabat-Zinn J. Full catastrophe living: using the wisdom of your body and mind to face stress, pain and illness. New York: Delta; 1990.

11. Salmon P, Sephton S, Weissbecker I, Hoover K, Ulmer C, Studts J. Mindfulness meditation in clinical practice. Cogn Behav Pract. 2004;11(4):434–46.

12. Ofri D. Medicine in translation: journeys with my patients. Boston: Beacon; 2010.

13. Irving AJ, Dobkin PL, Park J. Mindfulness-based medical practice: cultivating self-care and mindfulness in health care professionals. Investigating and integrating mindfulness in medicine, health care and society. Proceedings of the 7th International Scientific Conference for Clinicians, Researchers and Educators; 2009, March 18–22; Worcester, MA.

14. Gawande A. Complications: a surgeon's notes on an imperfect science. New York: Metropolitan Books; 2002.

15. Firth-Cozens J. Interventions to improve physicians' well-being and patient care. Soc Sci Med. 2001;52(2):215–22.

16. Shanafelt TD, Bradley KA, Wipf JE, Back AL. Burnout and self-reported patient care in an internal medicine residency program. Ann Intern Med. 2002;136(5):358–67.

17. Halbesleben JR, Rathert C. Linking physician burnout and patient outcomes: exploring the dyadic relationship between physicians and patients. Health Care Manage Rev. 2008;33(1): 29–39.

18. Boudreau D, Santen SA, Hemphill RR, Dobson J. Burnout in medical students: examining the prevalence and predisposing factors during the four years of medical school. Ann Emerg Med. 2004;44(4):S75–6.

19. Dobkin PL, Hutchinson TA. Primary prevention for future doctors: promoting well-being in medical trainees. Med Educ. 2010;44(3):224–6.

20. Jones JW, Barge BN, Steffy BD, Fay LM, Kunz LK, Wuebker LJ. Stress and medical malpractice: organizational risk assessment and intervention. J Appl Psychol. 1988;73(4):727–35.

21. Antonovsky A. Unraveling the mystery of health: how people manage stress and stay well. San Francisco: Jossey-Bass; 1987. p. 166.

22. Miller NM, McGowen RK. The painful truth: physicians are not invincible. South Med J. 2000;93(10):966–73.

23. Ratanawongsa N, Wright SM, Carrese JA. Well-being in residency: a time for temporary imbalance? Med Educ. 2007;41(3):273–80.

24. Hafferty FW, Levinson D. Moving beyond nostalgia and motives: towards a complexity science view of medical professionalism. Perspect Biol Med. 2008;51(4):599–615.

25. Dobkin PL, Zhao Q. Increased mindfulness – the active component of the mindfulness-based stress reduction program? Complement Ther Clin Pract. 2011;17(1):22–7.

26. Kabat-Zinn J. Participatory medicine. J Eur Acad Dermatol Venereol. 2000;14(4):239–40.

27. Puddester D. The Canadian Medical Association's Policy on physician health and well-being. West J Med. 2001;174(1):5–7.

28. Ruff KM, Mackenzie ER. The role of mindfulness in healthcare reform: a policy paper. Explore (NY). 2009;5(6):313–23.

Chapter 8
Healing, Wounding, and the Language of Medicine

Abraham Fuks

Every patient needs mouth-to-mouth resuscitation, for talk is the kiss of life.

Anatole Broyard [1].

Keywords Words • Language • Healing • Narrative • Doctor–patient relationship • Listen • Talk • Placebo • Sociolinguistics • Silence • Dementia • Military • Metaphor

If clinical medicine is, at least in part, the art of human interactions, then words are its stock in trade. The words we use form the mental models of our lived worlds and shape our perceptions, understandings, and meanings. Given the power of language to bend our thoughts and minds, it is hardly a surprise to discover the influence of verbal interactions on our affect, mindset, and physical and mental well being. Mother's words shape the development of her infant's brain, and lack of verbal stimulation leaves traces visible to the neuropathologist. A comforting word can light up a face, and a voodoo curse can cause cramps in the guts of a believer. The language of the clinical setting can lead to effects and outcomes as potent as those following the administration of pharmacologic agents, yet the powerful agency of words in healing or wounding receives scant attention in contemporary medicine – there is no linguistic *materia medica* in the library.

This is all the more surprising given the recurrent finding that "being listened to" is at the top of the lists of needs articulated by patients, and "the capacity to listen" is in their descriptions of the ideal physician, landing well above technical competence [2]. Perhaps correctly, patients presume their physicians have the competence to practice yet perceive that appropriate clinical communication skills are less common. This chapter explores the use of words in the clinical encounter with an emphasis on their meanings and impact. One might well describe this as "medical linguistics," a subset of sociolinguistics and a new field of study!

A. Fuks (✉)
Professor of Medicine, McGill University, 3647 Peel Street, Montreal, QC H3A 1X1, Canada
e-mail: abraham.fuks@mcgill.ca

T.A. Hutchinson (ed.), *Whole Person Care: A New Paradigm for the 21st Century*,
DOI 10.1007/978-1-4419-9440-0_8, © Springer Science+Business Media, LLC 2011

Whose Words?

The first question we need to address is "whose words do we have in mind?" We naturally think of the words spoken by the caregivers, while forgetting that patients ask to be *listened* to, not *spoken* to – a reminder that attending physicians can be understood to mean, those who listen to their patients (from the Latin, *attendere*, "give heed to"). The opportunity for a patient to share his/her fears, anxieties, and uncertainties in facing the threatening, as yet unclear, implications of an illness is the first step in the construction of the relationship that will entwine the patient and physician and that can become the arena for trust and healing. Indeed, the various forms of psychotherapy in both traditional and contemporary psychiatry revolve around the story told by the patient, sometimes developed over many years of treatment. Equally familiar is the refrain, "all we did was talk, and I feel better already" cited by countless patients after a single clinical encounter. Though it is not clear how such a "talking cure" provides its benefits, it seems recurrently demonstrated that the attitude, mindset, and behavior of the listener are significant in this regard. It is likely that the patient finds solace in sharing the facts of the illness as he/she understands them and, through talk, extends a feeler into the darkness to decipher the import of his/her symptoms. Through talk, the patient constructs a plausible story of his/her illness and looks to the physician to help "name" the illness through diagnosis. The physician's role in this arena is multifold. He must first learn to listen attentively, without interruption, and thereby signal to the patient a readiness to enter into the partnership that constitutes the clinical dyad. To quote John Scott, who identified a series of attributes of physician-healers, "It [healing] resides neither in the doctor nor the patient, but in the space created by the network of relationships that enfold both doctor and patient" [3]. Second, the physician must learn to listen to silence and determine whether that signals anger, grief, or dementia. Drawing out an uncommunicative patient is a skill that requires a great deal of experience for mastery. Finally, the initial words of the patient provide strong clues to the role that the patient needs the physician to play in the particular clinical event. A skilled clinician expressed this idea as follows:

> Is this a story of shame and they need you to listen? Is this a story of fear and they need you to be there with them? Is this a story of blame…or self-blame and they need to hear that it wasn't their fault? I mean, what is the story? So what role do they need you to be in? [4]

Playing an interlocutor's role that the patient requires presumes a level of attunement based on a practiced combination of active listening and emotional mindfulness – a capacity to "hear" the ideas behind the words, to decode the semiotics of the body, and to interpret the hermeneutics of silences.

A Half-Word to the Wise

A wonderful example of the effect of altering a single, apparently innocent, qualifier is available in the work by Heritage et al. carried out in offices of community-based physicians. The physicians were randomized to ask one of the two following questions once the initial history had been discussed with the patient: "Is there anything else you want to address in the visit today?" or "Is there something else you want to address in the visit today?" The readout was a measure of the extent to which patients shared concerns noted in previsit questionnaires but not yet expressed during the visit (unmet concerns). The "something" question elicited positive responses in 90% of instances and revealed 78% of unmet concerns, whereas the "anything" question elicited positive responses in 53% of instances and revealed no additional concerns beyond those presented by patients in a control group who had no research-driven question posed to them [5]. Thus, the use of the qualifier *some* (but not *any*) was a useful trigger in inducing patients to bring forward issues that were troubling them prior to the visit. Of note, the "something" question did not lead to longer visits yet arguably led to improved communication and perhaps greater patient satisfaction, though this was not measured. What is of interest to us is the reason for the differences in responses. The authors note that the word *any* has negative polarity and tends to be used in interrogatory forms for which a "no" response is expected. Whatever the sociolinguistic mechanism, this work certainly makes the point that a single word (or part of a word) can have an enormous clinical impact, and physicians must be aware of the importance of seemingly innocent choices.

(Almost) An Hour of Healing

The impact of talking with a patient and the power of words as a vehicle for recognition, attention, and clinical improvement are evident from a series of experiments conducted by Kaptchuk et al. [6] to decipher the components of the placebo effect. A group of patients with irritable bowel syndrome were randomized to one of three interventions: a waiting list group (also served as control group), sham acupuncture (six sessions over a 3 week period), or sham acupuncture (as above) with the addition of a 45-min structured interaction between the patient and the acupuncturist practitioner. This included a discussion of the patient's symptoms, his understanding of his illness as well as stipulated behavioral requirements for the practitioner of active listening, an articulation of empathy, and the transmission of a sense of confidence in the efficacy of acupuncture therapy. Improvements in symptom scores and quality-of-life indices were noted in all three groups after 3 and 6 weeks (compared to baseline measures). However, the degree of improvement showed an increasing trend line from the waiting list through the sham acupuncture group to the acupuncture plus interaction group. The latter group showed the greatest degree of improvement of the illness, and indeed, the trend followed the nature and the degree and intensity of interactions with the study team, that is, mere registration to a waiting list with its anticipation of future benefits is itself helpful. The actual interaction with practitioners who simply apply a sham therapy brings added benefits, and the provision of a positive discussion and words of empathy and encouragement provide the greatest benefits. The trend lines suggested to the authors that the practitioner interaction is the most potent of the amalgam of effects and that the percentage of patients in the third arm (ca. 60%) who demonstrated a beneficial clinical response is on the same order of magnitude seen in clinical trials of therapies for IBS. The suggestion from this interesting trial is that the benefits of a so-called *placebo* may reside in large part not in the pill and the ritual that attends its administration, but stems rather from the practitioner whose attention and words of support and confidence evince the requisite trust and belief by the patient whose own neurophysiologic mechanisms complete the cycle of improvement.

A Walking Placebo

These data open the door to the idea that all therapies, whether *verum* or *placebo*, are enabled or, at least, enhanced by the words of the practitioner who is the agent of caring and care. In fact, Benedetti et al. [7] have demonstrated the former, namely, the added benefit of open compared with the hidden administration of morphine for postoperative care. One group received the drug by machine administered infusion with no special announcement to the patient; the second group received the morphine by bedside infusion by a physician who informed the patient that a potent painkiller was being given. The pain suffered at 30 and 60 min after drug administration was significantly lower in the open administration group compared to the hidden administration group. The effect was extended in an interesting direction in another experimental group in which the interruption of morphine administration was announced or not. Again, knowledge by the patient of the cessation of the medication resulted in a more rapid recurrence of pain than in the second group in which the hidden interruption of medication permitted an extended therapeutic effect. There is no placebo in these trial designs, unless of course, we consider the physician a walking placebo (or nocebo) [8].

A highly cited paper that adds an interesting twist to the impact of the caregiver was carried out by Gracely et al. in a study of patients having dental extractions who were informed that they would be randomly assigned to receive placebo (saline), naloxone (an antagonist to narcotic agents), or fentanyl, a potent narcotic analgesic and that the pain levels, measured by questionnaire might increase, decrease, or not change. One subgroup of these individuals received their treatment and questionnaire administration from clinicians who were informed that their subjects would receive placebo or naloxone (PN group), and a second group received the same treatment and questionnaires from clinicians who were told they their patients would receive placebo or naloxone or fentanyl (PNF group). All drugs were administered double blind. At the end of 1 h, the members of the PN group who received placebo only reported an *increase* in pain while the members of the PNF group who received placebo only reported a *decrease* in pain – the two groups differed significantly in pain reports at 1 h. Please note that the only empirical difference between these two groups is the knowledge of the clinician of the range of possible treatments his subjects might receive. The clinicians did not know what treatments were actually given, and in these instances, it was placebo only in all subjects. And yet, the expectation of benefit (PNF group) or not (PN group) was somehow transmitted to the subjects despite the double blind nature of the design. This is a wonderful demonstration that the clinician's anticipation of benefit can induce a similar expectation in the patient through some subtle verbal or behavioral cues [9]. Thus, the power of words and language can be exceptionally cryptic and hidden yet transmissible all the same to the patient who can either be healed or harmed by verbal or body language, depending on the intent, mindset, and behavior of the clinician.

Soft Talk and Big Sticks

Caregivers often use innocent phrases to support patients and provide soothing words of concern. How often do we say, "This won't hurt a bit" or "It will feel like a bee sting," when about to administer an injection. The effect of such words was assessed by Lang et al. [10] in a study of interactions between patients and caregivers prior to and during interventional radiological procedures. Warning the patient with respect to pain or other undesirable experiences resulted in greater pain and greater anxiety than simply stating that the procedure was about to start. Furthermore, sympathizing with the patient using language that refers to negative experiences did not affect pain measures but did increase levels of anxiety. This effect is described by the authors as the nocebo effect and may stem from a phenomenon called negative affective priming, in which suggestions can produce the affect to which they refer, with even minimal input [11]. In fact, even the phrases, "you will feel no pain," "here is a prescription for your pain medicine," may evince paradoxical effects. This may be rather more common than suspected in medicine, where physicians may discuss side effects of medications, for example, even if to indicate how rare they are. Thus, words such as hurt, complication, pain, bleeding can be heard by the patient as expectations rather than rare occurrences.

An intriguing example of the import of a single word in healthcare education comes from a thesis project examining by interview the experiences of medical students in their third year of study and presented by Anna Romer for her doctoral work at Harvard University [12]. Romer noticed the recurrent use by the medical students of the word, "just," as in "I just sat there" or "I just talked to her" as deprecating their own activity by contrast with the active interventions of the residents who might, after all, do things such as lumbar punctures, bone marrow aspirations, and prescribe chemotherapy. Thus, the students reflected their learned presumptions that talk is, especially if they listen, particularly passive, nonmedical, and devalued by their mentors. Some students noted that their golden opportunity to talk with patients would evaporate when they entered the "real world" of medicine as they had observed from role models that talking with patients varies inversely with ability to provide care, place in the hierarchy and importance of rank and status. What was most interesting was the students' clear-eyed realization that what they are taught in classes on doctoring skills is often not supported, if not actively discouraged, when they reached the hospital wards. They learn quickly that the ability to reel off a differential diagnosis with arcane diseases receives more recognition and higher grades than their burgeoning "relational knowledge."

As Romer notes in her discussion, "relational concerns are simultaneously idealized and devalued (just talk)." Despite these pressures, the students understood that these interludes of talking with patients were moments of healing. A major admonition to teachers of medicine is to remember the paraphrase of the old saw, "students learn what we practice, not what we preach."

Silence is Golden

Hippocrates taught us to listen to the silences as well as the words. By that, he meant many things. Pauses, changes in breathing patterns, body shifts, paralanguage, facial expressions all communicate content and affect, and the skilled listener uses the silences to pay particular attention to these [13]. Silence can also mean that the patient is having difficulty in articulating a concern that may be laden with emotion and, indeed, may be particularly important. Hence, such silences must not be interrupted as they can be preludes to the most significant concern the patient is bringing to the particular encounter. Of course, silent pauses are spaces for reflection and can provide time for moments of mindfulness for the clinician.

Respect for silence is also a reminder that words must be measured and not abused, neither in number nor in kind. Is it possible to be too talkative? Is there such a thing as too much communication? The answer to this pair of questions stems from understanding that talk is not necessarily communicative. Some talk is mindless, at best. A study by McDaniel et al. [14] examined the frequency of physician self-disclosure in just over a hundred unannounced visits by standardized patients to primary care physicians; that is, how often did doctors talk about themselves? The researchers were "shocked" to find physicians talking about their own concerns, illnesses, and families in a third of patient visits [15]. In fact, the conversation returned to a patient-centered concern only 21% of the time, and the evaluators estimated that 85% of such self-disclosures were not useful to the patient and the purpose of the visit. There was no apparent benefit to the patients from such revelations by physicians of their own personal experiences.

Now, it may be the case that a physician can express a sense of understanding by noting, for example, that he too is a diabetic and forming a bond with the patient. However, this study reminds us that if we find ourselves talking instead of listening, and especially talking about ourselves, to be mindful of that and remember that we are there for the patient, not the converse.

Elderspeak: Geriatric Baby Talk

An interesting phenomenon that seems to accompany the growing numbers of individuals in our society over the age of 70 is the advent of elderspeak. In a word, this is the use of what would otherwise pass for baby talk in communicating with the frail, and not so frail, elderly. This form of speech is especially common in settings where older individuals require care, such as hospitals, nursing homes, and institutions caring for those with dementia [16]. In some strange sense, once we provide care for those who are, like children, at least in part dependent, we use the same simplified word choice and syntax at both ends of the span of life. The examples are endless – dear, sweetie, young lady (for a woman of 68) – and the questions even more charming, e.g., the collective noun (How are we today?), check for comprehension (did you understand what I just told you?), directing the question to a son or daughter while ignoring the patient (please tell your father what I just told you), the breezy presumption of first name address (Hi, Mr. Bill!), and the quest for yesteryear (what did you used to be?). These forms of infantilizing discourse are very irritating and insulting to the elderly and undermine their sense of self-confidence and self-worth. Very few, if any, retirees find this language endearing or respectful. That alone would be a warning to change our mode of communication. However, the effects may be even more pernicious than at first thought.

A study of a patient with dementia in a nursing home demonstrated a correlation between the degree of elderspeak used in interacting with the patient and her "resistiveness to care," a measure of a series of behaviors that signal an aversive response to the interaction [17]. This initial finding was later replicated in a larger sample of 20 patients studied in 80 encounters [18]. Thus, even in an individual whose cognitive functions are diminished, the ability to distinguish between infantilizing and normal language appears to remain intact, and more significant, disrespectful language may lead the person to resist an intervention intended to be helpful.

A second perspective on the impact of language felt by the elderly recipient to be demeaning is afforded by an interesting longitudinal study of aging by Levy et al. [19] in a sample of 660 persons. They found "that older individuals with more positive self-perceptions of aging....lived 7.5 years longer than those with less positive self-perceptions of aging." This finding was a complement to a parallel longitudinal assessment that demonstrated that functional health among the elderly over a two decade span was influenced by their self-perceptions of aging at the outset of the period [20]. Together, those aging persons who have positive attitudes and views about growing old do so in better health and live longer than their peers who have a negative outlook. The tantalizing (and depressing) conclusion is that by undermining elderly persons' self-confidence and self-esteem by the use of elderspeak, we can transform them to patients who need more care because of poorer functional health status, resist the care when it is offered, and have a shorter life expectancy. Whoever said "it's only words" neglected the rich connections among social environment, mind, brain, and body!

The Gall Bladder in Room Six

Language can simultaneously shape our thoughts while revealing our mindsets and mental models. The words we choose to describe patients and diseases indicate a dramatic shift in the attention of the physician, that is, in what is important to him/her. A traditional focus on the patient with illness has been supplanted by a substitution of the patient by the disease. This has occurred in a stepwise fashion in which the first was the inordinate attention paid to diagnosis, in both the medical and popular imaginations. In medicine, the development of pathology and more precise imaging techniques permits physicians to use MRI machines to peer directly at disease processes so that patients have become transparent. An echocardiogram allows the cardiologist to examine the heart valves and diminishes the need for a stethoscope, which brought the doctor in direct physical contact with the patient. Now, a machine suffices, and the cardiologist examines computer screens and paper traces. This transition from person to disease was abetted by what Charles Rosenberg calls the "tyranny of diagnosis" [21], and indeed, the television heroes of the recent past are expert diagnosticians rather than inspired therapists. It is now presumed, and quite incorrectly, that once a diagnosis is established, treatment follows automatically and successfully. Just as the technically adept surgeon is the role model on a surgical service, the diagnostic "star" is emulated on internal medicine wards. With the advent of an increasingly technologized medicine over the past 25 years, more of the doctor's attention is channeled toward modalities that mediate between him/her and the patient, and less direct contact with the individual is evident in both inpatient and outpatient medicine. The effect of all these forces has been the reification of disease, that is, a thing that stands by itself, rather than a process of illness that happens to a patient. As Levenstein et al. [22] have aptly noted, "In the process of differential diagnosis there is a well-tried clinical method for understanding diseases, but no equivalent method for understanding patients." This, in turn, leads to a dissociation between the needs of physicians and those of patients, and these two partners in the clinical dyad now have different objectives, with the doctor developing a relationship to the disease which he intends to identify and eliminate, while the patient seeks attention, understanding, comfort, and a return to health. As expressed so aptly by Pauline Chen in her column in the New York Times, "...we see ourselves on opposite sides of a divide. There is this sense that we're facing off with each other and we're not working together. It's a tragedy" [23].

A second step in this evolution is the disappearance of the patient and the metonymic substitution by the disease or the afflicted organ. Hence, the phrases heard on wards, "the gall bladder in room six," or "the heart failure in the coronary care unit." These habits are of course disrespectful and inconsonant with any sense of civility or dignity – they are also clinically dangerous as all attention is focused with laser like intensity on a single locus that may have little to do with the source of suffering afflicting the individual patient. And woe betide the patient who has no diagnostic label – he becomes either "a poor historian," "idiopathic," "nonspecific," or one who simply disappears in a blind spot of clinicians who do not know what to call him/her and thus call him/her not at all.

Military Metaphors: Whose War Are We Fighting?

A clear indication of the reification of disease comes from the military metaphors that are so pervasive in the discourse of and about medicine [24]. We speak of the war on cancer, the battle against disease, the therapeutic armamentarium; we use silver bullets, magic bullets, and targeted therapies; we eradicate, eliminate, destroy, and issue doctor's orders. By turning disease into the enemy, we again emphasize its status as a "thing," independent of the patient, and establish a new, though adversarial, relationship between the protagonist physician and the disease. It is then a matter of an additional rhetorical and functional flourish to replace the patient with the disease. The doctor's interlocutor is now the disease, and while the battle rages, the patient has become the battlefield, not even an ally. This substitution may explain the limited communication with the preoperative patient who has become a vessel bearing the disease and the field of combat onto which the surgeon leads his troops. Not by accident does the old term for operating room, the operating theater, foreshadow the twentieth-century phrase, theater of war.

In this construct, the patient as a counterparty who is recognized and respected disappears, and the lessons of attentive listening become mooted victims of a new social order in which bodies are scanned or probed to find the disease lurking in little corners, much like the devil in Presbyterian churches. Illness, the patient's experience of being sick, is made irrelevant, and therapy is geared to extirpation. Diagnosis becomes agent-centered, not patient-centered, and public health is transformed into a barrier to the immigration of strange foreign agents, SARS, for example.

The metaphors we use not only reflect our beliefs and the meaning we attach to the objects of our worlds, but they also shape our thoughts and by placing emphasis on one feature of an object may obliterate another. Hence, the celebration of diagnosis as an end in itself and the reification of disease turn the patient into an increasingly passive object, one that is almost superfluous to the technologized physician. Indeed, the hierarchical structure of the medical team of a teaching hospital ward provides a perverse figure in which the "lower" on the team, the more likely you are to recognize the patient as an individual. Medical students report that they have much more contact with the patients they look after than the residents who in turn provide more hands on care than the attending staff. It seems that once you attain the status of a mature attending physician, you are able to provide care vicariously and perform the magic trick of patient-centered care while not ever seeing the actual person. Little wonder we speak of the hidden curriculum as a powerful teaching tool. Our students, thus, learn that the further a physician advances in training, the less he talks with patients [25]. Of course, this is in part the skewed perspective of inpatient medicine, but its influence is strong, as we have learnt in previous sections of this chapter.

Winners and Losers

The usual structure of the military metaphor is that physicians are engaged in fighting the enemy disease. However, the advocacy for patient involvement in care has placed an additional burden on the shoulders of some patients by insisting that they fight whatever illness afflicts them. Two unintended consequences have followed in the wake of such an expectation. Some patients have elaborated a different mental model of illness and healing that entails equilibrium and restoration of harmony and balance as the aims of medicine. Such individuals can become very upset by the aggressive language they hear from their caregivers and from friends and neighbors [26]. Even Lance Armstrong, a world-renowned athlete and cyclist who "fights his way" to the tops of French mountains and who might be expected to be quite comfortable with a military metaphor was in "shell shock" when confronted with the martial images and incendiary language of one oncologist to whom he was referred. He immediately left and sought care from a team with whom he could build a trusting relationship.[1] Another patient with cancer found the discourse of fighting and winning less than palatable. He had already experienced real war in Vietnam and "was not anxious to repeat anything closely resembling that." Listen to this question from a patient living with a malignancy and receiving chemotherapy, "But can you fight your disease and not yourself?" [27]. This person understood keenly what too many physicians have forgotten – disease cannot be psychologically removed from a patient's body and mind and placed somewhere "out there" where it can be ignored, let alone fought without collateral damage. For that matter, patients are all too aware that when physicians take up arms against disease, the collateral damage is painful and many know stories of the casualties of "friendly fire."

The second and more serious result of all the Web sites telling patients to fight and admonishing them to "think positively" is the entailed idea that winning the war (defeating the cancer) is only a matter of fighting hard enough. This in turn leads to the commonly expressed notion that so-and-so became "too tired to fight" and "gave up." Obituaries are filled with descriptions of patients who were defeated "after a courageous battle." Note the shift in agency: physicians are winners when things go well yet patients are losers when physicians cannot "win." Sontag [28] describes aptly how the words of war can evolve into the language of guilt ascribed to patients.

When All Else Fails, Blame the Patient

The mindless statement too often heard in oncology settings is, "the patient failed chemotherapy." What a peculiar syntax to express the fact that chemotherapy failed to help the patient! Why then do we use it? Why do we say, as Donnelly pointed out 25 years ago, that the patient "threw an embolus" or "dropped his blood pressure"? The language structure of the hospital and clinic assigns agency to the patient when things go awry. It creates a neat split that permits physicians to claim credit when treatment succeeds yet assign blame to patients when therapy fails or complications arise. This is of course not a self-conscious action or intent to disparage.

---

[1]Despite this, the Web site of the Lance Armstrong Foundation tells us to "Find out how you can get involved in the fight against cancer."

This interesting and widespread phenomenon is rooted in part in the military metaphors of medicine described above and the entailment of winners and losers. A second source is the advent of the modern pharmacopeia. When physicians select active therapeutic interventions, they thereby permit themselves to declare victory should the patient get better. However, to maintain the self-confidence needed to "fight another day" for the next patient, physicians have developed this linguistic mechanism of ascribing failure to patients. This takes many forms: poor historian, poor compliance, communication barrier, lack of will to live, lack of energy to fight, and as noted above, the patient gave up.[2]

These phrases demonstrate that we are far from a form of medical care in which patients are partners and respected as autonomous individuals. This evident lack of regard for our patients' abilities to understand when we are clear in our explanations, and their desires to live longer and well when we listen carefully to their hopes and dreams serves to undermine the doctor–patient dyadic relationship without which medicine is bankrupt.

There are many studies of the barriers to clear communications between caregivers and patients that also document the deleterious consequences of such lapses. However, too many of them again conclude that patients are at fault in some fashion. One recent example comes from a careful study by Engel et al. [29] who studied the ability of English-speaking patients to understand the information and instructions they received in an emergency room. They noted that "Seventy-eight percent of patients demonstrated deficient comprehension" and furthermore found that "most patients appear to be unaware of their lack of understanding and report inappropriate confidence in their comprehension and recall." In other words, most patients did not comprehend what they were told and indeed, were not aware of their gaps in understanding. What is of interest to our question of blame is the fact that while the authors consider various barriers to comprehension, they ascribe the failures solely to the patients. It is quite remarkable that the possibilities that the physicians or other caregivers were less than clear in their instructions or insensitive to the need for extreme clarity in such high-stakes settings for their interlocutors were virtually ignored in the publication. Once again, if we fail to communicate, the listeners, our patients, are at fault.

Words, Words, Words

If words fall into disrepair, what will substitute? They are all we have.

Tony Judt [30].

---

[2]The most egregious example that I have heard was related by a colleague in gynecology who heard the following statement at a conference: "the patient perforated her uterus during the procedure."

Language in the clinical situation is a means to an end. It is the modality of attunement in the clinical dyad and forges a bond of trust. Words create the conduit between physician and patient that channels bilateral recognition of worth and respect that in turn make possible the intimacy necessary for truth. Narratives are needed to make sense of sickness, and their partnered coconstruction can repair the breach in a life story whose rending is the onset of illness and whose mending is the aim of therapy. Finally, the skein of recognition, commitment, and directedness toward the other that can relieve suffering and permit healing is spun by language and knotted by words [31].

References

1. Broyard A. Intoxicated by my illness: and other writings on life and death. New York: C. Potter; 1992.
2. Boudreau JD, Jagosh J, Slee R, Macdonald ME, Steinert Y. Patients' perspectives on physicians' roles: implications for curricular reform. Acad Med. 2008;83:744–53.
3. Parker-Pope T. Doctors and patients, on stage. New York Times [Internet]. 16 Oct 2008; JG Scott, Comment 10. http://well.blogs.nytimes.com/2008/10/16/doctors-and-patients-on-stage/?scp=13&sq=October+16%2C+2008+health&st=nyt.
4. Scott JG, Cohen D, Dicicco-Bloom B, Miller WL, Stange KC, Crabtree BF. Understanding healing relationships in primary care. Ann Fam Med. 2008;6:315–22.
5. Heritage J, Robinson J, Elliott M, Beckett M, Wilkes M. Reducing patients unmet concerns in primary care: the difference one word can make. J Gen Intern Med. 2007;22:1429–33.
6. Kaptchuk TJ, Kelley JM, Conboy LA, et al. Components of placebo effect: randomised controlled trial in patients with irritable bowel syndrome. BMJ. 2008;336:999–1003.
7. Benedetti F, Maggi G, Lopiano L, et al. Open versus hidden medical treatments: the patient's knowledge about a therapy affects the therapy outcome. Prev Treat [Internet]. 23 Jun 2003. http://psycnet.apa.org/journals/pre/6/1/1a.pdf.
8. Brody H. The doctor as therapeutic agent: a placebo effect research agenda. In: Harrington A, editor. The placebo effect. Cambridge: Harvard University Press; 1997. p. 77.
9. Gracely RH, Dubner R, Deeter WR, Wolskee PS. Clinician's expectations influence placebo analgesia. Lancet. 1985;1(8419):43.
10. Lang EV, Hatsiopoulou O, Koch T, et al. Can words hurt? Patient-provider interactions during invasive procedures. Pain. 2005;114:303–9.
11. Zajonc RB. Feeling and thinking: references need no inferences. Am Psychol. 1980;35:151–75.
12. Romer AL. Healing and curing: a psychological exploration of patient-doctor relationships through the experiences of third-year medical students [Ed. D. thesis]. Denver, CO: Harvard Graduate School of Education; 1994.
13. Cassell E. Talking with patients. Vol 1, the theory of doctor-patient communication. Cambridge: MIT Press; 1985.
14. McDaniel SH, Beckman HB, Morse DS, Silberman J, Seaburn DB, Epstein RM. Physician self-disclosure in primary care visits: enough about you, what about me? Arch Intern Med. 2007;167:1321–6.
15. Kolata G. Study says chatty doctors forget patients. New York Times [Internet]. 26 Jun 2007. http://www.nytimes.com/2007/06/26/health/26doctors.html?scp=10&sq=June%2026,%20 2007&st=cse.
16. Leland J. In 'sweetie' and 'dear,' a hurt for the elderly. New York Times [Internet]. 6 Oct 2008. http://www.nytimes.com/2008/10/07/us/07aging.html?_r=1.

17. Cunningham J, Williams KN. A case study of resistiveness to care and elderspeak. Res Theory Nurs Pract. 2007;21(1):45–56.
18. Williams KN, Herman R, Gajewski B, Wilson K. Elderspeak communication: impact on dementia care. Am J Alzheimers Dis Other Demen. 2009;24(1):11–20.
19. Levy BR, Slade MD, Kunkel SR, Kasl SV. Longevity increased by positive self-perceptions of aging. J Pers Soc Psychol. 2002;83(2):261–70.
20. Levy BR, Zonderman AB, Slade MD, Ferrucci L. Age stereotypes held earlier in life predict cardiovascular events in later life. Psychol Sci. 2009;20:296–8.
21. Rosenberg CE. Our present complaint: American medicine, then and now. Baltimore: Johns Hopkins University Press; 2007.
22. Levenstein JH, McCracken EF, McWhinney IR, Stewart MA, Brown JB. The patient-centred clinical method. Fam Pract. 1986;3(1):24–30.
23. Parker-Pope T. WELL; doctor and patient, now at odds. New York Times [Internet]. 29 Jul 2008. http://query.nytimes.com/gst/fullpage.html?res=9B07E5D8133AF93AA15754C0A96 E9C8B63&scp=83&sq=PAULINE+CHEN&st=nyt.
24. Fuks A. The military metaphors of modern medicine. In: Li Z, Long TL, editors. The meaning management challenge. Volume 124 of the Probing the boundaries series, health, illness and disease [eBook]. Oxford: Inter-Disciplinary Press; 2010. p. 57–68. http://www.inter-disciplinary. net/publishing/id-press/ebooks/the-meaning-management-challenge/.
25. Hafferty FW, Franks R. The hidden curriculum, ethics teaching, and the structure of medical education. Acad Med. 1994;69:861–71.
26. Reisfield GM, Wilson GR. Use of metaphor in the discourse on cancer. J Clin Oncol. 2004;22:4024–7.
27. Hoffman J. When thumbs up is no comfort. New York Times [Internet]. 1 Jun 2008. http://query.nytimes.com/gst/fullpage.html?res=9A07E5DF123CF932A35755C0A96E9C8B63&sc p=3&sq=June+1%2C+2008+chemotherapy&st=nyt.
28. Sontag S. AIDS and its metaphors. New York: Farrar, Straus, Giroux; 1989.
29. Engel KG, Heisler M, Smith DM, Robinson CH, Forman JH, Ubel PA. Patient comprehension of emergency department care and instructions: are patients aware of when they do not understand? Ann Emerg Med. 2009;53:454–61.
30. Judt T. Words. New York Review of Books. 15 Jul 2010. Vol. LVII, No. 12. p. 4.
31. Morgan ML. Discovering Levinas. New York: Cambridge University Press; 2007.

Chapter 9
Death Anxiety: The Challenge and the Promise of Whole Person Care

Sheldon Solomon and Krista Lawlor

> *Happy the hare at morning, for she cannot read*
> *The hunter's waking thoughts, lucky the leaf*
> *Unable to predict the fall, lucky indeed*
> *The rampant suffering suffocating jelly*
> *Burgeoning in pools, lapping the grits of the desert.*
> *But what shall man do, who can whistle tunes by heart,*
> *Knows to the bar when death shall cut him short like the cry of the shearwater,*
> *What can he do but defend himself from his knowledge?*
>
> W.H. Auden, The Cultural Presupposition
>
> *There is only one liberty, to come to terms with death. After which, everything is possible.*
>
> Albert Camus, Notebooks

Keywords Death anxiety • Terror management • Mortality salience • Defenses (proximal and distal) • Medical culture

In *The Denial of Death* [1], cultural anthropologist Ernest Becker proposed that while humans share with all forms of life a basic biological predisposition toward self-preservation in the service of survival and reproduction, we are exceptional in our capacity for symbolic thought, which enables us to ponder the past, plan for the future, and transform the products of our imagination into concrete reality. We are also aware of our existence, which according to the Danish philosopher Søren Kierkegaard gives rise to two uniquely human emotions, awe and dread. It is awesome to be alive and to know it, to recognize that we are each descended from the first form of life, and are thus related (albeit distantly) to everything that has ever been alive, is currently alive, or will be alive in the future, and be sublimely appreciative

S. Solomon (✉)
Department of Psychology, Skidmore College, 815 N. Broadway,
Saratoga Springs, NY 12866, USA
e-mail: ssolomon@skidmore.edu

T.A. Hutchinson (ed.), *Whole Person Care: A New Paradigm for the 21st Century*,
DOI 10.1007/978-1-4419-9440-0_9, © Springer Science+Business Media, LLC 2011

of the chance to carry the baton for a lap in the relay race of life! Yet, it is dreadful to be alive and to know it, to recognize that we are, like all living things, of finite duration, that our death can occur at any time for reasons that cannot be anticipated or controlled, and that we are, from a purely biological perspective, no more noteworthy or enduring than worms or walnuts.

According to Becker and like-minded thinkers (e.g., Sigmund Freud, Otto Rank, Norman O. Brown, Robert Jay Lifton, Irvin Yalom), the unvarnished awareness of death and tragedy gives rise to potentially debilitating dread that our ancestors very ingeniously, though quite unconsciously, mitigated through the creation of culture: humanly constructed beliefs about reality that reduces death anxiety by affording opportunities for individuals to perceive themselves as valuable members of a meaningful universe. Specifically, all cultures elucidate the origin of the universe, prescribe appropriate behavior, and offer literal (e.g., heaven or reincarnation) or symbolic (e.g., by having children, amassing vast fortunes, noteworthy achievements, being part of a great nation) immortality. People, thus, manage existential terror by believing that life is meaningful, and from self-esteem obtained by meeting or exceeding cultural values [2].

A considerable body of empirical research provides convergent support for Becker's assertion that cultural beliefs and self-esteem serve a terror management function [4]. Specifically, momentarily elevated or dispositionally high self-esteem reduced self-reported anxiety in response to graphic depictions of death, and physiological arousal in response to threat of electrical shock. Additionally, inducing mortality salience (MS) by having people think about themselves dying (or completing a death anxiety scale, being interviewed in front of a cemetery or funeral parlor, or subliminal exposure to the word "death") increased efforts to defend cherished cultural beliefs and bolster self-esteem. In one study for example, Christian students reminded of their mortality had more favorable reactions to Christian students and less favorable reactions to Jewish students. In other studies, German participants sat closer to a German and further away from a Turk after MS, and Americans were more physically aggressive against someone who did not share their political beliefs after MS. Death reminders also intensify self-esteem striving. People who derive self-esteem from their physical appearance rated their bodies as more integral to their self-concepts in response to MS [5].

Subsequent research has established that conscious and unconscious death thoughts instigate different psychological defenses [6]. *Proximal defenses* serve to remove death thoughts from conscious awareness, either by suppressing them, often assisted by various distractions, or by pushing the problem of death into the future through psychological contortions to deny one's vulnerability. People asked to stick their hands in a bucket of ice water for as long as they could kept them immersed a lot longer if they were told that high tolerance for cold is associated with longevity. Others told that low tolerance for cold is associated with longevity took a much shorter dip. Proximal defenses are "rational" in the sense that they entail seemingly logical analyses to support the belief that death is not imminent.

In contrast, unconscious thoughts of death instigate *distal defenses,*[1] which have no logical or semantic relation to the problem of death. Derogating others who repudiate cultural values or boosting self-esteem has little or no direct bearing on the brute fact that one will someday die. Nevertheless, such reactions diminish mortal terror by enabling people to view themselves as valuable members of a meaningful universe and thus eligible for literal or symbolic immortality.

Most people are, thus, shielded from existential terror by proximal defenses to eradicate conscious death thoughts and deriving a sense of meaning and value from their culture to keep unconscious death thoughts from becoming conscious. Others, however, by virtue of their genetic predisposition, neuroanatomical or biochemical anomalies, and stressful life experiences, cannot successfully deploy these means to quell death anxiety. Although the resultant psychological disorders come in many forms and stem from multiple causes, Irvin Yalom (in *Existential Psychotherapy*, p. 110–111) [7] argues that death anxiety often plays a role:

> All individuals are confronted with death anxiety; most develop adaptive coping modes – modes that consist of denial-based strategies such as suppression, repression, displacement, belief in personal omnipotence, acceptance of socially sanctioned religious beliefs that "detoxify" death, or personal efforts to overcome death through a wide variety of strategies that aim at achieving symbolic immortality. Either because of extraordinary stress or because of an inadequacy of available defensive strategies, the individual who enters the realm called "patienthood" has found insufficient the universal modes of dealing with death fear and has been driven to extreme modes of defense. These defensive maneuvers, often clumsy modes of dealing with terror, constitute the presenting clinical picture.

In accordance with this view, in response to MS, spider phobics found spiders more threatening and avoided them more assiduously; compulsive hand washers used more soap and water to remove electrode cream from their fingers, and people high in social anxiety spent less time with others [8]. Additionally, MS increased psychological dissociation and anxiety sensitivity (i.e., being anxious about becoming anxious), which are precursors of post-traumatic stress disorder (PTSD) and anxiety disorders, respectively [9].

Death anxiety also affects a host of health-related behaviors. Although people sometimes "do the right thing" to keep themselves alive and well, such as avoiding large trees in a hurricane or getting flu vaccines, they also often undermine their health through risky activities such as smoking and unsafe sex. To better understand why this is the case, Jamie Goldenberg and Jamie Arndt [10] proposed that people are primarily motivated to mitigate existential terror rather than take care of themselves per se. Conscious and unconscious death thoughts may consequently engender different health-related attitudes and behaviors. Proximal and distal reactions can improve physical well-being, but they can also kill you.

---

[1] The terms *proximal* and *distal* have a variety of connotations in psychological discourse, but here we are using them in the vernacular sense of the psychological distance (proximal = near; distal = far) from consciousness.

Some proximal defenses foster health. Worried about succumbing to athero-sclerosis? Eat a carrot stick instead of that fried cheese stick. It gets death off your mind and clumps of fat off the walls of your arteries. Immediately after MS,[2] when death thoughts are presumably still conscious, people planned to exercise more and buy more potent sunblock for the beach [11, 12]. Similarly, immediately after MS, smokers intended to cut back on cigarettes [13]. Other proximal defenses can, however, have pernicious consequences. "That fried cheese chick would be bad for me if I was fat, but luckily I'm just big-boned, so I'll have a dozen." This kind of "not-me" tactic gets death thoughts out of mind but undermines prospects for doing anything to promote physical well-being. Diminished self-awareness also helps purge death thoughts from consciousness, and overeating, excessive drinking, cigarette smoking, and long stints in front of the television all reduce self-awareness. Nothing like a gigantic pizza washed down with a case of Molson's topped off by a pack of Marlboro's in the midst of a Law and Order marathon to stifle self-consciousness. That such maneuvers serve as proximal defenses has been established experimentally. Right after MS, cigarette smokers increased the amount of nicotine they inhaled when they smoked [13].

What happens to health-related attitudes and behaviors when unconscious death thoughts provoke distal defenses to shore up self-esteem and uphold cultural beliefs? Recall that immediately after MS, people intended to exercise more, buy more potent sunscreen before hitting the beach, and cut down on smoking – as proximal reactions to remove death thoughts from consciousness. But a very different picture emerges a few minutes after a death reminder, when mortal matters are no longer conscious. Now, only people who based their self-esteem on being fit reported increased intentions of exercising, but those whose self-esteem was derived from other sources did not. And although just about everyone intended to buy more powerful sunscreen immediately after MS, a few minutes later, people who based their self-esteem on being tan opted for a *less* powerful sunscreen and expressed *greater* interest in going to a tanning salon. Similarly, a few minutes after MS, people who based their self-esteem on their driving prowess drove more rapidly and recklessly on a realistic car simulator. A few minutes after MS, males were more eager to engage in unprotected sex, and they yearned for more sexual partners in the future.

Affirming important cultural values as a distal response to unconscious death thoughts can also have striking effects on health-related decisions. People who

---

[2]In all of the studies described to this point, there were a few minutes between reminding people of their mortality and asking them to evaluate others or rate their self-esteem (i.e., distal defenses). Research (summarized in [6]) has shown that conscious death thoughts are actively suppressed during this time, and distal defenses are not instigated until death thoughts are unconscious (and highly accessible). Consequently, measures obtained immediately after a mortality salience (MS) induction reflect proximal defenses in response to conscious death thoughts, while measures obtained a few minutes later (or in some studies, in response to subliminal death reminders) reflect distal defenses in response to unconscious death thoughts.

believe in the power of modern medicine, that getting regular physical exams and seeing the doctor immediately when anything appears amiss is the best way to stay healthy, should embrace such views more ardently and behave in accordance with them in response to unconscious death thoughts. But what about people who rely more on religious faith than modern medicine when they are ill? For example, some Christian fundamentalists believe that all physical maladies result from fear, ignorance, or sin, and only God has the power to cure them. Consequently, believers are urged to refuse medical treatment for themselves and their families, resulting in fatalities from conditions that, when treated, have survival rates of over 90%. Such religious-based medical noncompliance is amplified in response to unconscious death thoughts. A few minutes after MS, Christian fundamentalists in USA increased their support for prayer as a substitute for medical treatment, rated prayer as more effective then medical treatment, were more supportive of religiously motivated refusals of medical treatment, rated themselves as more willing to rely on faith alone for recovering from a physical ailment, and were more confident of the power of divine intervention to cure medical problems [14].

Unconscious death thoughts can also, ironically, be provoked by our bodies. Humans are occasionally uncomfortable with their bodies because being ensconced in a fleshy carcass that eats and excretes and breeds and bleeds and breaks is a constant reminder that we are finite animals. This fact is often most salient in the course of medical treatment. For men, there is "turn your head and cough" as an unwelcome prelude to the "bend over, this won't hurt much" prostate exam. Women are poked, prodded, and smeared in the "stirrups" at their annual physicals. Such glaring reminders that we are pretty much "talking sausages" can generate substantial health risks. Reminded of this fact by reading an essay including the statement "… our bodies work in pretty much the same way as the bodies of all other animals. Whether you're talking about lizards, cows, horses, insects, or humans, we're all made up of the same basic biological products," female college students were less inclined to conduct breast self-examinations in the future. In another experiment, a reminder of people's similarity to animals reduced the amount of time women spent conducting an exam on a breast model [15].

Hopefully, recognizing that conscious and unconscious death thoughts can produce very different health-related outcomes will enable medical practitioners to develop more effective strategies to promote physical well-being. In situations where conscious death thoughts are likely to be aroused, fostering healthy proximal reactions is the best way to go. A heavy-handed graphic depiction of AIDS as a pernicious and fatal disease should increase people's willingness to be tested for AIDS, but only if opportunities to do so are provided while death thoughts are still conscious. Waiting until death thoughts are unconscious to offer AIDS tests could be ineffective or counterproductive, in that people would then be more motivated to shore up their self-esteem and faith in the culture. People who derive self-esteem from their sexual prowess might consequently have unprotected sex with multiple partners as a distal reaction to unconscious death thoughts.

In situations where death thoughts are unconscious, changes in social values should be reflected in people's health decisions in efforts to meet cultural standards.

A few minutes after MS, South Florida beach patrons who read a fashion article with the statement "Bronze is beautiful" favored a less potent sunscreen and estimated they had spent more time in the sun (like the study described earlier). However, other beachgoers who read an article with the statement "Pale is pretty" favored a more potent sunscreen and estimated they had spent less time in the sun a few minutes after MS [16].

Death Anxiety and the Caregiver

> Dr. M, an experienced palliative care physician, found herself planning for another intervention to prolong the life of a young woman actively dying of advanced breast cancer. The patient's family desperately wanted "everything possible" be done to have more time with her although the patient herself had recently expressed her wish to "let go". Dr. M. was aware of the growing distress of the patient and her family, as well as that of the palliative care nurses who were feeling increasingly uncomfortable with the interventions undertaken each day in an effort to prolong the patient's life, often at the expense of her comfort. She was also increasingly aware of her own distress at having come to see death as the enemy.

Does death anxiety influence medical practice and treatment outcomes, given that medical settings are saturated with subtle and blatant intimations of mortality? Although there is currently a paucity of relevant research,[3] existing evidence suggests that death anxiety does indeed influence healthcare providers and patients in medical settings. For example, a few minutes after a MS or control induction, American medical students[4] inspected emergency room admittance forms for either a Muslim or Christian patient complaining of chest pain, and subsequently estimated the risk for coronary artery disease and myocardial infarction. Although risk estimates did not differ as a function of the religion of the patient in the control condition (as it should be given that the presenting symptoms were identical), after MS, medical students reported higher cardiac risk estimates for a Christian patient (which could result in unnecessary medical treatment) and lower risk estimates for

---

[3] There are dozens of studies examining the relationship between death anxiety and a host of medical outcomes (e.g., death anxiety and choice of medical specialty; death anxiety and stress in various hospital settings). This work, while interesting and important, is generally uninformative for present purposes for two reasons. First, correlational studies do not allow inferences of causality; e.g., perhaps death anxiety leads to stress in emergency rooms or intensive care units, but it is also possible that emergency room or ICU stress leads to death anxiety. Second, self reports of death anxiety conflate (and possibly confound) conscious and unconscious death anxiety. So for example, Greenberg et al. [3] found that people who reported the lowest levels of death anxiety actually responded most vigorously in defense of their cultural worldviews following a mortality salience induction, suggesting that (in this case at least) low conscious death anxiety was a defensive manifestation of high unconscious death anxiety.

[4] There were no Muslim participants in this experiment.

a Muslim patient (which could result in a lack of necessary medical treatment) [17]. This suggests that healthcare providers use their cultural identification to manage their own unconscious death anxiety.

In another study, fourth year American medical students read the following case after a MS or control induction:

> You are a family practitioner who is taking care of a 65-year old man who has severe lung disease. You have known him for about 15 years. His lung disease has gotten progressively worse. Over the last 18 months he has been hospitalized three times. Each time he is hospitalized he has required mechanical respiratory support (a respirator). Each time he improves enough to go home. At home, however, he must be on 24 hours a day oxygen therapy. He can't leave the house without his oxygen; he can do nothing without his oxygen. He has made it clear to you (with an Advanced Directive) that he doesn't want any aggressive therapy that would not result in curing him or reversing all the things he doesn't like about the way his life currently is. He deteriorated further. His family panicked and concerned, take him to the emergency room. You meet him and the family at the emergency room. You are now confronted with the concerns of the family, the wishes of the patient and the resources of the emergency department. The patient appears to you to be coherent and understands the situation. He reiterates his treatment philosophy.

Everyone was then asked how much they supported trying to convince the patient that this was a minor setback and to accept therapy even it included a respirator. The medical students (especially those high in neuroticism) reminded of their mortality were more supportive of aggressive treatment despite it being against the patient's wishes. This suggests that healthcare providers may strive to keep their patients alive to assuage their own death fears. Consistent with this notion, in another group of medical students in the same cohort who participated in this study after a 4-day rotation in palliative care[5] where they worked with hospice professionals to come to terms with their own mortality, MS no longer increased support for aggressive treatment [18].

Healthcare providers are, thus, surrounded by reminders of death, and this influences their medical decision making. What about terminally ill patients, for whom death is imminent?

> Mr. H. was a 44 year old avid cook and wine connoisseur who was the obvious axis around which a large and loving group of friends and family revolved. He was admitted to the palliative care unit with pain and shortness of breath caused by his advancing lymphoma. On admission he stated that he would want to be euthanized as death approached, in order to avoid the suffering he felt would otherwise be inescapable. With time, good symptom control, skilled support and an environment that was able to contain and explore his distress as well as his family's, he began to write his first short story, and explore his experience of illness and approaching death, with the treating team and with his loved ones. With candor and courage as he discussed living fully in the awareness of his approaching death, he said "this dying business is hard work, but I can't imagine doing this any other way…this time has been a gift."

In Chap. 1, we learned about palliative care physicians Balfour Mount's and Michael Kearney's observation that "The improvement they often saw in dying

---

[5]The first group of medical students participated in the study just before the palliative care rotation.

patients' quality of life did not appear to depend on control of disease, improvement in function, or even control of symptoms." Given that people manage the existential terror engendered by the awareness of death by confident subscription to world-views that provide a sense that life is meaningful and that they are valuable members of their culture, dying patients' quality of life should vary as a function of their ability to sustain (or augment) a sense of meaning and value in the wake of their impending demise. It does. In one study of religious patients with end-stage congestive heart failure (CHF), depression was associated with death concerns that undermined their faith. The researchers concluded that "religious struggle is a breakdown in the terror management system that leaves the individual vulnerable to the terror of death, and that properly functioning religious worldviews offer comfort by buffering the individual against death concerns" [19]. Other studies of cancer survivors find that efforts to derive meaning from their experiences are associated with declines in depressive symptoms and cancer-related distress, and increases in self reports of physical and psychological vitality [20, 21].

Death Anxiety: How Can We Respond?

How does death anxiety affect our attitudes and behavior as healthcare profes-sionals? How does it affect how we perceive and treat patients and their loved ones? And how we perceive our own mortality and live our lives? These questions are vital to our understanding of the care we provide and the potential for healing or wounding in the relationships we develop with those for whom we provide that care.

We suggest that unexamined and unexplored death anxiety affects our profes-sional and personal lives in the following ways:

1. Unexamined death anxiety may increase the likelihood that healthcare profes-sionals adhere unquestioningly to the medical culture in which they have been trained and practice. The predominant Western medical culture remains one that elevates curing/fixing/"doing to" over healing/bearing witness/"being with." In this culture, our unconscious death anxiety may well lead us to prescribe yet one more round of antibiotics in an attempt to stave off death when what may be needed is an acknowledgement that death is imminent, inevitable, and perhaps timely.
2. Unexamined death anxiety promotes dualistic thinking and may increase the likelihood that healthcare professionals begin to see patients (and their families) as "other" in the same way that the students mentioned previously [5] sat further away from someone of a different culture after being reminded of their mortality. How much simpler and less terrifying to reduce the patient to their risk factors, disease, or pathology, rather than to acknowledge their humanity and similarity to ourselves (and thereby acknowledge our own vulnerability and mortality). How difficult to remain fully present, to resist the urge to flee, physically, emo-tionally, and psychologically, in the face of deep suffering and fear...the patient's and our own.

If one accepts the implications of death anxiety and its effects on our behavior and actions, does that condemn us to a life of largely unconscious death denial and terror management? A colleague reported the following experience:

> Soon after beginning work in Palliative Care when interacting with dying patients he noticed an inclination to avoid or skate away from the topic of death. However, when he decided not to go with this avoidance but was willing to discuss whatever fears or concerns the patient had about dying now or in the future, a strange phenomenon occurred. Time seemed to slow down, and he felt completely present without concerns for the past or future. His compassion, even for those for whom he normally had little time appeared to enlarge rather than to narrow - the opposite to what might be expected.

And there is precedence for this experience [22]. We have the impression that frequent opportunities to confront mortality are the primary reason why palliative care is both so difficult and so rewarding an experience. This is not to question the validity of the research showing that our proximal and distal defenses to death anxiety are pervasive, powerful, and probably universal. We need to stay aware of these inbuilt reactions to prevent our care being affected and possibly controlled by them. However, as with all natural unconscious reactions, a different learned response may also be possible. One possible way of describing our colleague's experience is that he became mindful. Meditation on death plays a very prominent role in Buddhist meditation [23]. Balfour Mount would say that this is part of the process of healing [24]. Our colleague noticed the same phenomenon in the patients that he treated. Those patients willing to face the reality of their own death appeared to have a different (healing) trajectory.

Death anxiety: The Challenge and the Promise of Whole Person Care

The uniquely human awareness of death gives rise to potentially paralyzing dread that is assuaged by perceiving oneself to be a valuable member of meaningful universe. Intimations of mortality stimulate efforts to remove thoughts of death from awareness, and nonconscious death thoughts instigate efforts to shore up self-esteem and reaffirm faith in cherished cultural values. Existing evidence (more is sorely needed) suggests that existential concerns affect patient outcomes as well as medical practitioner's diagnostic and treatment decisions.

We believe these ideas accentuate the challenge and the promise of whole person care in the twenty-first century. In addition to mastering an enormous body of (rapidly burgeoning) information and acquiring and maintaining a host of sophisticated clinical skills, healthcare professionals devoted to the whole person care paradigm must also consider how illnesses (especially unexpected, severe, and terminal) threaten to puncture the delicate fabric of meaning necessary for constructive and satisfying human activity. This is a challenge for both healthcare professionals and patients. There is also another challenge for health professionals themselves. They need to recognize how their own nonconscious death fears, combined with the abundant reminders of death that are typical of medical practice, especially in highly technologically focused academic/tertiary care hospital settings, influence how they diagnose and treat their patients. Healthcare providers are socialized into and eventually immersed in a "medical culture" that predisposes them to "do more" – more investigations, more interventions, more technology. This is often good medicine. However, sometimes healthcare professionals grappling (largely unconsciously) with their own death anxiety, and responding (largely unconsciously) to the suffering they see around them, are driven to "fix" the often unfixable, to "do more" in the face of their own anguished powerlessness. This is bad medicine. Recognizing when death fears may turn good medicine bad is a challenge.

There is also a promise for both patients and healthcare practitioners. Part of this is the ability to recognize when we are being driven by our own unconscious death anxiety and being free to make other choices. Perhaps as a patient we do need to use stronger sunblock even if our self-esteem is bolstered by a tan, or as physicians we do not need to do that extra procedure because we realize we are treating our own death anxiety and not the patient. As healthcare providers, there is also the humility and self-compassion that comes with becoming aware that we, like our patients, are easily and unconsciously driven by our own fear of death. And there is a deeper level to the promise: the expansion of awareness and compassion that comes with being willing to stand in the face of death and overwhelming threat. Since antiquity, wisdom traditions from diverse parts of the world have found that a genuine confrontation with one's mortality yields a greater appreciation for life, the capacity to be fully involved in the moment rather than constantly preoccupied with the past or obsessed with the future, and dignified efforts to improve the human condition. In this sense, whole person care in the twenty-first century involves some very old wine in a very new bottle. Part of the challenge will be to provide the right contexts outside palliative medicine in which healthcare workers can learn to experience this transforming response to death and overwhelming vulnerability. But we believe the effort will be worth it. Because it is a fine wine: "...come to terms with death. After which, everything is possible."

References

1. Becker E. The denial of death. New York: The Free Press; 1973.
2. Solomon S, Greenberg J, Pyszczynski T. A terror management theory of social behavior: the psychological functions of self-esteem and cultural worldviews. In: Zanna M, editor. Advances in experimental social psychology, vol. 24. Orlando: Academic Press; 1991. p. 93–159.
3. Greenberg J, Simon L, Harmon-Jones E, Solomon S, Pyszczynski T, & Lyon D. Testing alternative explanations for mortality salience effects: Terror management, value accessibility, or worrisome thoughts? Eur J Soc Psychol. (1995);25(4):417–33. doi: 10.1002/ejsp.2420250406.
4. Greenberg J, Solomon S, Arndt J. A basic but uniquely human motivation: terror management. In: Shah JY, Gardner WL, editors. Handbook of motivation science. New York: Guilford; 2008.

5. Goldenberg J, McCoy S, Pyszczynski T, Greenberg J, Solomon S. The body as a source of self-esteem: the effect of mortality salience on identification with one's body, interest in sex, and appearance monitoring. J Pers Soc Psychol. 2000;79(1):118–30.
6. Pyszczynski T, Greenberg J, Solomon S. A dual-process model of defense against conscious and unconscious death-related thoughts: an extension of terror management theory. Psychol Rev. 1999;106(4):835–45.
7. Yalom ID. Existential psychotherapy. New York: Basic Books; 1980.
8. Strachan E, Schimel J, Arndt J, et al. Terror mismanagement: evidence that mortality salience exacerbates phobic and compulsive behaviors. Pers Soc Psychol Bull. 2007;33(8):1137–51.
9. Kosloff S, Solomon S, Greenberg J, et al. Fatal distraction: the impact of mortality salience on dissociative responses to 9/11 and subsequent anxiety sensitivity. Basic Appl Soc Psychol. 2006;28(4):349–56.
10. Goldenberg J, Arndt J. The implications of death for health: a terror management health model for behavioral health promotion. Psychol Rev [serial online]. 2008;115(4):1032–53.
11. Arndt J, Schimel J, Goldenberg JL. Death can be good for your health: fitness intentions as a proximal and distal defense against mortality salience. J Appl Soc Psychol. 2003;33:1726–46.
12. Routledge C, Arndt J, Goldenberg JL. A time to tan: proximal and distal effects of mortality salience on sun exposure intentions. Pers Soc Psychol Bull. 2004;30:1347–58.
13. Cox CR, Arndt J, Goldenberg JL, Piasecki T. The effect of mortality salience on smoking intensity among habitual and occasional smokers. University of Missouri, Columbia; 2009. Manuscript in preparation.
14. Vess M, Arndt J, Cox C, Routledge C, Goldenberg J. Exploring the existential function of religion: the effect of religious fundamentalism and mortality salience on faith-based medical refusals. J Pers Soc Psychol [serial online]. 2009;97(2):334–50.
15. Goldenberg J, Arndt J, Hart J, Routledge C. Uncovering an existential barrier to breast self-exam behavior. J Exp Soc Psychol [serial online]. 2008;44(2):260–74.
16. Cox C, Cooper D, Vess M, Arndt J, Goldenberg J, Routledge C. Bronze is beautiful but pale can be pretty: the effects of appearance standards and mortality salience on sun-tanning outcomes. Health Psychol. 2009;28(6):746–52.
17. Arndt J, Vess M, Cox C, Goldenberg J, Lagle S. The psychosocial effect of thoughts of personal mortality on cardiac risk assessment. Med Decis Making. 2009;29(2):175–81.
18. Solomon S. The effects of mortality salience and neuroticism on medical students' treatment preferences for patients with terminal illnesses. Unpublished pilot data. Skidmore College; 1999.
19. Edmondson D, Park C, Chaudoir S, Wortmann J. Death without God: religious struggle, death concerns, and depression in the terminally ill. Psychol Sci. 2008;19(8):754–8.
20. Park C, Edmondson D, Fenster J, Blank T. Meaning making and psychological adjustment following cancer: the mediating roles of growth, life meaning, and restored just-world beliefs. J Consult Clin Psychol. 2008;76(5):863–75.
21. Yanez B, Edmondson D, Stanton A, Park C, Kwan L, Ganz P, et al. Facets of spirituality as predictors of adjustment to cancer: relative contributions of having faith and finding meaning. J Consult Clin Psychol. 2009;77(4):730–41.
22. Kearney M, Weiniger R, Vachon M, Harrison R, Mount B. Self-care of physicians caring for patients at the end of life. JAMA. 2009;301(11):1155–64.
23. Wallis G. Sutta 16, the application of present-moment awareness. In: Basic teachings of the Buddha. New York: The Modern Library; 2007. p. 57–67.
24. Mount BM. The 10 commandments of healing. J Cancer Educ. 2006;21(1):50–1.

Chapter 10
Whole Person Self-Care: Self-Care from the Inside Out

Michael Kearney and Radhule Weininger

Keywords Self-care • Burnout • Compassion fatigue • Empathic engagement • Exquisite empathy • Wounded healer • Soul and role • Clinician self-awareness • Mindfulness meditation

A discussion of self-care normally begins by focusing on topics such as stress, ways of protecting ourselves from the traumas of the workplace, and encouragement to find sources of self-renewal outside of work. We would like to start with a different focus, one that is offered by Tibetan Buddhist teacher Chögyam Trungpa when he writes the following:

> We are in touch with basic health all the time. Although the usual dictionary definition of *health* is, roughly speaking, "free from sickness," we should look at health as something more than that. According to the Buddhist tradition, people inherently possess Buddha-nature; that is, they are basically and intrinsically good. From this point of view, health is intrinsic. That is, health comes first: sickness is secondary. Health *is*. So, being healthy is being fundamentally wholesome, with body and mind synchronized in a state of being which is indestructible and good. This attitude is not recommended exclusively for patients but also for the helpers and doctors. It can be adopted mutually because this intrinsic basic goodness is always present in any interaction of one human being with another [1].

What if self-care is not so much about stress management and damage limitation as about finding ways of remembering and staying connected in the workplace with the wholeness that is already there? And what might self-care look like if it is true, as psychoanalyst Michael Balint puts it, that "we are the medicine" [2]? If, as Balint suggests, we are the most powerful medicine we will ever give our patients, then who we are as persons matters as much as how knowledgeable and skilled we are as professionals. The quality of our lives affects the quality of our patients' lives. As clinicians, therefore, the question "what is the quality of my life?" has both personal and professional consequences. At a personal level, it speaks to the

M. Kearney (✉)
Santa Barbara Cottage Hospital, Visiting Nurse and Hospice Care,
Santa Barbara, CA 93105, USA
e-mail: mkkearney@cox.net

T.A. Hutchinson (ed.), *Whole Person Care: A New Paradigm for the 21st Century*,
DOI 10.1007/978-1-4419-9440-0_10, © Springer Science+Business Media, LLC 2011

possibilities of being happy, of flourishing, of growing in our work. Professionally, it speaks to our quality of presence and to our resilience and effectiveness as clinicians.

If there is such a thing as "Whole Person Self-Care" what might it look like in clinical practice and in our secular lives? In this chapter, we explore this question by sharing stories, reflections, and ideas. We tell one of our own personal stories as illustrative of the two syndromes of clinician stress, Compassion Fatigue and Burnout, and reflect on this against the backdrop of two universal stories: that of the Wounded Healer and that of the Rainmaker of Kiao-chau. And we present a model of self-care based on clinician self-awareness, which, we suggest, offers a positive, whole person approach to self-care.

The Story Then

In the summer of 1980, having decided that "Hospice Medicine," as it was then called, was what I (MK) wanted to specialize in, I began working at St Christopher's Hospice in London. This gave me the opportunity to work alongside and learn from some of the pioneers of the modern hospice movement, including Dame Cicely Saunders, Professor John Hinton, and Dr Colin Murray Parkes. I felt lucky to be doing something that was congruent with my soul, with who I was, and to have such wonderful teachers and colleagues. While I learnt a lot professionally during my time at St Christopher's, I believe I learnt even more at a personal level. There was one particular event that proved a turning point in this regard.

I had just completed my first 3 months at St Christopher's. I looked forward to coming to work each day and happily gave my patients and their families my all. While there were obvious limits to what I could offer in terms of my clinical and communication skills, I tried to make up for this by being as openhearted as possible. Listening attentively, taking it all in, the pain, the fear, the joy, the tenderness, the regrets, the sadness, and leaving work each day feeling simultaneously depleted and enriched. As I walked those couple of hundred yards between the hospice and the apartment where I was living with my wife and our baby daughter, I felt like I was walking in a silent landscape that had been blasted by a hurricane, flattened by a tsunami. Yet I simultaneously felt centered and, in some curious way, fulfilled.

On this particular morning, I was to attend a family meeting with the husband and children of a young woman with a glioblastoma who was very close to death. Elizabeth, the social worker, the patient's nurse, Alison, and I, were to meet with the patient Julia's husband John, and their three children John, aged 7, Matt, aged 5, and Rosie who was 3.

By then, Julia was very weak, drowsy, and at times confused – evidence, we felt, that death was imminent. When Elizabeth had met previously with John, he had told her that he had spoken to the children about their mum being "very ill" but not that she was dying. He had said that he wanted to protect them as much as possible for as long as possible. Nonetheless, he had gratefully accepted Elizabeth's offer of a family meeting to help him talk to the children about this as he realized it could not wait any longer.

All three children knelt at the low table in the middle of the family meeting room, drawing with waxed crayons on large pieces of white paper. "Why don't you draw your family?" Elizabeth had suggested. Matt began to draw a house with his dad and the children standing by the front door, his mum standing alone and by herself at the extreme left-hand side of the paper. John drew his mum upstairs in bed, his dad and brother and sister down in the kitchen, and himself walking down the stairs. Rosie started drawing a round figure whose arms were wrapped around a tiny little figure on her belly. "That's me and mummy," she said.

Ever so gently, Elizabeth told them that we had asked them to come in today because we wanted to talk with them about their mum. She said she would really like to hear from them about how they thought their mum was doing.

After a short silence, Matt spoke. "I know mummy is dying. I have not wanted to talk about it because I did not want to upset daddy." The others did not look up from their drawing. It seemed that these words came as no surprise to them, or perhaps in Rosie's case that she did not understand what they meant. Turning to me, Elizabeth said, "Perhaps Dr Michael can tell us all just how your mum is doing these days."

I don't remember what words I used. What I do recall is the way the two boys paused as I began to speak and turned to look in my direction, still leaning on the table, crayons in their hands, faces wide-open in expectation. Rosie, meanwhile, continued to draw. I began to speak because I knew I had to, not because I knew what to say. I fumbled to find the kindest words I could to say the impossible.

As I finished speaking, I was aware that John was sobbing quietly. The children had all returned to their drawing. Then, Matt looked up and asked, "Do you mean that mummy will never come home again?" I replied that I was terribly sorry to say that I did not think so. At that, Rosie left her drawing, walked over to her dad and put her arms around him. The boys followed, one at a time.

Meanwhile, I continued to sit, as did my colleagues, witness to this family held in a single embrace of grief. I felt part of it and yet separate. I had wanted so badly to say something that would make the children feel better, yet my words had just inflicted more pain. My heart ached. I felt a failure.

The following day, I came to work in a fog. This sensation lingered through the day and I noticed that I could not easily concentrate. I was aware of a sense of dread in my chest and I became more and more apprehensive. Then, as I sat listening to a colleague talking about a patient, a strong sense of déjà vu wafted from nowhere into my consciousness. It immediately captured my complete attention. I felt panicked, "What was this?" "What did it mean?" "Was I having a nervous breakdown?" In the midst of this whirlwind of images, feelings, and questions, I was suddenly aware that my colleague was still speaking to me, now with a look of concern on her face. I felt disorientated and confused. I could not make sense of what she was talking about. Then, the rumbling sense of dread in my chest swelled to a wave that seemed to crash right through me. I excused myself and left the office bumping into Tom West, the then Medical Director of St Christopher's, who was walking down the corridor. I asked if I could speak with him. He led me to his office.

Tom listened attentively as I described how I was feeling. "You sound exhausted," he said, "You have been here three months now and you have not had a break. You've thrown yourself into the work and you're doing a great job, but I think you may not have learned yet that you also need to take care of yourself. Two suggestions: One that you take this Friday off. Make it a long weekend and go away somewhere nice with your family. Second, I can recommend someone you could meet and talk with from time to time. I have been doing this myself for years and I would not have survived in this work without it."

My head was still reeling, but I felt relieved. I heard Tom saying that he understood what I was talking about and, more importantly to me at that moment, that he did not think I was crazy to be feeling this way.

Early the following week, I met with a counselor, whom I immediately liked. We agreed to meet on a weekly basis for the coming 3 months. Little did I then realize that I was experiencing an acute case of what I would later understand to be "Compassion Fatigue." And little did I realize that I was on the threshold of what PW Martin calls "An Experiment in Depth" [3], that I was unwittingly heeding Jung's advice "to dive, not drown."

Compassion Fatigue

The term "Compassion Fatigue" (CF) is used to describe a syndrome of clinician stress that evolves from *the relationship between the clinician and the patient* [4]. Compassion Fatigue is also known as Secondary Traumatic Stress Disorder, the hypothesis being that clinicians may be vicariously traumatized by their patients' suffering [4]. In the process, a clinician's own unresolved trauma material and unconscious unresolved childhood conflicts may be stimulated [5].

The symptoms of CF include those of Post-Traumatic Stress Disorder (PTSD): hyperarousal, reexperiencing, and avoidance. Chronic CF may lead to burnout, the other and better-known syndrome of clinician stress, which is discussed below, and "symptoms of burnout may be the final common pathway of continual exposure to traumatic material that cannot be assimilated or worked through" [6].

There are several theories for the mechanism of transmission of traumatic stress from one individual to another. Useful information may be gained by focusing on the nature and practice of empathy [7]. Figley has hypothesized that the caregiver's empathy level with the traumatized individual plays a significant role in this transmission [4]. The concept of "Vicarious Traumatization" (VT) is very similar to that of CF and is defined as "the cumulative transformative effects upon therapists resulting from empathic engagement with traumatized clients" [6].

Exquisite Empathy

Recent research calls into question existing assumptions about the presumed causal relationship between caregiver empathy and VT. In a phenomenological study, Harrison and Westwood [8] looked at a group of peer-nominated, exemplary mental health therapists who were thriving in their work with traumatized clients. They identified a variety of protective practices that enhance caregiver's professional satisfaction and help prevent or mitigate VT. Of particular interest to us here, they noted that trauma therapists who engaged in a form of empathic engagement they called *exquisite empathy* were "invigorated rather than depleted by their intimate professional connections with traumatized clients" [8]. Harrison and Westwood define exquisite empathy as "highly present, sensitively attuned, well-boundaried and heartfelt empathic engagement" [8] and note that "moment-by-moment embodied awareness of self and surroundings helps therapists develop the kind of interpersonal presence and clarity crucial to the practice of exquisite empathy" [8].

The Wounded Healer

Judith Lewis Herman summarizes the recovery from trauma as follows: "The core experiences of psychological trauma are disempowerment and disconnection from others. Recovery, therefore, is based upon the empowerment of the individual and the creation of new connections" [9]. For me, the process of recovery from the CF I experienced during my early months at St Christopher's Hospice began with the counseling I started at that time. Within the secure container of that therapeutic relationship, I was committing myself to what I now understand to be a life-long process of self-knowledge and to the realization that my true power as a clinician is found, paradoxically, in an acceptance of my limits and, at times, my powerlessness in the face of another's suffering.

The image of the wounded healer is ancient and universal, dating back to the shamanic healers of early tribal cultures. A shaman is an individual who has been initiated into an underworld of suffering by a wounding or illness and returned with knowledge and wisdom gleaned from that experience to serve their tribe. In Western culture, the image of the wounded healer is found in the Greek mythological figure of Chiron:

> Chiron was a centaur, half-human and half-horse. Being a demi-god he did not die when he was wounded in the leg by a poisoned arrow. Rather, he lived on with a painful un-healable wound. Day after day, he limped around the slopes of Mount Pelion searching for herbs anything that might ease his pain and cure his wound. While he became knowledge-able in healing plants and herbs he was unable to heal himself. He was, however, able to heal others. Those suffering all manner of ailments came to him from far and wide. Each received a remedy that helped. Furthermore, Chiron's understanding and compassion touched something within them. As they walked away they knew that a deeper healing had also taken place.

"Know Thyself!" – The Dynamics of the Wounded Healer Relationship

The psychodynamics of the wounded healer have important implications for clinician self-care. They give an insight into the power dynamics of the therapeutic relationship and contrast two kinds of clinical encounter, one that is a liability to the clinician and another that is potentially protective and restorative.

In his book, "Power in the Helping Professions," depth psychologist Adolf Guggenbühl Craig [10] describes the archetype of the wounded healer as a universal, unconscious psychological structure, which is "dyadic," meaning that it encompasses both a wounded part and a healer part. As an archetype, it exists in what depth psychologist Carl G. Jung calls the "Collective Unconscious" of all, clinicians and patients alike, where it remains in a latent state until it is activated by specific external circumstances.

Since clinicians are expected to be problem solvers, they tend to exclusively identify with the "healer" part of the wounded healer archetype, repressing the "wounded" part in their unconscious. With patients, on the contrary, the opposite is the case. They tend to identify exclusively with the "wounded" part of the archetype and repress the "healer" part. A therapeutic relationship based on this dynamic is one that holds the clinician as the sole active therapeutic agent and the patient as the passive recipient of treatment. While a therapeutic alliance based on this premise can and often does have a successful outcome, it also has significant implications for clinician self-care. In such a relationship, empathy is flowing in one direction only, from clinician to patient, while simultaneously the clinician is receptive to information about the patient's problems and associated distress. Within this dynamic, which Guggenbühl Craig [10] calls "the power dynamic," empathy is a potential liability, a one-way street that can lead to vicarious traumatization, CF, and emotional depletion of the clinician. This may be extremely stressful for the clinician and trigger survival reactions of fight, flight or freeze, which may be seen in overtreatment, abandonment, or emotional numbing or disassociation.

According to Guggenbühl Craig [10], there is another possibility, what he calls "the wounded healer dynamic." Here, while the clinician continues to do all that can be done to solve the patients' problems and alleviate their suffering, he or she does so with an awareness that he or she is not omnipotent, that there are limits to what he or she can do. In other words, the clinician begins to allow into consciousness the "wounded" part of the archetype, which up until now has been repressed in the unconscious. The clinician also realizes that patients have within themselves innate capacities to heal physically, psychologically, and spiritually. In other words, the clinician understands that patients also carry within themselves the "healer" part of the wounded healer archetype, and he or she then strives to find a way to awaken this innate potential in the patient.

What this looks like in clinical practice becomes clear by considering some of the insoluble issues a clinician may encounter. Let us consider, as an example, an actively dying patient in profound existential anguish who says to his clinician, "promise me you won't let me die." As the clinician realizes and begins to accept that he or she is "wounded," in the sense that he or she cannot give this patient what he is asking for, the previously repressed wounded part of the archetype comes into consciousness, and a process of psychological integration begins to take place. The clinician may experience this as a mix of emotions, for example, feelings of frustration and failure, as well as feelings of relief and self-compassion.

Further implications of the dynamics of the wounded healer for clinician self-care are understood by considering the impact this process has for the patient. A clinician who chooses to stay empathically present in the therapeutic relationship, despite being unable to solve the patient's problem, encourages the patient to stay with his or her experience of suffering. As the patient does so, he or she may begin to realize that, like it or not, "this is how it is." With this, a subtle yet significant shift may occur in his or her experience. He or she may notice more spaciousness within their suffering, and, possibly, a lessening of its intensity, and articulate this with a phrase such as "the pain is still there, but I can live with it now." What is happening here is that the patient is experiencing the reality of his or her own "inner healer." He or she has also now become a wounded healer. In contrast to the earlier power dynamic, the empathic flow is now moving in both directions, clinician to patient and patient to clinician; and, as each realizes that the other is wounded, and human, both may experience the transformative power of profound human connection.

To live as a wounded healer necessitates a high degree of self-knowledge on the part of the clinician; we need to know ourselves well enough to recognize that we have reached that place of powerlessness, to prevent ourselves reacting impulsively, and to consciously respond in the most appropriate way, including the possibility of calling "time-out," or choosing to remain compassionately present without acting, despite possibly painful feelings of failure or impotence. For the clinician, the rewards of the path of the wounded healer include finding healing and meaning within his or her empathic connection with patients.

The Story a Year Ago

By this time last year, I had been in the field of end-of-life care for 29 years. I was working as a physician with a hospital and community-based palliative care service, and with a community and inpatient hospice program in Santa Barbara, CA. While I was truly grateful to be working with good people in good palliative care and hospice programs, I had become aware that I was no longer happy in my work. I noticed that I was not excited, as I had been in my early days in hospice and palliative care, to go to work each morning. In fact, I was feeling emotionally and physically pretty run down much of the time. I no longer had that inner "hum," that inner "knowing" that was there in the past, and that came from sensing that I was in and doing the right work. Instead, I had a pervasive feeling that I was not doing what I really wanted to do and was doing too much of what I did not want to do anymore. I realized that I was burnt out.

As I reflected on how this might have happened, and talked about it with my clinical supervisor, I came to see that this was probably at least in part due to the 29 years of almost daily exposure to profound human suffering that came from working in end-of-life care; burnout as a result of chronic vicarious traumatization and compassion fatigue, in other words. However, I concluded that this was neither the only nor possibly the main reason. When Harrison and Westwood [8] described exquisite empathy in the way they did, they described something that I was familiar with. I could relate to the protective and renewing power of this way of being with others in their suffering. Indeed, when I did an inventory of those aspects of my work that were most meaningful and replenishing for me, I identified just such occasions of being with another in a mutuality of suffering and healing, wounded healers together.

I concluded that the other significant contributor to these feelings of burnout was a growing mismatch between who I was, or had become, and the role and tasks I was expected, needed to, and was paid to perform in my work every day. Burnout as a result of the slow grinding down that comes from being "a square peg in a round hole," in other words. I knew that long-term sustainability in our work is dependent on there being at least a "good-enough" fit between our calling and our responsibilities. I realized that I needed to pay attention to this and that I would need to make some changes. I asked myself how much of this was about inner, subjective change; if I didn't have much flexibility in *what* I was doing at that time, were there changes in *how* I was doing what I was doing that could make a difference? And how much was it about needing to try to change external, objective circumstances so that what I was doing in my work, whether in my current or some other work setting, would be more aligned with who I was?

Burnout

Burnout (BO) results from stresses that arise *between the clinician and his or her work environment.* The syndrome of BO may present as overwhelming exhaustion – emotional and physical – as feelings of cynicism and detachment from the job, and/ or as a sense of ineffectiveness and lack of personal accomplishment [11, 12]. BO results from frustration, powerlessness, and inability to achieve work goals [13].

Other symptoms of BO may be apparent at an individual or at a team level. For example, an individual may experience poor judgment, overidentification or overinvolvement, boundary violations, perfectionism and rigidity, interpersonal conflicts, addictive behaviors, frequent illnesses that include headaches and gastrointestinal disturbances, and immune system impairment [14]. A team that is experiencing BO may have chronically low morale, poor job retention, impaired job performance, and frequent staff conflict [15].

Maslach et al. [14] suggest that a "mismatch" between the individual and the organization may lead to BO. They identify six areas of worklife, namely, workload, control, reward, community, fairness, and values, and postulate that BO arises when there are chronic mismatches between individuals and their work settings in some or all of these areas. On the contrary, the better the match or fit between the individual and their work environment, the greater will be their job engagement and satisfaction.

The Rainmaker

There is story of a Rainmaker of Kiao-chau that was told to Carl Jung by his friend, Richard Wilhelm. Wilhelm, a Christian minister, Sinologist, and the author who introduced the West to the *I Ching* [16] witnessed this incident during his time in China. Jung was very taken by the story. His students describe how he told them never to teach a seminar without including the story of the rainmaker [17]. Here is Jung's own version of the story [18]:

> There was a great drought where Wilhelm lived; for months, there had not been a drop of rain and the situation became catastrophic. The Catholics made processions, the Protestants made prayers, and the Chinese burned joss sticks and shot off guns to frighten away the demons of the drought, but with no result.
>
> Finally, the Chinese said, "We will fetch the rain-maker." And from another province, a dried-up old man appeared. The only thing he asked for was a quiet little house somewhere, and there he locked himself in for three days.
>
> On the fourth day, the clouds gathered and there was a great snowstorm at the time of the year when no snow was expected, an unusual amount, and the town was so full of rumors about the wonderful rainmaker that Wilhelm went to ask the man how he did it. In true European fashion, he said: "They call you the rain-maker, will you tell me how you made the snow?"
>
> And the little Chinese man said: "I did not make the snow, I am not responsible."
>
> "But what have you done these three days?" Wilhelm asked.
>
> "Oh, I can explain that. I come from another country where things are in order. Here they are out of order, they are not as they should be by the ordinance of heaven. Therefore the whole country is not in Tao, and I also am not in the natural order of things because I am in a disordered country. So I had to wait three days until I was back in Tao and then, naturally, … the rain came."

Becoming Rainmakers

The story of the rainmaker could be read as a story of burnout, in this case, the parched lands, dying animals, and suffering humans in a drought-ridden part of China, which had not seen replenishing rains for some time. It tells of how burnout is a consequence of being "out of Tao," that is, of being disconnected from our deepest selves, which, the story implies are contiguous with the rhythms of the natural world, and how *the primary move* in addressing burnout is to do whatever it is we need to do to "come into Tao," for "then, naturally, the rain comes."

"To be in Tao" brings healing to ourselves and to the other (in this case the drought-ridden land and its peoples). And yet we note that the rainmaker did not "do" this, in the sense of willing and acting to make it happen in a causal way. Rather, the resolution of the drought, the weather's once again coming "into order," was in some mysterious, noncausal way related to the inner work he did, his own coming into Tao, for "healing begets healing begets healing ..." [19]. This story suggests that if we want to achieve healing in our own lives, including the healing of burnout, and if we want to be healers to others, we, like the rainmaker, must first come into balance, into order, "into Tao."

Soul and Role

Educator and author Parker Palmer offers a helpful way of thinking about how we might do this when he speaks of the importance of aligning "soul and role" [20]. Writing of the sense of calling or vocation in our work, Palmer observes, "Vocation does not mean a goal that I pursue. It means a calling that I hear. Before I can tell my life what I want to do with it, I must listen to my life telling me who I am. I must listen for the truths and values at the heart of my own identity, not the standards by which I *must* live – but the standards by which I cannot help but live if I am living my own life" [21].

Palmer suggests that vocation is an expression of soul, which "wants to keep us rooted in the ground of our own being" [20]. The consequences of a disconnection between soul and role is what Palmer calls a "divided life" leading to psychological pain that we "try to numb ... with an anesthetic of choice, be it substance abuse, overwork, consumerism, or mindless media noise" [20]. While a disconnection between the calling of our core or deepest selves and what we do in our work may lead to burnout, a realignment of soul and role may lead to an experience of joy and flourishing. And our personal choice to realign our lives in such a way may have more than purely personal consequences because our individual soul is contiguous with a wider and deeper web of connectedness. As I attend to my soul, I am simultaneously tending *Anima Mundi*, the soul of the world, and my act of personal responsibility becomes one of service. As Palmer puts it, "As we [align soul and role], we will not only find the joy that every human being seeks – we will also find our path to authentic service in the world. True vocation joins self and service, as Frederick Buechner asserts when he defines vocation as "the place where our deep gladness meets the world's deep need" [21, 22].

Healing Connections and Meaning-Based Coping

In a phenomenological study, Mount and his colleagues interviewed 21 patients with life-threatening illness who were experiencing either existential anguish or, conversely, integrity and wholeness, in an attempt to identify "inner life" and existential contributors to suffering and subjective well-being in advanced illness [23]. In their discussion of their findings, they state: "A sense of meaning was evident in those able to find a sense of well-being and wholeness in facing serious illness, while a sense of meaninglessness was common to those experiencing suffering and anguish. Meaning-based coping was associated with a capacity to form bonds of connection, what we came to call healing connections in response to the evident revitalization, sense of security, and equanimity that accompanied them" [23]. Mount et al. [23] identify these healing connections as being in one of four areas: "Connection with self, others, the phenomenal world experienced through the five senses, and with God or ultimate meaning, however conceived by that person," and continue, "The experience of healing connections, in large part, characterized the striking difference between those with 'positive' and 'negative' coping patterns."

The implications of these findings in the prevention and mitigation of both BO and CF are evident. Healing connections bring a sense of meaning, which allows us to not only survive but also thrive in our work. Exquisite empathy offers a roadmap on how this might be possible in even the most challenging of circumstances. As Harrison and Westwood put it, "exquisite empathy … affords clinicians opportunity to ethically benefit from 'healing connections' [23] with clients, without sacrificing clients' needs to their own. In this sense, exquisite empathy may constitute a form of mutual, reciprocal, healing connection, in which clients and clinicians alike benefit from the latter's caring, well-boundaried, ethical attunement to the client" [8].

How each of us establishes healing connections is a highly individual process. The four domains identified by Mount et al. offer us a useful framework to consider some possibilities:

1. *Within the Individual*: Meditation, Reflective writing, Dream work
2. *With Others:* Quality time with significant others, Humor
3. *With the Phenomenal World:* Exercise, Yoga, Massage, Nature, Music
4. *With Ultimate Meaning:* Spiritual and religious practice, Creative expression

Developing Clinician Self-Awareness

We suggest that clinician self-awareness is the key to a whole person approach to self-care. Clinician self-awareness can mitigate CF and BO. Clinician self-awareness can enable us to practice exquisite empathy, to make choices that align soul and role, and to establish healing connections. We identify four overlapping and complementary aspects of clinician self-awareness: self-knowledge, self-empathy, preparing the mind through the practice of mindfulness, and contemplative awareness.

Self-knowledge lays the foundation for clinical awareness. This means becoming familiar with our family history, our cultural, racial, and religious history, as well as our individual strengths and limitations. Having an insight into our background allows us to work through emotional challenges so that these will not get repressed or projected onto others. This allows us to recognize "Transference" (the unconscious redirection of feelings from one person to another, for example, from patient to clinician) and "Countertransference" (the clinician's unconscious projection onto the patient and/or his or her reaction to the patient) [24], enabling the clinician to engage in the therapeutic encounter with more awareness and less reactivity. Some possible ways for the clinician to increase self-knowledge include counseling or psychotherapy, peer-group or individual clinical supervision, and reflective writing.

Self-empathy is an essential complement to self-knowledge. As we become more familiar with ourselves through the practice of self-knowledge, we may not like what we see and become self-critical and judgmental. Self-empathy includes noticing how hard it is for us to accept our imperfections and mistakes with an attitude of warmth and self-acceptance while simultaneously being committed to finding a way to become more forgiving and compassionate toward ourselves. Certain practices from the Buddhist tradition are especially helpful in developing self-empathy. Metta or Loving-Kindness Meditation is an explicit practice of opening the heart with empathy and compassion towards oneself and others [25].

Preparing the Mind involves developing three specific cognitive skills: focused-awareness, mindful-self awareness, and dual-awareness. Mindfulness Meditation practice can be used to cultivate these three cognitive skills, which are synergistic with one another. Meditation teacher and author Jon Kabat-Zinn describes Mindfulness Meditation as a process of developing careful attention to minute shifts in body, mind, emotions, and environment while holding a kind, nonjudgmental attitude toward self and others [26]. *Focused awareness* is the platform from which we prepare the mind and is taken here to mean the stabilization and direction of attention. Tibetan Buddhist teacher and author Alan Wallace emphasizes the importance of deep relaxation, stabilization of the mind, and an attitude of vividness in his method of teaching mindfulness of breathing to focus the mind [27]. *Mindful self-awareness* arises naturally from focused awareness. It means being able to witness the stream of our thoughts, physical symptoms, and feelings without commentary, reaction, or comparison. *Dual awareness* is a cognitive stance that permits the clinician to simultaneously attend to and monitor his or her own subjective experience and the needs of the patient and/or the work environment. It is the ability to be simultaneously aware of our inner and outer experience without reactivity, or at least with the ability to be conscious of our reactivity. Dual awareness builds on the practices of focused awareness and mindful self-awareness. Through focused and mindful self-awareness, we attend to and witness our experience in a nonjudgmental way. As we do so, we may notice moments of expanded awareness, when we are aware that we are aware of the object of our focused mindfulness, or possibly that we have just been distracted by a thought. With time and practice, we can deliberately choose dual-awareness, use it to monitor the quality of our attention in meditation practice, and, in time, begin to include it in clinical and social contacts as a means of self-monitoring. This can help to prevent us from getting trapped in reactivity or self-preoccupation and allow us to respond to the patient with more flexibility and greater sensitivity.

Contemplative Awareness is awareness that we as individuals are situated in a larger field of relationships. Psychologically, this includes the recognition of the intersubjective field in the therapeutic encounter, and of an archetypal or universally shared dimension to our experience. Spiritually, it can be understood as the experience of our relationship to the sacred. It includes becoming aware how we find meaning through our values, our cosmology, and our philosophy of life. Practices to develop contemplative awareness will be unique to each of us as individuals. They may include some of the methods of establishing "healing connections" outlined above.

A Proposed Self-Awareness-Based Model of Self-Care

In Fig. 10.1, a proposed Self-Awareness-Based Model of Self-care and its consequences builds on the hypothesis that clinician self-awareness enhances self-care [28] and is supported by recent empirical data [29].

In the proposed model, two adjacent, symmetrical circles represent contrasting pathways in response to occupational challenges for the clinician in his or her interactions with the work environment and the patient's suffering. The circle to the left illustrates possible negative consequences of the clinician's interactions. The circle to the right represents possible positive consequences of the same interactions.

The amount of self-awareness determines which route the clinician travels. When functioning with less self-awareness, clinicians are more likely to lose perspective, suffer more from stress in interactions with their work environment,

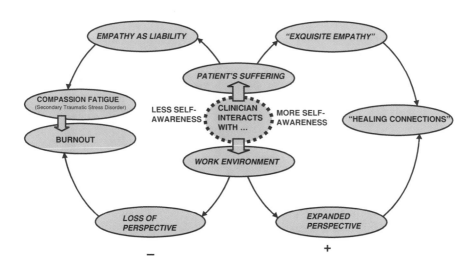

Fig. 10.1 A proposed self-awareness based model of self-care

experience empathy as a liability, and have a greater likelihood of compassion fatigue and burnout. On the contrary, clinicians functioning with greater self-awareness are more likely to have an expanded perspective, experience less stress and more satisfaction in interactions with their work environment, experience exquisite empathy in their interactions with their patients, and promote healing connections with themselves, their patients, their family, and their colleagues.

Self-care may be practiced with or without enhanced self-awareness. Methods of self-care that do not specifically increase self-awareness, such as maintaining clear professional boundaries, can offer protection at work and renewal outside of work. Self-awareness-based methods of self-care, however, offer the additional possibility of finding regeneration *within* the work environment and clinical encounters, for example, through the practice of exquisite empathy and by establishing healing connections.

Organizational Benefits of a Self-Awareness-Based Model of Self-Care

The successful implementation of a self-awareness-based model of self-care depends on the choices, commitment, and practices undertaken by the individual clinician. However, unless there is also support from the organization within which that individual works, this may simply become another source of frustration and stress. While it would be nice to think our organizations would choose to support such initiatives for altruistic reasons, it is unlikely that this will happen. Organizations need to be persuaded that there are potential tangible benefits from such practices for the organization and its bottom line. These may include increased staff retention and reduced absenteeism, increased employee morale and job satisfaction, reduced employee conflicts, employees who are present, empathic, and effective, and increased patient and family satisfaction. If our organizations understand this, they will realize that an investment in encouraging and facilitating clinician self-awareness and self-care is a sound business strategy that benefits staff, clients, and the healthcare organization. They may, then, accept that this is a joint responsibility of *both* organization and employees.

The Story Now

One year later, and now 30 years in end-of-life care, I continue to work full-time as a physician in palliative care and hospice. The external circumstances of my work have not changed, in part, because it is not possible for me to do so at this time. Over the past 12 months, I have continued to reflect, individually and in dialog with others, on what it means to live with the daily reality of compassion fatigue and burnout as I continue to work with my colleagues in trying to alleviate suffering and promote healing in those we care for. I have come to certain insights that are sustaining me in work. While I realize they are personal and individual, I share them in the hope that they may have some resonance for others:

- Self-care is not a luxury. It is an ethical and clinical imperative. It affects both my sustainability as a clinician and the quality of my work.
- Clinician self-awareness is the key. It allows me to survive, maybe even to thrive, in even the most adverse of circumstances. It is like a psychophysiological process that generates the oxygen I need to breathe underwater.
- Self-care is an ongoing process that needs to become as integral a life practice as eating or sleeping.
- From time to time, I will make an inventory of those aspects of *my work* that are most meaningful and satisfying by asking myself, "Where and when am I most myself and most awake, alive, and connected in my work?" I will try to include as many of these aspects of my work as I can and, ideally, have them written into my job description at the expense of those parts of the job that are most depleting.
- From time to time, I will make an inventory of those aspects of *my life* that are most meaningful and satisfying by asking myself, "With whom, where, doing what, am I most awake, alive, and connected and most myself?" I will commit to making space and time for those relationships, activities, practices, and places that are most nourishing to me and that bring the deepest sense of healing connectedness.
- If, despite making what changes I can in and outside my work, I become increasingly burnt out, I will consider either a partial or complete job change to allow for a greater soul-role alignment when circumstances allow.

Practicing Clinician Self-Awareness

The wholeness is already there. Our task as healers, of ourselves as well as others, is to remember this, to radically re-member this, and to do so both *inside* as well as *outside* of the workplace. This is not as easy as it sounds, but it is possible if we develop clinician self-awareness. Clinician self-awareness involves a commitment to deepening in self-knowledge, the practice of self-empathy and mindfulness, and experiencing connectedness and the sacred through the practice of contemplative awareness.

Practicing clinician self-awareness makes whole person self-care possible. Clinician self-awareness in the workplace allows us to engage in exquisite empathy with the possibility of protection from traumatization while simultaneously finding sources of nourishment and renewal in the work itself. But this alone is not enough. We also need times of retreat, times when we step back and completely away from our work and immerse ourselves in whatever is most deeply meaningful for us. Such times of retreat allow us to see our work from a different perspective, to sense the bigger picture and to discern if soul and role are in alignment. This allows us to experience healing connectedness, to rest in the source, to be in Tao, and then, naturally, it rains.

References

1. Gimian CR. The collected works of Chögyam Trungpa. The Path is the Goal – Training the Mind – Glimpses of Abhidharma – Glimpses of Shunyata – Glimpses of Mahayana – Selected Writings, vol. 2. Boston: Shambala; 2003. p. 532.
2. Balint M. The doctor, his patient and the illness. London: Churchill Livingstone; 2000.
3. Martin PW. An experiment in depth: a study of the work of Jung, Eliot and Toynbee. London: Routledge & Kegan Paul; 1987.
4. Figley CR, editor. Compassion fatigue: coping with secondary traumatic stress disorder in those who treat the traumatized. New York: Brunner/Mazel; 1995.
5. Hayes JA. Therapist know thyself: recent research on countertransference. Psychother Bull. 2004;39:6–12.
6. McCann IL, Perlman LA. Vicarious traumatization: a contextual model for understanding the effects of trauma on helpers. J Traum Stress. 1990;3:134.
7. Hojat M, Gonnella JS, Nasca TJ, Mangione S, Vergare M, Magee M. Physician empathy: definition, components, measurement, and relationship to gender and specialty. Am J Psychiatry. 2002;159(9):1563–9.
8. Harrison RL, Westwood MJ. Preventing vicarious traumatization of mental health therapists: identifying protective practices. Psychother Theor Res Pract Train. 2009;46(2):203–19.
9. Herman LJ. Trauma and recovery. New York: Basic Books; 1997. p. 133.
10. Guggenbühl Craig A. Power in the helping professions. Putnam: Spring Publications; 2009. p. 79–92.
11. Maslach C, Leiter MP. Early predictors of job burnout and engagement. J Appl Psychol. 2008;93(3):498–512.
12. Maslach C. Job burnout: new directions in research and intervention. Curr Dir Psychol Sci. 2003;12(5):189–92.
13. Valent P. Diagnosis and treatment of helper stresses, traumas, and illnesses. In: Figley CR, editor. Treating compassion fatigue. New York: Brunner-Routledge; 2002. p. 17–37.
14. Maslach C, Schaufeli WB, Leiter MP. Job burnout. Annu Rev Psychol. 2001;52:397–422.
15. Vachon MLS. Staff stress in hospice/palliative care: a review. Palliat Med. 1995;9(2):91–122.
16. Wilhelm R, Baynes CF. The I Ching or book of changes. Princeton: Princeton University Press; 1967.
17. Hanna B. Active imagination. Wilmette: Chiron Publications; 2001. p. 13–4.
18. Jung CG. Vision: notes on the seminars given 1930-34. In: Douglas C, editor. Psychiatric studies, vol. 1. Princeton: Princeton University Press; 1997. p. 333–5.
19. Mount B, Kearney M. Healing and palliative care: charting our way forward [editorial]. Palliat Med. 2003;17:657–8.
20. Palmer PJ. A hidden wholeness: the journey to an undivided life. San Francisco: Jossey Bass; 2004. p. 13.
21. Palmer PJ. Let your life speak: listening for the voice of vocation. San Francisco: Jossey Bass; 2000. p. 4–5.
22. Buechner F. Wishful thinking: a seeker's ABC. San Francisco: Harper San Francisco; 1993. p. 119.
23. Mount BM, Boston PH, Cohen RS. Healing connections: on moving from suffering to a sense of well-being. J Pain Symptom Manage. 2007;33(4):372–88.
24. Kearney M. A place of healing: working with nature and soul at the end-of-life. New Orleans: Spring Journal Books; 2009.
25. Kornfield J. The wise heart: a guide to the universal teachings of Buddhist psychology. New York: Bantam Books; 2009. p. 386.
26. Kabatt-Zinn J. Mindfulness-based interventions in context: past, present, and future. Clin Psychol Sci Proc. 2003;10(2):144–55.
27. Wallace BA. The attention revolution: unlocking the power of the focused mind. Somerville: Wisdom Publications; 2006.

28. Kearney MK, Weininger RB, Vachon MLS, Harrison RL, Mount BM. Self-care of physicians caring for patients at the end of life. JAMA. 2009;301(11):1155–64.
29. Krasner MS, Epstein RM, Beckman H, et al. Association of an educational program in mindful communication with burnout, empathy, and attitudes among primary care physicians. JAMA. 2009;302(12):1284–93.

Chapter 11
Prevention and Whole Person Care

Tom A. Hutchinson

Keywords Whole body • Whole person • Primary prevention • Secondary prevention • Prevention paradox • Randomized trials • Exercise • Diet • Sleep • Stress • Well-being • Quality of life • Meaning • Connection • Hippocratic • Asklepian • Mindful

Prevention of disease always seems like a good idea. Who could argue against taking measures to prevent a heart attack or detecting cancer early (at a stage when it can be removed or effectively treated)? These disease-focused measures aimed at prevention make such good common sense that it is hard to argue against them and we would not do so because they really can work. And yet, there are problems with these approaches that often elude common sense. We believe that these limitations need to be appreciated and the preventative measures aimed at disease need to bolstered by complementary measures based on the whole body and the whole person.

What are the limitations of disease-based prevention? First, the limitation of *primary* prevention [1] aimed at stopping disease before it occurs (as in taking cholesterol-lowering drugs to prevent a heart attack) is that we need to target appropriately those whose risk of disease is sufficiently high to justify the side effects and costs of the intervention or medication. This is fairly straightforward if we limit ourselves to those at the highest risk levels in whom the individual benefit will be substantial. However, if we restrict our interventions in this way, we will miss most of the disease occurring in the population, which will continue to come from the much larger numbers of people whose individual risk is not high – a phenomenon known as the prevention paradox [2]. It is not clear if we can prevent the majority of disease by primary means because as we begin to extend our preventative measures to those at lower risk, the overall costs (both financial costs and the costs of side-effects) will increase and the benefits to individuals will decrease.

T.A. Hutchinson (✉)
Professor, Faculty of Medicine, Director, Programs in Whole Person Care, McGill University, 546 Pine Avenue West, Montreal, QC H2W 1S6, Canada
e-mail: tom.hutchinson@mcgill.ca

T.A. Hutchinson (ed.), *Whole Person Care: A New Paradigm for the 21st Century*, DOI 10.1007/978-1-4419-9440-0_11, © Springer Science+Business Media, LLC 2011

However, there are other factors at play. The studies to establish the cost–benefit ratio for individual patients will need to become larger and more complex. Large pharmaceutical companies, unlike individual patients, or governments and other third parties who may pay for the medications, necessarily benefit the wider the preventative treatment is disseminated. The high costs of the necessary studies are usually borne by these companies because only they can afford to fund them. What trials are done and how the results are publicized to affect prescribing may be more determined by concerns for profit rather than what is best for individual patients or the public health [3]. We need to be cognizant of these influences unrelated to public or individual health when we make decisions about primary prevention.

Next, the limitation of *secondary* prevention [1] aimed at early detection and treatment of disease is the tendency of detection methods to overrepresent mild and even insignificant disease. Why does this happen? For illustrative purposes, let us take two cases with the same kind of cancer. Case 1 is a patient with very aggressive and rapidly progressing cancer. The time from first appearance of detectable cancer to the onset of symptoms necessitating a doctor's visit is 3 months. Case 2 is a patient with the same kind of cancer but not so aggressive or rapidly growing. The time from first appearance of detectable cancer to symptoms severe enough to prompt a doctor's visit is 3 years. What kind of cancer do you believe will be most likely to be detected by screening? The answer is the second kind, and the difference of their representation in those detected by screening is a factor of 12! It is difficult to test often enough to detect the really severe cases, and more sensitive diagnostic methods do not help, leading mainly to the detection of more and more of the mild cases [4] with slowly progressive disease.

Clinical epidemiologists have long been aware of this problem [1], and the resultant effect that screening always appears to look good because the cases detected tend to be mild from the outset. For this reason, researchers insist on randomized trials to evaluate screening methods. And the results are sometimes very surprising. In one famous study from the Mayo Clinic [5], smokers were randomized to be screened by 4 monthly chest X-rays and sputum tests compared to a similar group who were randomized to regular care. As expected, the group randomized to regular X-rays and sputum tests had more cancers detected, more surgery to remove them, and a better survival in those with cancer detected. But here is the surprising result. The overall mortality and the mortality due to lung cancer was identical in the two groups. It appears that the regular testing swelled the number of those labeled as having lung cancer but did not change the number of patients dying from lung cancer in the screened group. And the results remained the same after 20 further years of follow-up [6].

Does this mean that screening is useless? No, but we need good randomized studies and perhaps to look again at our simple model of disease. The model of disease upon which most prevention is based is that disease (cancer or other) starts with small changes, progresses to a point where it is detectable but not symptomatic, and continues to progress until it produces symptoms, dysfunction, and possibly death. But, surprisingly, there is evidence that a significant proportion of cancers detected by screening are not life threatening [7], or progressive [8], and some detected cancers appear to regress spontaneously [9]. The varied spectrum of biologic behavior in cancer and other diseases, combined with the costs and side effects of testing and follow-up interventions, explains why disease-based prevention based on early detection may be useful for some diseases but not for all diseases in all patients. We need to target our detection and intervention more precisely to diseases and people at risk for those diseases who stand to benefit from screening. This is an ongoing process that has resulted in recommendations, for instance, that routine mammography screening is worthwhile in women between 50 and 74 years of age but not in younger women, or older women [10]. There is an analogous need for very precise targeting in primary prevention where, for instance, how seriously we should take and treat a high cholesterol value depends not just on the level of the abnormality but also on the balance of other risk factors for heart disease in the person being evaluated [11]. The complexity of our bodies and different disease processes that makes disease-aimed prevention not always the clear answer for most people has another implication – we may need a complementary method that fills the gaps in our preventative armamentarium.

We suggest that an approach based on the whole body and the whole person is what is needed. Whole-body prevention is doing things that have multiple beneficial effects on the whole complex organism that is our body. A good example is regular exercise that appears to: help prevent obesity, control lipid abnormalities, diabetes, and blood pressure, improve psychological functioning and prevent depression, decrease the risk of major diseases such as heart disease and some cancers, slow the development of osteoporosis, and keep people more functional and mobile for longer. A short list of things we can do, which appear to be good for the whole body, are get regular exercise [12], eat a healthy diet (good food, not supplements) [13], sleep enough [14], manage stress [15] (e.g., mindfulness [16] and other approaches), avoid injurious habits (e.g., smoking). You will notice that every one of these measures not only has multiple and complex beneficial effects but also tends to improve quality of life and well-being, which might be an equally good reason for doing them. We tend to think of prevention as aimed primarily at future survival but should not preventing or reversing a decrease in quality of life also be important. And in these whole-body preventative measures, we appear to be able to have it both ways. What then is whole person prevention and does it have the same attractive properties?

Whole person prevention is aimed at preventing a loss of meaning [17] or increasing the depth of meaning and connection [18, 19] in our lives. So it might be said that while disease-based prevention is aimed at survival, whole-body prevention is directed toward survival and quality of life, and whole person prevention is concerned with meaning and the effect that has on our survival and quality of life at a deeper level. And interestingly, the measures we might take based on these three approaches do not always seem to agree. Consider the following story about Viktor Frankl from the film "The Choice is Yours" [20].

Frankl is living in Vienna, and the Nazis have invaded Austria and the writing is on the wall for Jewish citizens like Frankl and his family. He has applied for a visa to go to USA that arrives, making everyone including his parents happy. He at least will be saved. But this will leave his parents in Vienna to the mercy of the Nazis. He does not know what to do and asks the world for a sign. That night he notices that his father has brought home a piece of marble from a destroyed synagogue. It is a piece of one of the Ten Commandments. His father asks him "And do you know which commandment this marble is from?" The answer is "Honor father and mother and stay in the land". Frankl stays and ends up surviving Auschwitz and writing "Man's search for meaning" within months of his release. His parents and wife die in the camps.

Our natural first thought is that the surest way for Frankl to have preserved his life was to take the visa to USA. But that might have meant going against his deepest values. What does "his life" mean in this context? Is it just his body or is there a larger meaning to this term that includes the whole person and the values, meaning, and relationships that are important to that person. Did Frankl take the only option open to him to preserve his life in this larger sense while risking his body? In our desire to prevent bad outcomes, do we need to take our values into consideration?

There is a clear relationship here to the two sides of the Hippocratic/Asklepian dichotomy. In the Hippocratic mode, we should do everything to preserve the body and control the future. In the Asklepian mode, we may need to focus more on preserving our values, which includes what we enjoy in life, and lessen our grip on the future survival of the body. One way of getting at this is to ask ourselves why we may want to live a long time. The answers would differ for each person, but for myself I might say, for instance, that I want to continue to enjoy life, to see and nurture my grandchildren, and to leave a legacy. The next question is whether I am living my life in line with those goals right now. Am I enjoying life fully right now? Am I doing everything I can to nurture my future grandchildren? Am I actively working on my legacy? And so on. I find that this is a strangely and surprisingly healing process. The truth is that none of us know what is in store for us. The best preventative measures may not foresee or avoid what is actually in the cards. But we can do something about the present. For instance, when I ask myself the three questions that I posed earlier, the answers are surprising. Am I enjoying life to the full right now? Well not really because I am waiting for something to happen (to retire? to get older? for something else but for what?). Am I doing everything I can to nurture my future grandchildren? Not really because although I know that it is very important to me, I hardly ever think about it. Am I working on my legacy? Indirectly, but mostly, I am not aware of it one way or the other. It is not that achieving those goals is important for their own sake but confronting those questions has a profound effect on my being in the current moment. I have a sense of calm energy when I ask myself those questions that I believe may be the best tool we have to optimize our current health and well-being, to prepare ourselves for whatever the future may bring, and possibly even to preserve our lives.

Does this mean that we should stop exercising? No, but perhaps we should take it on with more flexibility, and in ways that fit the rest of our lives and that we enjoy more for their own sake. It might mean joining a tennis club rather than taking regular solitary visits to the gym. Perhaps we should do it less out of duty or fear and more out of enthusiasm or love for whatever the exercise activity in which we are engaged.

Perhaps our better diet becomes less a matter of restriction and more a focus on mindful enjoyment of foods that we thoroughly savor. One advantage here is that we are much more likely to continue an activity that we really enjoy. But at a deeper level, I believe that deep enjoyment of the present moment is our best preparation for the future. Why? Because the future is inherently uncertain, things will happen that we did not expect, and our challenge will be to get the most out of whatever happens. Our best prevention may be to learn how to enjoy the present moment and by extension all future present moments. Focusing primarily on trying to avoid "bad" things happening is ultimately doomed to failure with the added complication that what we thought would be "bad" events can turn into "good" events – turning points in our lives that open us to a deeper and more meaningful experience of being alive, a report that we hear from patients with serious illness [21].

Where does this leave us? We would conclude the following:

1. Disease-based prevention methods should be continued but only in those situations where there is clear evidence based on randomized trials that they work to prevent significant disease in the persons targeted.
2. Whole-body-based prevention methods are almost always a good idea because they work on multiple systems at the same time and generally have immediate effects on quality of life and well-being.
3. Taking whole person concerns into account may significantly modify how 1 and 2 are best implemented in different people.

Lastly, since the extent to which people are in touch with their deep values may determine their quality of life now and in the future, this should be an overriding concern in prevention, especially given the inevitable uncertainties in people's very complex and changeable lives. Because patients are whole persons in which all the parts are connected, we cannot limit ourselves to the Hippocratic side of the medical dichotomy in prevention any more than in treatment. We are just beginning to scratch the surface of what good preventative measures mean in whole person care.

References

1. Fletcher RH, Fletcher SW, Wagner EH. Prevention (Chapter 8). In: Clinical epidemiology. The essentials. 3rd ed. Baltimore, MD: Williams & Wilkins; 1996. p. 165–85.
2. Rose G. Strategy of prevention: lessons from cardiovascular disease [Occasional Review]. Br Med J (Clin Res Ed). 1981;282:1847–51.
3. Brophy JM, Costa V. Statin wars following coronary revascularization – evidence-based clinical practice? Can J Cardiol. 2006;22(1):54–8.
4. Black WC, Welch HG. Advances in diagnostic imaging and overestimations of disease prevalence and the benefits of therapy. N Engl J Med. 1993;328(17):1237–43.
5. Taylor WF, Fontana RS, Uhlenhopp MA, Davis CS. Some results of screening for early lung cancer. Cancer. 1981;47:1114–20.
6. Marcus PM, Bergstralh EJ, Fagerstrom RM, Williams DE, Fontana R, Taylor WF, et al. Lung cancer mortality in the Mayo Lung Project: impact of extended follow-up. J Natl Cancer Inst. 2000;92(16):1308–16.

7. Helgesen F, Holmeberg L, Johansson JE, et al. Trends in prostate cancer survival in Sweden, 1960 through 1988: evidence of increasing diagnosis of nonlethal tumors. J Nat Cancer Inst. 1996;88(7):1216–21.

8. Hakama M, Holli K, Visakorpi T, Pekola M, Kallioniemi O-P. Low biological aggressiveness of screen-detected lung cancers may indicate over-diagnosis. Int J Cancer. 1996;66:6–10.

9. Zahl PH, Maehlen J, Welch HG. The natural history of invasive breast cancers detected by screening mammography. Arch Intern Med. 2008;168(21):2311–6.

10. U.S Preventive Services Task Force. Screening for breast cancer: U.S. preventive services task force recommendation statement. Ann Intern Med. 2009;151(10):716–26.

11. Hayward RA, Krumholz HM, Zulman DM, Timble JW, Vijan S. Optimizing statin treatment for primary prevention of coronary artery disease. Ann Intern Med. 2010;152:69–77.

12. Fletcher GF, Balady G, Blair SN, Blumenthal J, Caspersen C, Chaitman B, et al. Statement on Exercise: Benefits and Recommendations for Physical Activity Programs for All Americans. Circulation. 1996;94:857–62.

13. Cassileth BR, Heitzer M, Wesa K. The public health impact of herbs and nutritional supplements. Pharm Biol. 2009;47(8):761–7.

14. Zee PC, Turek FW. Sleep and health: everywhere and in both directions. Arch Intern Med. 2006;66(16):1686–8.

15. Selye H. Stress and the general adaptation syndrome. BM J. 1950;4667:1383–92.

16. Kabat-Zinn J. Full catastrophe living. Using the wisdom of your body and mind to face stress, pain, and illness. 15th ed. New York, NY: Delta Trade Paperback; 1995.

17. Frankl V. Man's searching for meaning. Boston: Beacon; 2006.

18. Harrington A. Healing ties (Chapter 5). In: The cure within. A history of mind-body medicine. New York, NY: W. W. Norton; 2008. p. 175–204.

19. Mount B, Boston P. Healing connections: a phenomenological study of suffering, wellness and quality of life. J Pain Symptom Manage. 2007;33:372–88.

20. Drazen RY. The Choice Is Yours [DVD]. Drazen Productions; 2001. Distributed by the American Board of Internal Medicine Foundation.

21. Smith K. Chapter 14. In: Philips D, editor. Heroes. 100 Stories of living with kidney failure. Montreal, QC: Grosvenor House; 1998. p. 43–47.

Chapter 12
Whole Person Care and Complementary and Alternative Therapies

Mary Grossman

> *Natural Forces within us are the true healers of disease ....*
> *It is far more important to know what person the disease has than what disease the person has.*
>
> Hippocrates

Keywords Integrative medicine • Complementary modalities or therapies • Whole person care • Holistic • Healing • Placebo effect • Mind–body therapies • Health-related expectations • Health beliefs • Reductionist methods • Stress management • Spiritual growth

Introduction

Patients have been the huge beneficiaries of medicine's singular focus on curing disease. Assisted by the combined forces of the scientific method and health-related technologies, medical science has effectively advanced the diagnostic and treatment capabilities of the medical profession [1]. In the past century, more diseases have been cured or effectively managed than in the previous 2,000 years combined [1]. Yet, the past decade has witnessed a groundswell of patients across North America who are calling upon health care practitioners to care/treat the whole person, and not just their illness. This demand for a more comprehensive approach that would respond to the individual needs of the whole person may explain why so many people are turning to complementary therapies (CT) before, during, and after their medical treatment, the majority having neither informed nor consulted with their treating oncologist [2–4]. This growing trend has begun to

M. Grossman (✉)
Director, Lung Cancer Brojde Centre, Segal Cancer Centre, Jewish General Hospital,
3755 Côte-Ste-Catherine Road, Montreal, QC H3T 1E2, Canada
e-mail: mgrossman@jgh.mcgill.ca

T.A. Hutchinson (ed.), *Whole Person Care: A New Paradigm for the 21st Century*,
DOI 10.1007/978-1-4419-9440-0_12, © Springer Science+Business Media, LLC 2011
     133

challenge underlying assumptions about health and illness traditionally held by health care practitioners. It has led to the development of a new philosophy of practice known as integrative medicine.

The purpose of this paper is to explore patient perceptions of conventional medicine and complementary therapy use in facilitating their health and healing to underscore the need for a new model of integrative medicine in whole person care.

Medical Treatment and the Patient

Before antibiotics, the practice of medicine was shaped as much by the art as the science of its discipline. With a paucity of known effective treatments, both patient and doctor valued the relationship that evolved from their shared hope in the healing capabilities of the patient. In the absence of proven remedies, the physician was viewed as a knowledgeable and caring practitioner whose professional demeanor was apt to instill an expectation that the patient could get better, often with the pleasing result that many seemingly improved without treatment [5]. And when there was nothing more to do, the physician was there to help the family come to terms with the inevitable.

> When Evelyn lost her fight with pneumonia just short of her second birthday, there was little that could be done medically to save her in 1903. What the town's doctor could do was be there for the young mother and father, supporting them as they comforted their dying daughter. With compassion, he showed them how to position their child in bed to ease her labored breathing, what to do to lower their daughter's fever, to offer sips of water and ensure a clean and warm environment. And when Evelyn's exhausted being gave up, it was the doctor who filled the tragic void with comforting words and frequent home visits. Although he was helpless to save Evelyn's life, by his caring and his presence, he encouraged Evelyn's parents to talk about their sadness and their loss in a way that helped them to move forward with their lives.

As more medical discoveries were made, the former wait-and-see medical approach to illness increasingly gave way to scientifically based clinical decisions. By the 1950s, healing was associated less with the patient's innate capabilities than with the medical intervention itself. Healing was the result of what the physician did to eliminate an infection, contain a virus, and close a physical wound. For the first time in medical history, physicians could speak with greater conviction about curing the patient. This remarkable achievement was, in large part, attributed to medicine's use of the scientific method that consisted of diverse research designs, but especially, the randomized controlled trial (RCT), for evaluating the efficacy and effectiveness of proposed medical treatments.

To this day, the RCT reductionist model is the preferred scientific method of clinical medicine. Remedies, treatments, and, most recently, CT that have not been subjected to the same rigorous scientific evaluation are generally discredited. Yet, the reductionist approach, upon which the practice of clinical medicine is based, divides the whole into objective measurable parts [6], that is, a given treatment tends to be evaluated in terms of measures that can be easily quantified, such as the presence or absence of illness, living or deceased, the size of the tumor in centimeters, and so on. The unfortunate consequence is that health care providers lack scientific knowledge of the whole being that limits their ability to respond medically to the whole patient. Because a scientific understanding of the whole person is lacking, the message may inadvertently be conveyed that the whole is of lesser import medically than the particular disease under investigation.

> Eleanor Johnson had never been sick a day in her 45 years. So when her arm accidentally brushed against a solid lump lying along the outer aspect of her left breast, during her exercises that evening, she was momentarily incredulous but also knew instinctively that she was in trouble. When the doctor removed the aspiration needle from the center of the huge lump the next morning, she did not need to be told the significance of the empty syringe. A swell of anxiety and fear overcame her normally collected composure. She was going to die. 'You know what this means,' the doctor said, oblivious to the fact that she was struggling to concentrate on what he was saying. 'You have cancer. You need a biopsy. You'll need to be booked for surgery and then chemotherapy. Come back in a couple of weeks for the biopsy results.' And that was that.

Similar stories tend to occur when the health care provider is overly centered on the diagnosis and treatment, with the unfortunate result that the patient is frequently left to his or her own means to sort out emotions and develop a strategy for navigating the health care system. But it is understandable in that "reductionist" methods, upon which the practice of medicine is based, pay scant attention to the overall well-being, sense of meaning, and quality of life of the patient, which are subjective measures of the *person* as opposed to the illness [6]. Accordingly, thoughts, feelings, and beliefs are deemed "subjective" because they are filtered through the biased "lens" of the patient, thereby rendering the information, presumably, noncredible. While patient perceptions may be subjective, they are no less real to the person merely because the philosophic underpinnings of the scientific method are incompatible with a subjective way of "knowing" the whole person.

Nonetheless, research on the potential impact of medical treatments (or the disease) on the psychological, socioemotional, and spiritual dimensions of the whole person, and vice versa, is still rare. Medical studies exploring the bidirectional impact of emotions and beliefs on biological health remain underinvestigated. As a consequence, empirical knowledge of the complex world of patient beliefs, thoughts, and feelings has not been integral to evidence-based clinical decisions. In particular, the potential role of patient beliefs and expectations about getting well and facilitating their healing capabilities has largely remained beyond the scope of medical practice, arguably, with important clinical implications within the context of the physician–patient relationship [5, 7].

> Even now 10 years after his wife succumbed to pancreatic cancer, Mr. Brown continues to relive over and over again, like a surreal dream, the moment they learned 'she was doomed'. He remembers something streaming out of the doctor's mouth like unravelling, tumbling letters of the alphabet, constructing nonsensical meanings, which suddenly dropped from sight with the doctor's words' 'there is nothing I can do'. It was a death sentence from which there was no escape. He sealed her fate. 'I know, I know the statistics aren't great. I tell you she could have lived a little longer with hope'.

There is documented evidence that our innate capability to heal has to do with the positive expectations we hold about our health and what we need to do to get well [8–10]. According to Benson [5], these beliefs, which are deposited as memories throughout the body, are reflected by the placebo effect. They are the result of a neuropsychophysiological phenomenon that he calls "remembered wellness," in which previous health-related experiences are associated with feelings of well-being [11]. These positive memories, when evoked, can activate the body's physiological healing capabilities.

In contrast, when negative expectations about wellness have been established in memory through previous experiences, the potential effectiveness of the placebo is dramatically reduced [11]. When a health care professional expresses doubt or skepticism about a patient's belief in a mode of treatment, the placebo effect may be seriously impaired. Benson and Friedman [11] argue that the quality of the physician or health care provider relationship with the patient is of utmost importance in either activating or deactivating the body's healing response as a function of whether the patient, physician, or both believe in a proposed treatment.

The effectiveness of the placebo highlights the importance of conceptualizing the patient as a whole person with an illness as opposed to honing in on the disease and its medical treatment as if the other interrelated parts of the person played no role in the patient's health and healing. It suggests that what the physician or health care provider says to the patient and how it is conveyed may be as important as the medical treatment itself; it may in fact exert a profound impact, for better or worse, on the patient's innate healing capabilities.

There is another concern, however, about the reductionist model that occurs each time a patient is prescribed a medication or assigned to a medical protocol. These standardized treatments are derived from RCTs that were done to evaluate the efficacy of the pharmacological agent or surgical intervention. However, the inclusion and exclusion criteria that determine which patients are eligible to participate also raise legitimate concerns about the extent to which the research findings may be generalized to subsequent clinic patients suffering from the same cancer [6]. Moreover, when mean values are reported, the results reflect the group average and not the actual value obtained by each patient. Even data reported as intent-to-treat results, which can identify the actual patients in the study who benefited from the standardized treatment, can say little about the clinical relevance of the treatment for a given patient in the clinic, as no two persons are biologically the same.

The inherent weaknesses of protocols derived from a reductionist method may explain why some patients do better than others on a given protocol when both are suffering from the same cancer type, stage, and grade. It may be that uncertainty about the treatment's efficacy along with frequently endured toxic symptoms contributes to the patient's sense of vulnerability and growing dissatisfaction, resulting in an understandable expectation that the health care provider should look beyond the disease and the treatment to address the needs of the whole person.

When Eleanor received the biopsy report, she learned that the news was extremely grim, stage 4 of an extremely aggressive tumor that had a poor prognosis. She made the decision to find an oncologist with a team approach. 'Yes, it is aggressive but there are things we can do. Remember that a prognosis is about the natural trajectory of the illness before the medical intervention. Statistics say nothing about how you personally will respond to treatment.' With that, the load of fear and anxiety started to lift. 'Don't forget,' the oncologist added, 'there is a whole team behind you. We have an idea of what we want to do- but we also are consulting with colleagues at several leading cancer centers.' For the first time, Eleanor began to feel safe. But there was still something else she needed to understand. 'But I don't fit a protocol? Her anxiety soaring again. 'True, but we have something else- your cancer to help direct us to the best combination of treatments. We think the surgery should be delayed until we try to make the tumor smaller- and then we can monitor its response to the chemotherapy.' 'Ok' she persisted. 'But I have a hard time just doing nothing.' 'Who says you have nothing to do? Your work is to eat healthy food, stay calm, and walk everyday. My job will be to take care of your treatment.' He could see she was hesitating, not totally convinced. 'I know you have a PhD in physiology- Are you interested in me sending you a key article before our next meeting so we can review the pros and cons of the options I'm considering?' And then Eleanor knew that she was fortunate. This was not for every patient, but it was perfect for her.

Regrettably, the built-in bias of the medical model has led health care providers, at times to unintentionally be dismissive of the patients' very "real" feelings and beliefs, especially about promoting their health and getting better. Research on beliefs, expectations, and remembered wellness highlights the importance of conceptualizing the patient as a whole person with an illness as opposed to focusing mainly on the disease and treatment. Patients seem to understand this, and increasingly are seeking to satisfy their need to optimize the wellness of their whole being. Perhaps it is no coincidence then that the use of CT among cancer and other patients has dramatically increased in the past decade.

The Potential Benefits of Complementary Therapy Use

CT are health-promoting practices associated with whole medical systems such as Traditional Chinese Medicine (TCM) and Ayurvedic Medicine (AM) that function outside conventional medicine and conceptualize the person in terms of the inseparability of the mind, body, and spirit. In contrast to the western medical system's emphasis on curing disease, the philosophy of TCM and AM is similar to that of nursing in its focus on the health and healing of the whole person who may be living with a terminal illness [12–14]. CT are used to optimize wellness by facilitating the person's innate healing capabilities. When the self, the self in relation to others, and the universe are in harmony and balance, optimal wellness is obtained [15].

An estimated 83–90% of patients turn to some form of complementary therapy following a cancer diagnosis, and more than half do this without the knowledge of their treating physician [4, 16, 17]. CT include naturopathy, homeopathy, oriental herbs, mushrooms, natural supplements, vitamins and minerals, mindful meditation, visualization, reflexology, massage yoga, qigong, therapeutic healing, acupuncture/acupressure, cognitive structural reframing, counseling, and spiritual practices that are typically grouped into one of the following domains of practice: mind–body, biologically-based, manipulative and body-based, and energy or biofield therapies [3, 12, 18–20].

Daphne Smith was only 35 when she was first diagnosed with advanced colorectal cancer. Married with two pre-adolescent children, Daphne was a teacher who had never smoked.

As described by her husband, Daphne was the heart and soul of the family. But she completely unraveled following the diagnosis. Unable to sleep or make decisions for herself or her children, her husband stepped up, but nothing seemed to help. Devastated, Daphne gave herself over to the health care team; she underwent chemotherapy and radiation to kill the tumor and manage the bone metastases; she took anti depressants and saw a psychiatrist in the hope of overcoming the deep feelings of sadness and despair that seemed to overwhelm her. Even when she was told that her cancer was in remission, she remained dispirited, until one day a friend encouraged her to drop by the Ayurveda center in town. That day, she explained, changed her life.

Reasons for CT use vary. Cancer patients typically hope to reduce treatment-related symptoms, increase their immune response, prevent a recurrence, slow down the spread of cancer, use a holistic approach, help the body heal, support the medical treatment, control symptoms, have more control over medical decisions, feel hopeful, and increase the well-being of the whole person [3, 16, 17, 21–23]. These explanations reveal some of the beliefs, hopes, and expectations people have about getting better.

I first met Daphne 9 months after she had begun to follow Ayurvedic practices. Daphne was on a program of daily meditation, walks, yoga, and a health-promoting diet. She was taking herbs to strengthen her immune response and acupuncture to help manage her bone pain. Daphne looked thin but exuded energy and an aura of peacefulness. By her own account, Daphne was a new person who attributed the profound change in her well being to the Arurvedic practices that had helped to 'heal her whole being'. Because of the Ayurvedic practitioner, Daphne now felt that there was someone caring for her while the oncology team 'looked after' the cancer. Daphne was convinced that the Ayurvedic practices with the medical treatment had been essential in promoting her current state of health. As evidence, she rather proudly revealed that she no longer took anti -depressant medication; she had resumed her mothering role with renewed purpose, and had reconnected more meaning-fully with her husband. On reflection, her quality of life, she felt, was in many ways better now than ever. She had learned to live fully in the present.

CT use has been found to improve wellness and quality of life by addressing, at the physiological level, the interrelated physical, psychosocial, emotional, and spiritual needs of the patient. CT that promote regular exercise, stress management, spiritual growth, and a health-promoting diet are thought to synergistically enhance the health and healing of the whole person.

Health-Promoting Diet

A diet of green and cruciferous vegetables, carrots, berries, fruits, fish, olive oil, legumes, shiitake and other mushrooms, whole grain cereals and flaxseed not only improves physical and mental fitness but also enhances quality of life and lowers the risk of cancer [24, 25]. These foods strengthen the immune system, decrease inflammation, promote cancer cell suicide, and detoxify the body of carcinogens [24, 26].

Green tea, for example, inhibits tumor cell growth and its spread by blocking the proinflammatory action of nuclear factor kappa-B produced by cancer cells and by inhibiting angiogenesis or the creation of blood vessels needed to nourish the developing tumor [24, 27, 28]. Cruciferous vegetables such as broccoli, cabbage, and spinach prevent precancerous cells from developing into malignant tumors. Nonfleshy fruits such as blueberries, raspberries, and strawberries contain active molecules such as ellagic acid and proanthocyanidins that stimulate cancer cell death, inhibit blood vessel growth, and eliminate carcinogenic substances from the body [24, 26].

Health-promoting foods provide a multifocal biological approach that enhances wellness while creating "a hostile physiological environment for cancer cells," as Dr. Richard Beliveau is fond of saying. Thus, for newly diagnosed cancer patients of normal weight and energy, the research findings suggest the value of patients adopting a healthy diet as described above. At a minimum, it seems to promote wellness [29]. As a result, the AICR [25] also recommends that cancer survivors follow this diet to promote their health and well-being.

Physical Exercise

Regular exercise improves physical strength, stamina, mood, and overall well-being [25, 30]. In addition, there are significant physiological effects of exercising regularly. Walking, tai chi, yoga, and qigong appear to decrease proinflammatory cytokine and blood sugar levels, improve immune activity, stimulate natural killer cell activity, decrease tumor growth, and reduce the treatment-related toxicities of fatigue [30–32]. Doing exercise during chemotherapy also has been found to improve physical functioning, aerobic capacity and strength, raising the possibility that it may protect the patient longer from the debilitating effects of the disease and treatment [33]. In fact, there is scientific evidence that exercise may help to prolong survival in cancer patients [25, 30, 34, 35].

Stress Management

Managing stress is one of the main reasons that patients turn to mind–body therapies such as mindful meditation, hatha yoga, relaxation techniques, guided imagery, hypnosis, cognitive-behavioral therapy, and counseling. This is particularly true for patients with a life-threatening illness, depression, or loss [36, 37]. Chronic distress has been linked to proinflammatory mechanisms that create the physiological conditions within which cancer is thought to flourish [38, 39]. Moreover, a psychosomatic, neuropeptide-receptor network that connects the emotional brain with virtually all body systems, organs, and cells serves as the physiological mechanism for emotions and body systems, including the immune system, to affect one another [40]. Thus, patients who are chronically stressed, depressed, or feel helpless have significantly reduced immune responses such as deactivated natural killer cells [26].

By contrast, when patients feel hopeful, a sense of personal control, or feel supported, they do better physically, as evidenced by a strengthened immune response and elevated natural killer cell activity [41]. Mind–body practices are thought to stimulate the psychoneuropeptide network resulting in significant reductions in anxiety, mood disturbance, and depression, as well as improvements in coping skills, and emotional and social well-being [41, 42].

Of these, regular practice of mindful meditation offers several health benefits including significant reductions in stress, cortisol and blood sugar levels, and improvements in mood, quality of life, immune activity and autonomic nervous system (ANS) coherence, a reputed, physiological key to well-being [43–46]. Chronically elevated cortisol and blood sugar levels have been implicated in promoting inflammation.

The issue of whether mind–body therapies can slow down the spread of cancer, thereby potentially improving survival, is still unknown. However, numerous studies attest to the benefits of these complementary practices on the cancer patient's psychological well-being and quality of life. Those findings are consistent with what we know about the psychoneuroimmunological interrelationships among a person's emotions and beliefs, and the body's immune response. Those physiological interconnections are thought to account for the so-called placebo effect discussed in the previous section [7, 11]. This may account in part for Daphne's seeming well-being. Through daily mindful meditation and yoga, she had found an inner strength and meaning to her life that projected an aura of wellness that her health care providers could not have anticipated.

Symptom Management

Increasingly, patients with cancer and other chronic conditions are turning to CT for relief from symptoms associated with their disease or treatment. Energy-based practices such as acupuncture, healing touch, and reiki strive to restore the flow of energy throughout the body, thereby helping to reduce fatigue and enhance a person's normal vitality [12]. There is documented evidence of acupuncture's effectiveness as a treatment for pain, dry mouth, neuropathies, nausea, and vomiting [47–50]. However, acupuncture also has been associated with significant increases in levels of leukocytes, white blood cells, and other related factors of the immune system [51, 52]. There seems to be several potential therapeutic benefits for patients in using acupuncture before, during, and/or after medical treatments.

Mind–body therapies such as guided imagery, hypnosis, mindful meditation, counseling, support groups and cognitive-structural reframing are thought to restore a person's sense of harmony and balance [12]. In contrast, manipulative body-based practices such as massage and reflexology stimulate circulatory and lymphatic systems that promote health and healing [12]. Often used in combination, these CT have been effective in reducing discomfort, pain, nausea, vomiting, and anxiety according to numerous controlled studies [37, 41, 53–55].

Patients also rely on natural supplements to effectively treat a host of symptoms. Carnitine, for example, has been found to improve cancer-induced fatigue [2]. Ginger can effectively reduce feelings of nausea [56]. Selenium can improve symptoms of lymphedema [2]. Other studies suggest that glutamine may be helpful in managing diarrhea, neuropathies, and stomatitis [57], and omega-3 has become a popular supplement for the treatment of fatigue as well as to prevent the loss of appetite, weight, and muscle strength [58].

Over-the-counter supplements reviewed by this paper only reflect a small proportion of biologic remedies being accessed by the public. The possibility of drug interactions when the health care team is unaware of the supplements being taken by the patient under conventional treatment is a serious medical concern. Making CT an integral part of clinical practice would go a long way in meeting the needs of the whole person while providing comprehensive care that is effective and safe.

Spiritual Growth

A life-threatening illness, profound loss, or unrelieved suffering may initiate a spiritual quest in the hope of making sense of a situation from which there is no relief, no escape. In those moments, patients may turn inward drawing support from the contemplative practices of prayer, meditation, yoga, communing with nature, or labyrinth walking. By helping patients shift their attention toward the inner world of being, these CT help to liberate patients from their previous ways of thinking and feeling. In so doing, they may feel free to embark on an existential search leading to a new sense of self and purpose [13, 59].

Spiritual growth looks beyond earth-bound considerations to embrace the infinite possibilities of the being within the universe [13]. Spiritual growth is the culmination of an existential quest that goes to the core of the patient's true, essential self. It is related to psychosocial-emotional healing in that both are innate and intertwining developmental processes through which the person grows toward wholeness, fulfillment, and acceptance [13]. Both move the person to a deeper understanding of the self within a greater more meaningful context. The insights gleaned from this process of self-discovery can provide profound comfort to patients in the throes of an incurable disease. CT, such as mindful meditation, may be an invaluable support for patients grappling with matters of life and death for which feelings of serenity and acceptance would be a welcomed release.

The first time we met, it was hard to accept the fact that Daphne's cancer had returned; she was not on active treatment, she radiated energy, and she was managing this potentially traumatizing return of her cancer with emotional serenity. As she explained, 'Thanks to meditation, I have come closer to knowing who I am than I ever understood before. I am a mother first and a wife. What I know with certainty is that we are all connected; I am part of nature and nature is part of me. My energy will go on; it will continue to be a part of my children's lives. They just need to talk to me silently to know that I am there, in their heart.'

Mindful meditation may have helped to stir Daphne's spiritual growth in which her despair and sadness were able to yield to feelings of acceptance, love, and purpose. Although the role of spirituality in the survival of cancer patients has yet to be scientifically demonstrated [60], several studies show significant relationships between spiritual well-being and quality of life notwithstanding the presence of pain or fatigue [61].

Despite accumulating scientific evidence that complementary practices benefit patients we do not know the frequency, duration, or "best" complementary blend of therapies to promote wellness. Notwithstanding the need for further research, the findings, nonetheless, offer ample reasons why patients are likely to continue to use CT with or without input from their health care providers. That would seem to be reason enough for bringing CT "out of the cold" and into mainstream practice.

Integrative Medicine, a Philosophy of Whole Person Care

Integrative medicine combines relevant complementary practices and medical treatments to achieve the optimal health and healing of the whole person [62]. CT that promote physical activity, health-promoting diets, symptom management, and stress reduction enhance the wellness of the whole person by reestablishing balance and coherence among the biological systems of the mind and body, including the ANS [26, 29]. CT assist the body in regaining an optimal level of health and healing, which may be leveraged synergistically to help withstand and actively "fight" the disease alongside mainstream treatment.

Important core values of integrative medicine include comprehensive and compassionate care, tailored to the needs of the whole person [62]. Integrative practice is about promoting the wellness, health, and innate healing capabilities of the person while providing effective medical treatments. Interdisciplinary professional relationships are nonhierarchical, mutually respectful, and collaborative between complementary and medical practitioners, and between practitioners and the patient, who is welcomed as an equal "partner" in decisions about the treatment plan and care [63].

Combining complementary and medical treatments is in the early stages of clinical implementation. In fact, the practice of integrative medicine is still mainly a theoretical exercise, lacking scientific evidence [62, 64, 65]. Nonetheless, as a first phase, a few leading university-teaching hospitals have created affiliated wellness centers, usually off-site, in an acknowledgment of the potentially important role that CT may play in the health, healing, and well-being of patients. One such example is the Hope and Cope Wellness Center of the Jewish General Hospital of Montreal. Typically, patients from these hospitals and their family are welcome to participate in any of the health-promoting services being offered at the wellness center. For patients who are not on active treatment, the opportunity to make their own health-related selections is likely therapeutic in itself by enhancing their sense of personal control over decisions concerning their well-being.

Some hospital-based health care teams refer their patients to wellness centers for a specific medical purpose, such as reducing anxiety, increasing physical fitness, or learning how to make nourishing meals. In a few hospitals, dedicated complementary therapy teams respond to medical and nursing requests to see patients. However, the notion that the medical treating team would consist of relevant complementary as well as conventional practitioners is still a novel idea. At the Jewish General Hospital, the Cancer and Nutrition Rehabilitation program and, in particular, the newly established Peter Brojde Lung Cancer Center consist of health care teams that include TCM practitioners with expertise in Chinese herbs, acupuncture, and qigong, one of whom is also a physiotherapist as well as nurses acquiring training in reflexology, acupressure, deep relaxation techniques, and visualization.

A model of integrative medicine and whole person care can be useful in providing a framework for implementing and evaluating clinical programs. However, proposed models are only beginning to emerge in the literature with a current emphasis now on arriving at a consensus of key characteristics, structures, values, processes, and outcomes [62, 64, 65]. There are numerous structural and organizational issues that need to be sorted out to effectively shift to a new medical paradigm of practice in a hospital setting. For starters, there are multiple layers of "integration" to consider across clinical, research, educational, and administrative practices of a hospital that may have profound implications for the implementation of integrative medicine and whole patient care. Depending on the scope of practice, this paradigm shift will eventually impact professional associations, government policies, medical and other health-based university programs, as well as provincial and hospital budgets. These issues will need to be systematically addressed if integrative medicine is going to be the practice model of all health care professionals.

Of equal import is the need to change the research paradigm of evidence-based practice from a reductionist model to a more encompassing methodology that will more effectively capture the complexities of the whole person with an illness. As previously discussed, RCTs cannot account for the individualized, synergistic, and holistic effects of blended complementary and conventional treatments [63]. A mixed method approach combining quantitative and qualitative data, depending on the study objective, seems an appropriate approach to more fully represent the potential health and healing effects of an integrated intervention [6]. However, as pointed out by Leis and colleagues [63], what also needs to be considered is a whole systems research framework to evaluate the overall practice of integrative medicine in a clinical environment. There is much to do.

While there is scientific evidence of the health and healing benefits of many CT based on individual effects, knowledge about dosing, frequency, and the optimal blending of complementary modalities before, during, and after medical treatment is still lacking. Moreover, caring and treating the whole patient is extremely complex, more often than not, necessitating a multiple rather than single therapeutic approach. As the health care team acquires the scientific evidence to propose truly holistic and tailored treatments, it is likely to assume a blended and synergistic multimodal approach to the whole patient to intervene effectively at multiple psychosocial and biological targets.

Even so, there likely will continue to be differences in opinion between the health care team and the patient regarding the "best" CT to include in the treatment plan. In keeping with the values of integrative medicine, the patient's opinions must be respectfully and carefully addressed, keeping in mind that the beliefs and expectations that patients hold about their health may affect their healing capabilities. Those beliefs also may be influenced by the nature of the physician's and other health care provider relationships with the patient [11]. According to Benson [5], what the physician says and how he says it may be instrumental in either activating or deactivating the healing capabilities of the patient.

Thus, central to the practice of integrative medicine is the quality of the relationship between the patient and the health care provider. It is the health care provider who creates the therapeutic context within which the patient's healing capabilities may be supported. Thus, a therapeutic relationship is a healing relationship.

To be truly healing depends on the health care provider's ability to be open, nonjudgmental, sensitive, and, above all, fully present to the thoughts, feelings, behaviors, and attitudes of the person being treated/cared for [13, 59]. Being fully present means respecting the patient's beliefs about his or her health and healing, and including ideas about promoting wellness. It means finding ways to support the patient's personal capabilities, strengths, purpose, and innate healing capabilities within the current realities of his or her illness [13, 59].

In conclusion, integrative medicine strives to redress the shortcomings of the medical model by reestablishing a professional legacy that focuses on the whole person, not just the illness, by recognizing the centrality of the physician–patient relationship in facilitating the healing capabilities of the patient, and by acknowledging the value of optimizing the patient's wellness and treatment efficacy via a blended, evidence-based approach of relevant complementary and conventional treatments. In doing so, integrative medicine reaffirms comprehensive, compassionate, and individualized care and treatment as the basis of whole person care.

References

1. Cruse JM. History of medicine: the metamorphosis of scientific medicine in the ever-present past. Am J Med Sci. 1999;318(3):171–80.
2. Hardy ML. Dietary supplement use in cancer care: help or harm. Hematol Oncol Clin North Am. 2008;22(4):581–617, vii.
3. Gupta D, Lis CG, Birdsall TC, Grutsch JF. The use of dietary supplements in a community hospital comprehensive cancer center: implications for conventional cancer care. Supp Care Cancer. 2005;13(11):912–9.
4. Yates JS, Mustian KM, Morrow GR, et al. Prevalence of complementary and alternative medicine use in cancer patients during treatment. Supp Care Cancer. 2005;13(10):806–11.
5. Benson H. Timeless healing. New York, NY: Simon & Schuster; 1997.
6. Verhoef MJ, Leis A. From studying patient treatment to studying patient care: arriving at methodologic crossroads. Hematol Oncol Clin North Am. 2008;22(4):671–82, viii–ix.
7. Roberts A, Kewman D, Mercier L, Hovell M. The power of non-specific effects in healing: Implications for psychosocial and biological treatments. Clin Psychol Rev. 1993;13:375–91.

8. Butler C, Steptoe A. Placebo responses: an experimental study of psychophysiological processes in asthmatic volunteers. Br J Clin Psychol. 1986;25(Pt 3):173–83.

9. Benson H, McCallie Jr DP. Angina pectoris and the placebo effect. N Engl J Med. 1979;300(25):1424–9.

10. Horowitz R, Visoli L, Berkman R, et al. Treatment adherence and risk of death after myocardial infarction. Lancet. 1990;336:542–5.

11. Benson H, Friedman R. Harnessing the power of the placebo effect and renaming it 'remembered wellness'. Annu Rev Med. 1996;47:193–9.

12. NCCAM. What is CAM. National Center for Complementary and Alternative Medicine. http://nccam.nih.gov/health/whatiscam. Accessed 22 January 2010.

13. Erickson H. Modeling and role-modeling: a view from the client's world. Cedar Park, TX: Unicorns Unlimited; 2006.

14. Gottlieb L, Rowat K. The McGill model of nursing: a practice-derived model. ANS Adv Nurs Sci. 1987;9(4):51–61.

15. Erickson HL. Philosophy and theory of holism. Nurs Clin North Am. 2007;42(2):139–63, v.

16. Richardson MA, Masse LC, Nanny K, Sanders C. Discrepant views of oncologists and cancer patients on complementary/alternative medicine. Support Care Cancer. 2004;12(11):797–804.

17. Richardson MA, Sanders T, Palmer JL, Greisinger A, Singletary SE. Complementary/alternative medicine use in a comprehensive cancer center and the implications for oncology. J Clin Oncol. 2000;18(13):2505–14.

18. Miller P, Demark-Wahnefried W, Snyder DC, et al. Dietary supplement use among elderly, long-term cancer survivors. J Cancer Surviv. 2008;2(3):138–48.

19. Wells M, Sarna L, Cooley ME, et al. Use of complementary and alternative medicine therapies to control symptoms in women living with lung cancer. Cancer Nurs. 2007;30(1):45–55; quiz 56–47.

20. Velicer CM, Ulrich CM. Vitamin and mineral supplement use among US adults after cancer diagnosis: a systematic review. J Clin Oncol. 2008;26(4):665–73.

21. Shen J, Andersen R, Albert PS, et al. Use of complementary/alternative therapies by women with advanced-stage breast cancer. BMC Complement Altern Med. 2002;2:8.

22. Boon H, Stewart M, Kennard MA, et al. Use of complementary/alternative medicine by breast cancer survivors in Ontario: prevalence and perceptions. J Clin Oncol. 2000;18(13):2515–21.

23. Helyer LK, Chin S, Chui BK, et al. The use of complementary and alternative medicines among patients with locally advanced breast cancer – a descriptive study. BMC Cancer. 2006;6:39.

24. Beliveau R, Gingras D. Foods that fight cancer. Toronto, ON: McClelland & Stewart; 2006.

25. WCRF/AICR. Food, nutrition, physical activity, and the prevention of cancer: a global perspective. Washington, DC: World Cancer Research Fund/American Institute for Cancer Research; 2009.

26. Servan-Schreiber D. Anticancer. Toronto, ON: HarperCollins; 2008.

27. Aggarwal B, Ichikawa P, Garodia P, et al. From traditional Ayurvedic medicine to modern medicine: identification of therapeutic targets for suppressing inflammation and cancer. Expert Opin Ther Targets. 2006;10(1):87–118.

28. Block K. Nutritional interventions in cancer. In: Weil A, editor. Integrative oncology. New York, NY: Oxford University Press; 2009. p. 75–103.

29. Block KI. Nutritional interventions in cancer. In: Abrams DI, Weil AT, editors. Integrative oncology. New York, NY: Oxford University Press; 2009. p. 75–103.

30. Stevinson C, Courneya K. Physical activity and cancer. In: Weil A, editor. Integrative oncology. New York, NY: Oxford University Press; 2009. p. 215–31.

31. Colbert LH, Visser M, Simonsick EM, et al. Physical activity, exercise, and inflammatory markers in older adults: findings from the health, aging and body composition study. J Am Geriatr Soc. 2004;52(7):1098–104.

32. Chen K, Yeung R. Exploratory studies of Qigong therapy for cancer in China. Integr Cancer Ther. 2002;1(4):345–70.

33. Adamsen L, Quist M, Andersen C, et al. Effect of a multimodal high intensity exercise intervention in cancer patients undergoing chemotherapy: randomised controlled trial. BMJ. 2009;339:b3410.
34. Meyerhardt JA, Heseltine D, Niedzwiecki D, et al. Impact of physical activity on cancer recurrence and survival in patients with stage III colon cancer: findings from CALGB 89803. J Clin Oncol. 2006;24(22):3535–41.
35. Holmes MD, Chen WY, Feskanich D, Kroenke CH, Colditz GA. Physical activity and survival after breast cancer diagnosis. JAMA. 2005;293(20):2479–86.
36. Zahourek RP. Integrative holism in psychiatric-mental health nursing. J Psychosoc Nurs Ment Health Serv. 2008;46(10):31–7.
37. Cassileth BR, Deng GE, Gomez JE, Johnstone PA, Kumar N, Vickers AJ. Complementary therapies and integrative oncology in lung cancer: ACCP evidence-based clinical practice guidelines (2nd edition). Chest. 2007;132(3 Suppl):340S–54.
38. Coussens LM, Werb Z. Inflammation and cancer. Nature. 2002;420(6917):860–7.
39. Antoni MH, Lutgendorf SK, Cole SW, et al. The influence of bio-behavioural factors on tumour biology: pathways and mechanisms. Nat Rev Cancer. 2006;6(3):240–8.
40. Pert CB, Dreher HE, Ruff MR. The psychosomatic network: foundations of mind-body medicine. Altern Ther Health Med. 1998;4(4):30–41.
41. Gordon JS. Mind-body medicine and cancer. Hematol Oncol Clin North Am. 2008;22(4):683–708, ix.
42. Devine EC, Westlake SK. The effects of psychoeducational care provided to adults with cancer: meta-analysis of 116 studies. Oncol Nurs Forum. 1995;22(9):1369–81.
43. Speca M, Carlson LE, Goodey E, Angen M. A randomized, wait-list controlled clinical trial: the effect of a mindfulness meditation-based stress reduction program on mood and symptoms of stress in cancer outpatients. Psychosom Med. 2000;62(5):613–22.
44. Carlson LE, Bultz BD. Mind-body interventions in oncology. Curr Treat Options Oncol. 2008;9(2–3):127–34.
45. Thayer ZC, Johnson BW. Cerebral processes during visuo-motor imagery of hands. Psychophysiology. 2006;43(4):401–12.
46. Devine EB, Hakim Z, Green J. A systematic review of patient-reported outcome instruments measuring sleep dysfunction in adults. Pharmacoeconomics. 2005;23(9):889–912.
47. Dundee JW, Ghaly RG, Fitzpatrick KT, Abram WP, Lynch GA. Acupuncture prophylaxis of cancer chemotherapy-induced sickness. J R Soc Med. 1989;82(5):268–71.
48. Roscoe JA, Morrow GR, Hickok JT, et al. The efficacy of acupressure and acustimulation wrist bands for the relief of chemotherapy-induced nausea and vomiting. A University of Rochester Cancer Center Community Clinical Oncology Program multicenter study. J Pain Symptom Manage. 2003;26(2):731–42.
49. Alimi D, Rubino C, Pichard-Leandri E, Fermand-Brule S, Dubreuil-Lemaire ML, Hill C. Analgesic effect of auricular acupuncture for cancer pain: a randomized, blinded, controlled trial. J Clin Oncol. 2003;21(22):4120–6.
50. Wong R, Sagar S. Acupuncture treatment for chemotherapy-induced peripheral neuropathy – a case series. Acupunct Med. 2006;24(2):87–91.
51. Lu W, Hu D, Dean-Clower E, et al. Acupuncture for chemotherapy-induced leukopenia: exploratory meta-analysis of randomized controlled trials. J Soc Integr Oncol. Winter 2007;5(1):1–10.
52. Zhao X, Wang H, Cao D. Influence of acupuncture and moxibustion on serum CSF activity of patients with leukopenia caused by chemotherapy. Zhen Ci Yan Jiu. 1999;24(1):17–9.
53. Myers CD, Walton T, Small BJ. The value of massage therapy in cancer care. Hematol Oncol Clin North Am. 2008;22(4):649–60, viii.
54. Grealish L, Lomasney A, Whiteman B. Foot massage. A nursing intervention to modify the distressing symptoms of pain and nausea in patients hospitalized with cancer. Cancer Nurs. 2000;23(3):237–43.
55. Syrjala KL, Cummings C, Donaldson GW. Hypnosis or cognitive behavioral training for the reduction of pain and nausea during cancer treatment: a controlled clinical trial. Pain. 1992;48(2):137–46.

56. Manusirivithaya S, Sripramote M, Tangjitgamol S, et al. Antiemetic effect of ginger in gynecologic oncology patients receiving cisplatin. Int J Gynecol Cancer. 2004;14(6):1063–9.
57. Savarese DM, Savy G, Vahdat L, Wischmeyer PE, Corey B. Prevention of chemotherapy and radiation toxicity with glutamine. Cancer Treat Rev. 2003;29(6):501–13.
58. Cerchietti LC, Navigante AH, Castro MA. Effects of eicosapentaenoic and docosahexaenoic n-3 fatty acids from fish oil and preferential Cox-2 inhibition on systemic syndromes in patients with advanced lung cancer. Nutr Cancer. 2007;59(1):14–20.
59. Remen R. Tending the spirit in cancer. In: Abrams D, Weil AT, editors. Integrative oncology. New York, NY: Oxford University Press; 2009. p. 384–95.
60. Stefanek M, McDonald PG, Hess S. Religion, spirituality and cancer: current status and methodological challenges. Psychooncology. 2004;14:450–63.
61. Brady M, Peterman A, Fitchett G, Mo M, Cella D. Case for including spirituality in quality of life measurement in oncology. Psychooncology. 1999;8:417–28.
62. Frenkel M, Cohen L. Incorporating complementary and integrative medicine in a comprehensive cancer center. Hematol Oncol Clin North Am. 2008;22:727–36.
63. Leis AM, Weeks LC, Verhoef MJ. Principles to guide integrative oncology and the development of an evidence base. Curr Oncol. 2008;15 Suppl 2:s83–7.
64. Boon H, Verhoef M, O'Hara D, Findlay B. From parallel practice to integrative health care: a conceptual framework. BMC Health Serv Res. 2004;4(1):15.
65. Geffen JR. Integrative oncology for the whole person: a multidimensional approach to cancer care. Integr Cancer Ther. 2010;9(1):105–21.

Chapter 13
Spiritual Dimensions of Whole Person Care

Abdu'l-Missagh Ghadirian

> *Nothing in life is more wonderful than faith – the one great moving force which we can neither weigh in the balance nor test in the crucible … Faith has always been an essential factor in the practice of medicine.*
>
> William Osler [1]

Keywords Spirituality • Values • Personhood • Medical education • Prayers • Suffering • Compassion • Death • Beliefs • Healing

Spirituality is an essential ingredient of whole person care. Although its role in health and healing is often neglected, spirituality is increasingly recognized for its relevance to personhood and creating a caring relationship with patients. As a result, its role in medical education has been emphasized to address the concerns of sick people, particularly those with life-threatening diseases, and those with diseases that affect quality of life (QOL). This chapter aims to outline the ways in which spirituality plays a role in whole person care.

Neglect of the Spiritual Dimension in Medicine

Throughout history, the healing profession has embraced the concept of mind–body and soul. In the ancient world, temples were not only places for worship but also centers for the healing of those who suffered from visible and invisible wounds of body and mind. In Middle Eastern and oriental countries, spiritual mindfulness was

A.-M. Ghadirian (✉)
Professor, Department of Psychiatry, McGill University, 1025 Pine Avenue West,
Montreal, QC H3A 1A1, Canada
e-mail: amghadirian@gmail.com

T.A. Hutchinson (ed.), *Whole Person Care: A New Paradigm for the 21st Century*,
DOI 10.1007/978-1-4419-9440-0_13, © Springer Science+Business Media, LLC 2011

one of the characteristics of scholars of science and medicine. This is exemplified by the life and work of great scholars such as Avicenna and Razi.

In the West, with the rise of industrialization, technology, and science, remarkable progress has been made in the advancement of medicine. However, the growth of a materialistic view of life that has sprung up in conjunction with the advancement of science has tended to create a divide between spirituality and medicine. Descartes in his work Treatise of Man viewed the body as a machine [2].

The view of Freud and his works such as "Civilization and Its Discontent" [3] have created doubts and skepticism with regard to spirituality/religion. Many psychiatrists, psychologists, as well as other health professionals, seem to have distanced themselves from spiritual matters in academic and clinical debates. As scientific and technological advancements were not complemented by greater acknowledgement of the important role of spirituality in the healing of patients, health sciences were not adequately equipped to address the needs of whole person care in a comprehensive way. Rosen stated, "[M]odern medicine seems to have lost sight of the art, the spirit, and the intangibles such as faith, hope and compassion that are essential to the healing process" [4].

Interest in reintegrating spirituality with medicine has begun to emerge during the past twenty years in North America [5]. Extensive research studies in recent years have demonstrated the positive and beneficial effects of spirituality on health, recovery from illness, QOL, palliative care, and other fields of medicine [6].

Obstacles to Spirituality in Medical Practice

However, the subject of spirituality is often avoided because of the following three major factors, which adversely influence physicians' pursuit of spirituality in their medical practice. One is scientific reductionism, which denies the existence of the transcendent and thus the spiritual nature of human reality. The second is a negative public impression of and attitude toward religion and spiritual beliefs due to critical publicity surrounding some organized religious institutions. This reinforces the denial of religion/spirituality as a viable phenomenon of humanity. The third is the industrialization of medicine, which reduces it to an economic enterprise, primarily concerned with efficiency and financial gain rather than the provision of compassionate care and treatment of the whole person. Put succinctly, "changes in health care are placing us under increasing pressure to become only physicians of the body and to abandon our responsibilities for the mind and soul ... The current health care system is globally insensitive to the psyche of patients, whatever the infirmities of their bodies ..." [7] These troubling developments in contemporary health care suggest the need to rethink the true goal of medicine with respect to saving lives and alleviating suffering. As Sulmasy stated, "no amount of scientific or economic transformation can alter the fundamental meaning and value of health care, nor can it ever eradicate the interpersonal nature of the healing relationship that begins when one person feels ill, and another highly skilled and socially authorized asks 'How can I help you?'" [8], demonstrating the original meaning of the word "psychiatry": physician/healer of the soul.

Spirituality and Healing

Spirituality is poorly understood and often avoided in the psychiatric and medical community. The word spirit is from the Latin word "spiritus" or breath and animating principle. One aspect of spirituality refers to the development of the capacity to acquire a deeper understanding of the purpose of life. Spirit is the inner reality of human beings, a nonmaterial entity that connects a material and mortal entity such as the human body to a universal transcendental power. Moreover, physical health and spiritual health are interconnected. In holistic terms, being healthy is a state of well-being of mind, body, and soul.

Healing is the art of restoration of hope and wholeness, and a healthy life goes beyond absence of disease. Some patients in palliative care and those near the end of life are overcome by a sense of hopelessness, which is not always characterized by other symptoms of clinical depression. The body may be perceived as an object that increasingly loses its meaning, and these patients may express the desire for hastened death. This strong feeling may be associated with loss of dignity and self-worth, which leads to demoralization. Demoralization is common among patients suffering from chronic medical illnesses and those with serious disabilities or who are terminally ill. It is a state of hopelessness, helplessness, existential despair, and meaninglessness, which arise from a feeling of being "trapped" and a desire to die [9]. Restoration of morale is vital in therapy.

Although science is able to alleviate physical pain and discomfort, it has limitations with respect to the meaning of life and the end-of-life experience. But spirituality can not only give meaning to this final stage of life but may also give a sense of hope, whatever the hope may be for the individual. This could be a specific belief that the journey of life goes beyond physical death or a more general trust or faith in life whatever the future may bring. One may perceive spirituality as a personalized feature of faith and religion as a structured and institutionalized expression of faith [6].

Prayer and Spirituality

One expression of faith is prayer. Prayer for the sick is the oldest means of alleviating anguish and suffering and is an assistance to recovery and healing used worldwide. However, it does not minimize or replace conventional treatment. In secular cultures, it may be difficult to comprehend the role of a nonmedical approach such as prayer in the healing process. Yet, there is increasing interest in the exploration of nonmaterial or nonphysical treatment as an alternative to traditional treatment. Among the 10 most frequent alternative medical procedures used in USA are prayers for oneself and for others (intercessory prayer).

Herbert Benson from Harvard University holds that prayer operates in the same way as a relaxation response [10]. It is believed that prayer can affect stress hormones, resulting in lower blood pressure and a moderation of pulse and respiration.

These are physiological findings that may not necessarily be related to prayer per se; however, the power of prayer goes beyond the physiological changes for healing the illness. Belief in the effect of prayer in health or illness was and still is taken as a matter of faith by many and traditionally did not require scientific confirmation of proof for efficacy as the majority of patients were and most still are religious people. A Gallup poll of American adults showed that 94% of them had a belief in God or a universal spirit. Among those surveyed, 87% admitted that religion was important in their lives. Many of those interviewed reported that they turned to prayer for assistance in overcoming disease. In another American study, 76% of those questioned professed that they prayed daily. Many said that they turned to prayer for assistance to overcome their disease, even though they tended to avoid direct affiliation with a religion [11].

Spirituality and Personhood

The term personhood reflects a holistic view of a person as well as a state or condition that encompasses an individual's essential meaning. Patients' beliefs and values are expressions of personhood that play a role in the treatment process and caring relationship. Personhood is not static, but is rather an evolving phenomenon that develops through life experiences. Likewise, the meaning of our life can change from day to day as we evolve. Mount stated "Our lives are shaped not by momentous events and huge crossroad decisions but by the thousands of little decisions that occur each day ... each of the little daily decisions shapes our lives to a greater extent than we may think" [12].

Maslow identified a hierarchy of needs that begin with basic biological requirements and end in self-actualization, which is the fulfillment of a human being's highest aspirations [13]. Spirituality is related to self-actualization and fulfillment of intrinsic values. The role of the physician as a healer is to facilitate this self-fulfillment through helping the patient to draw meaning from his or her suffering. Observation as well as research in the literature shows an important relationship between spirituality and well-being [14], which may have a nurturing effect in the development of personhood. It has been reported that spiritual well-being offers some protection against despair in those nearing the end of life [15]. Indeed, spiritual issues "lie at the very centre of the existential crisis that is terminal illness" [16]. This further underlines the role of a spiritual perspective in whole person care and in alleviating human suffering and despair.

Spiritual insight into a tragic event such as the death of a loved one may give new meaning to that event, possibly alleviating some of the grief. The following anecdote is a case in point. A mother asked a great spiritual sage to see her sick child because the efforts of doctors had yielded no results and the child was gravely ill. He came and brought two roses for the little girl as he visited her. Then, turning to her mother with a voice full of love told her that she must be patient. That evening, the child passed away. The mother was devastated and asked the wise man why this had happened.

He explained that the world of humanity is like a garden and the Creator is its Gardener. Human beings are like trees that grow in that garden. "When the Gardener sees a little tree in a place which is too small for its development, He prepares a suitable and more beautiful place where it may grow and bear fruit. Then He transplants that little tree. The other trees are surprised and say, 'This was a lovely tree. Why did the Gardener uproot it'? Only the Divine Gardener knows the reason. You are weeping, but if you could see the beauty of the place where your child is, you would no longer be sad…If you could see that sacred garden yourself, you would not be content to remain here on earth. Yet, this is where your duty now lies" [17]. This spiritual perspective on the meaning of death and the life after gave that mother, who was open to this perspective, a new vision of understanding that eased her sorrow.

Spirituality and intrinsic values are interrelated and reflect the essence of personhood in whole person care. In today's society, we need to reassess our concept of values to reach a deeper understanding of the meaning of life and its purpose. Intrinsic and personal values guide and propel individuals to fulfill their potential. These values are developed and nurtured through education, culture, and beliefs. According to Maslow, "human life will never be understood unless its highest aspirations are taken into account" [13]. Therefore, personal growth, self-actualization, and striving toward achieving a psychosocial and spiritual perspective on life are part of a universal human quest for fulfillment.

Spirituality and Medical Education

Since the 1990s, there has been an upsurge of educational programs in the curricula of medical schools in North America to familiarize physicians with the spiritual dimensions of health and healing [18]. A growing number of medical schools across USA have been offering courses on religion and spirituality in medicine and patient care. In 1994, only 17 of the 126 accredited medical schools in the country offered courses on spirituality as part of their medical education. By 1998, this number had increased to 39 [5]. By 2004, it had risen to 84 schools. Presently, 100 of the 150 US medical schools teach spirituality in medicine courses [18]. More than 75% of American medical schools teach subjects related to spirituality and health. Likewise, hospitals are initiating spirituality programs to promote compassionate care for their patients [14]. The Faculty of Medicine at McGill University was one of the first in Canada to introduce formal courses in the curriculum on spirituality and medicine. During the past ten years, there have been two courses on this subject: one, a required introductory course for first-year medical students, and the other, a comprehensive 4-week elective course on spirituality and ethics in medicine for the fourth-year medical students. Both have been well received, the students finding the courses to have contributed to their knowledge of the spiritual dimension of medicine.

In recent years, taking a spiritual history has been included in the spirituality courses of many medical schools. This may allow clinicians to have a broader understanding of their patients with different religious backgrounds. Spirituality in this context has a wide meaning. It may be perceived as transcendent experience that is often expressed as a relationship with God, but it may also have other meanings. Puchalski and Romer suggested that spirituality is whatever beliefs and values that give a sense of meaning and purpose to life [19]. Factors that may have contributed to integrating spirituality into medical education were a greater awareness of the role of spirituality in healing and a growing number of patients, especially in USA, who wanted to share their spiritual concerns with their physicians as they sought medical treatment.

Spiritual Needs and Concerns

An increasing number of patients, especially those with chronic or life-threatening diseases, come to physicians with spiritual needs and concerns to be answered. Serious illnesses and near-end-of-life conditions provoke questions about mortality, the purpose of life, the meaning of suffering, and whether there is a greater power and life beyond death. For many of these people, religious beliefs form a basis for understanding the mystery of death and the role of prayer in life-threatening situations. Fear of the unknown often leads to disturbing questions that call for understanding and comfort by those who have assumed the role of physicians as healers. Accepting the will of God is an experience commonly observed in those who have spiritual perspective near the end of life. In light of the fact that almost 90% of the world's population is reported to be involved in some form of religious practice [20], spiritual concerns of the patient population have worldwide implications in the work of medical and other health professionals.

In a study of hundreds of patients with advanced lung cancer, it was noted that when patients wanted to decide between different treatment options, their faith in God seems to have played an important part in making a decision, ranked second only to the recommendation of the medical oncologist. Conversely, their physicians thought that their patients' faith in God should rank as the least important factor to consider in their decision about treatment [21]. This underlines the importance of being mindful of patients' beliefs to make it easier for us to find a common ground for whole person care.

Spiritual/religious needs may vary across different cultures. These may include the need to be loved and remembered, to maintain personal dignity, to pray and to be loved by God, to have faith in the Creator and in the wisdom of suffering, to recognize the purpose of life, to be known to have lived a worthy and fulfilled life, to be reconciled to life challenges, to be forgiven, and to be obedient to religious principles. Patients may wish to discuss these and other needs with their caregivers and friends who can listen without being judgemental. They may want to have a safe environment where they can share some very personal thoughts of their lives. Such care may serve to fulfill real needs of the patient and is part of the healing process.

Among spiritual concerns are questions such as "Why do I have this disease?" Is it a punishment for sins of disobedience to God? "Why as a devoted believer should I suffer?" "Is there life after death?" Some terminally ill patients have a fear of dying and they wonder how to face the unknown, invisible world. Some view their imminent death as a liberation from suffering, like a bird being released from its cage. Others may wonder if death will be like a new birth into another world and if they will need to start learning again about the mystery of another world. Some may be tormented with thoughts of punishment by God for their misdeeds and transgressions. In patients with a history of mental disorder, this fear can be highly exaggerated and disturbing. Other patients who have faith in a merciful Creator may submit their will to God's and be content with whatever their destiny will be. Therefore, this point of transition can evoke a range of emotions, from fear and anxiety to transcendence with quiet and calm submission to a greater power. This is the domain of the spiritual world on which sacred writings have shed some light.

Spiritual beliefs may provide an existential framework through which grief is rapidly resolved. In a 14-month follow-up study of a population after the death of a loved one, the survivors and friends who had a stronger spiritual belief seemed to overcome their grief more rapidly and adequately as compared to those who had no spiritual belief [22].

In dealing with suffering due to life crises and disease, a spiritual outlook can be invaluable. In recent years, I have been in contact with a number of individuals who have gone through major crises in their lives. Among them were those who suffered from cancer. Some have risen above their pain and limitations, demonstrating a unique spirit of faith and resilience that surprised even their family and friends. Among them was a mother of two children who, at age 42 and at the height of her career, was diagnosed with breast cancer. She was devastated by this horrible news and could not believe what was happening to her. The surgeon advised a radical mastectomy to prevent relapse. After the surgical operation and chemotherapy, instead of feeling defeated or shattered, she decided to make a change in her life by becoming closer to her family and living life to the fullest. She wanted to discover her true purpose in life and move from resignation to affirmation.

A few years later, as she was recovering, she and two other cancer survivors created a support group called Hope to help and empower women cancer patients to see "the bright side of life." Her fear of dying was transformed into a celebration of life. Their Hope retreat became a success, attracting and inspiring many other cancer survivors.

After this organization was in existence for a few years, she and her coworkers received an award of distinction for their outstanding contribution in helping cancer patients to live with hope and to have a better QOL. About 10 years after her first cancer was diagnosed, she was shocked to learn that her cancer had returned in another form. She went through radiation treatment and persevered with faith and hope. Again, she recovered and was happy to resume the Hope project and become very active in promoting hope for cancer survivors. Her group won an award of recognition in the category "Health, Well-Being and Spirituality." This was another confirmation of her creative resilience helping others to fulfill their potential to the best of their ability. Unfortunately, a few years later further complications and metastasis revisited her, but her spirit remained unshaken.

In a letter she wrote that after 23 years of cancer and its challenges, she still tries to never give up hope and to be positive. Even though she had stage 4 cancer, she still responds to invitations from the College of Medicine in Saskatchewan to speak with medical and nursing students, telling them about the importance of hope in cancer patients.

In 2009, she wrote and published a book about her life and struggle with cancer called "A Rose Grows – Fighting Cancer, Finding Me." Like project Hope, her book became another source of inspiration that encouraged scores of cancer survivors to strive for a meaningful life. She wrote, "Cancer gave me a chance to become who I was really meant to be....There was a purpose in facing the challenges I faced. I have learned so much through my experience." She discovered what she was capable of after enduring cancer. Believing in spiritual strength she wrote "This was God's way of redirecting my life and making me see what life is really all about … and I will eternally be grateful for this journey" [23].

Her story shows how suffering can inspire people to pursue a creative life and to fulfill their latent potential and capacity of which they may not be aware. It also reflects how one can remain grateful for what one learns from adversity.

An illness can have different meanings: personal, social, and cultural. It can also have different meanings to the same person at different stages of life or in different circumstances. Our sociocultural beliefs about disease influence our perception of and attitude toward it. For example in some cultures, people's attitudes toward patients suffering from AIDS or mental illness are charged with negativism, stigma, and discrimination. On the contrary, a sickness can consume a patient's attention and like a sponge soak up his/her personal and social importance if there is no reliance on other forces of life that would give a deeper vision of meaning and purpose of creation [24]. Awareness of this dynamic may help a therapist to recognize the value of the patient as a whole person. Reflecting on the spiritual reality of the patient will make it easier for the physician to accept the patient unconditionally and to honour the essence of personhood within the person.

Spiritual Perspective on Death

Expectation for recovery and cure is not the only hope that seriously ill patients cherish. When cure is no longer possible, some patients reflect and hope that there will not be undue pain and suffering or that they will not be left abandoned. They strive to draw meaning from life crises and possibly to enjoy whatever time they have left with family and loved ones. They expect to be remembered by relatives and friends after death. During the near-end-of-life period, a sense of hopelessness and loss of meaning may precipitate depression. But for those who have found a spiritual perspective on life and its ultimate destiny, there is less likelihood of total despair and hopelessness. They may believe that the soul is not affected by physical and biological infirmities generated by disease, and therefore, they may be more prepared to let go. Death may be perceived as a transition to another world as was birth a transition into this world. They may envisage the journey of life as an organic process moving from one stage of growth to another and death as a gate to a new beginning. Death may also be viewed in the context of the evolution of the soul, leaving behind the physical frame as its vehicle while continuing its journey in a spiritual world. A metaphor that may be helpful to some people is the relationship between the computer (body) and the programmer (soul). The programmer, although closely associated with the computer, is not part of it and has a life of his own [25]. As the human soul or spirit is not a material entity, it is believed to be eternal and independent from the body. But human spirit is fully aware of the condition of the body, which is its instrument, just as the programmer is aware of the condition of the computer.

Viktor Frankl believed that traditional psychotherapy, which aimed at restoring one's capacity to work and enjoy life, was not sufficient and it should also include enabling the patient to regain his/her capacity to accept unavoidable suffering and to discover a meaning in it. "Man's main concern is not to gain pleasure or to avoid pain, but rather to see a meaning in his life" [26]. Frankl wrote about his interview with an elderly general practitioner who came to his office for treatment of a severe depression. He told Dr. Frankl that his depression began after the loss of his wife whom he loved dearly and who had died two years earlier. Dr. Frankl wondered how he could help this man and asked him the following question: "What would have happened, Doctor, if you had died first, and your wife would have had to survive you?" The man replied that this would have been terrible because his wife would have suffered so much. Then, Dr. Frankl commented, "You see, Doctor, such a suffering has been spared her, and it is you who have spared her this suffering, but now, you have to pay for it by surviving and mourning her" [26]. This explanation comforted and satisfied the patient because it gave a meaning to the tragic loss of his wife, which was consuming his mood and mind. Dr. Frankl wrote, "Suffering ceases to be suffering in some way at the moment it finds a meaning, such as the meaning of a sacrifice" [26].

When patients are valued as no more than physical entities, a disabling illness brings an end to their productivity and usefulness. In such an environment, patients are also deprived of the spiritual dimension of the therapeutic relationship and feel as though they are being treated like an object that is no longer of any value for society. This adds to patients' feeling of guilt for being a burden to family and friends. Living a life judged to be unproductive, sick, and useless is a recipe for hopelessness and self-destruction. Such patients may ask distressful questions such as what am I living for? What is the purpose or meaning of merely surviving? What is my value in a world immersed in selfish materialism? When I am disabled and no longer functional, what am I good for? These questions may lead to an impression that the physical body is a broken machine, a commodity or a product to be discarded if one so wishes. Such a pessimistic view becomes fertile ground for seeking out euthanasia or suicide. A spiritual perspective on life as a process of acquiring the capacity to learn from life struggles with faith and resilience gives a sense of hope to rise above limitations and to accept what cannot be changed.

Spirituality and Quality of Life

Although the QOL of individuals has been the subject of extensive studies, the spiritual dimension of that quality has not been explored as much as it deserves to be. This is partly because conducting research on spirituality is very complex, since it is concerned with the inner realm of human consciousness. Science has its limits with respect to exploring certain qualities that are not of a material nature such as the intrinsic values of an individual, the purpose and ultimate meaning in life, and the QOL based on personal values. These are issues that are deeply embedded in human consciousness and are influenced by spirituality.

In spite of the dearth of material on this subject and the complexity of studying it, there is a growing body of research findings and published reports on spirituality and QOL that suggest that spirituality and a better QOL are interrelated [6]. The US National Institutes of Health reported that in a study of population health, a 25% lower mortality rate was noted in those who attended religious services at least once a week. Some features of these services included meditation, social networking, and values that would discourage risky and unhealthy behaviour such as substance abuse, violence, and infidelity [6]. In addition, spiritual support and mindfulness enhanced coping skills in the face of anxiety and depression in believers.

In another study on international university students, it was noted that spirituality/religion was significantly correlated with psychological aspects of QOL. It was furthermore noted that spirituality/religion contributes to the development of the coping mechanisms of these students in dealing with cultural stressors [27]. However, the relationship between religiosity and QOL requires further exploration.

Spirituality not only influences QOL of individuals but also impacts quality of care and attitude of health professionals toward patients. In a large-scale survey on this subject, individuals were asked if they were to need treatment for cancer, what were the most important characteristics they would like to see in their treating physicians. A large majority of these individuals stated that it would be most important for them to have a doctor who would care about them, would recognize them as a person, and would be "spiritually attuned" to them. They valued these qualities more than technical medical expertise. This finding further supports the role of attitude and empathy in the doctor–patient relationship, especially at a time when patients face grave and life-threatening disease [28].

Conclusion

In conclusion, this chapter explores the importance of a spiritual perspective and intrinsic values in whole person care. Integrating spirituality into the mainstream of health sciences remains a challenge. This is partly because of misconceptions regarding spirituality among a large number of health professionals as well as the complexity of defining an abstract phenomenon such as spirituality. Nevertheless, there are a growing number of research studies and clinical observations that support the need for a role and implication of spirituality in addressing the well-being and QOL of patients [29]. Moreover, there are encouraging signs suggesting that science and spirituality could have complementary roles in enabling health professionals to have a more comprehensive approach to whole person care in society.

References

1. Osler W. The faith that heals. Br Med J. 1910;1910:1470.
2. Garber D (1998, 2003). Descartes, René. In Craig E, editor. Routledge encyclopedia of philosophy. London: Routledge. http://www.rep.routledge.com/article/DA026. Accessed 24 Nov 2010.
3. Freud S. Civilization and its discontent. New York, NY: W.W. Norton; 1961.
4. Rosen DH. Modern medicine and the healing process. Humane Med. 1989;5:18–23.
5. Puchalski CM, Larson DB. Developing curricula in spirituality and medicine. Acad Med. 1998;73:970–4.
6. Peterson M, Webb D. Religion and spirituality in quality of life studies. Appl Res Qual Life. 2006;1:107–16.
7. Andreasen NA. Body and soul. Am J Psychiatry. 1996;153(5):549.
8. Sulmasy DP. Is medicine a spiritual practice? Acad Med. 1999;74:1002–5.
9. Kissane DW, Clarke DM, Street AF. Demoralization syndrome – a relevant psychiatric diagnosis for palliative care. J Palliat Care. 2001;17(1):12–21.
10. Benson H, Stark M. The power and biology of belief. New York, NY: Simon & Schuster; 1997.
11. O'Hara DP. Is there a role for prayer and spirituality in health care? Med Clin North Am. 2002;86(1):33–46.
12. Mount B. Nurturing your personhood: a message for 1986 graduates. CMAJ. 1986;135:291–3.
13. Maslow AH. Motivation and personality. New York, NY: Harper; 1954.
14. Puchalski CM. Physicians and patients' spirituality. Ethical concerns and boundaries in spirituality and health. Virt Mentor. 2009;11(10):804–15.
15. McClain CS, Rosenfeld B, Breitbart W. Effects of spiritual well-being on end-of-life despair in terminally-ill cancer patients. Lancet. 2003;361:1603–7.
16. Kearney M, Mount B. Spiritual care of the dying patient. In: Chochinov H, Breitbart W, editors. Handbook of psychiatry in palliative medicine. New York, NY: Oxford University Press; 2000. p. 357–73.
17. Faizi G. Stories about Abdu'l-Baha. New Delhi: Baha'i Publishing Trust; 1981. p. 12.
18. LoboPrabhu S, Lomax J. The role of spirituality in medical school and psychiatry residency education. Int J Appl Psychoanal Stud. 2010;7(2):180–92.
19. Puchalski C, Romer A. Taking a spiritual history allows clinicians to understand patients more fully. J Palliat Med. 2000;3(1):129–37.
20. Koenig HG. Research on religion, spirituality, and mental health: a review. Can J Psychiatry. 2009;54(5):283–91.
21. Silvestri GA, Knittig S, Zoller J, Nietert PJ. Importance of faith on medical decisions regarding cancer care. J Clin Oncol. 2003;21:1379–82.
22. Walsh K, King M, Jones L, Tookman A, Blizard R. Spiritual beliefs may affect outcome of bereavement: prospective study. Br Med J. 2002;342:3.
23. Stefaniuk O. A rose grows – fighting cancer, finding me. Regina, SK: Your Nickel's Worth Publishing; 2009.

24. Kleinman A. The illness narratives: suffering, healing and the human condition. New York, NY: Basic Books; 1988. p. 31–2.
25. Ghadirian A-M. Creative dimensions of suffering. Wilmette, IL: Baha'i Publishing; 2009.
26. Frankl V. Man's search for meaning. 3rd ed. New York, NY: Pocket Books; 1975. p. 178–9.
27. Hsien-Chuan Hsu P, Krägeloh C, Shepherd D, Billington R. Religion/spirituality and quality of life of international tertiary students in New Zealand: an exploratory study. Ment Health Relig Cult. 2009;12(4):385–99.
28. Breitbart W. Spirituality and meaning in cancer. Rev Francoph Psycho-Oncologie. 2005;4: 237–40.
29. Ghadirian A-M. Is spirituality relevant to the practice of medicine? Med Law. 2008;27: 229–39.

Chapter 14
Whole Person Care and the Revolution in Genetics

David S. Rosenblatt and Jennifer Fitzpatrick

Keywords Genetics • Medical genetics • Genetic counseling • Genetic testing • Pharmacogenomics • GWAS (genome-wide association studies) • Choice • Prevention • PKU • Down syndrome • *BRCA* • Huntington disease

Setting the Stage

Barton Childs, the great medical geneticist and teacher, provides a perspective on the role of genetics in medicine when he contrasts the approaches of two of the giants of medicine, William Osler and Archibald Garrod, both of whom held the position of regius professor of medicine at Oxford. Whereas the Oslerian world was one of a body ravaged by disease, the one that of Garrod was of an organism in balance with its environment. An individual with a given genetic endowment interacted with the environment to maintain or perturb homeostasis [1].

Physicians, who have been largely educated by teachers immersed in the Oslerian model, often speak to their patients with metaphors that reflect this model of medicine. They will say, "You are like a broken car and we have (do not have) the tools to fix it." We have had friends who were offended by the reference to a loved one as a car! However, the metaphor fits the approach of many doctors; their patients are broken and it is their job to fix them. All efforts point to the finding of the cure. There are some areas, such as trauma, where the metaphor works to a certain extent, but even there the response to therapy is more than about good mechanics.

The Garrodian model of medicine understands that an organism is born with a set of genetic traits, and this is the basis of their variability. The environment in the form of diet, pathogens, drugs, and even behaviors and beliefs will interact with this genetic endowment. Not only must the physician seek to understand the proximate cause of the illness and find a treatment or, better still, a cure but he should also

J. Fitzpatrick (✉)
Director, Program, Department of Human Genetics, McGill University, Room N5-13, Stewart Biology Building, 1205 Dr Penfield Avenue, Montreal, QC H3A 1B1, Canada
e-mail: jennifer.fitzpatrick@mcgill.ca

T.A. Hutchinson (ed.), *Whole Person Care: A New Paradigm for the 21st Century*,
DOI 10.1007/978-1-4419-9440-0_14, © Springer Science+Business Media, LLC 2011

seek to understand the ethical and humanistic dimensions of the illness that are relevant to its etiology and essential to good management. The Garrodian model provides a good metaphor for whole person care in that the patient is not treated in isolation, as a broken machine that needs repair, but as one whose disease emerged as the result of a network of influencing factors, both familial and environmental and, hence, one whose medical care will necessarily include all of the dimensions of his family, social, ethical, and religious network.

Medical Genetics and Genetic Counseling

Medical genetics deals with patients across the life span. In the prenatal setting, women and their partners present for risk assessment, diagnosis, and counseling when a fetus is found to have a structural anomaly on ultrasound, when a screening test reveals an elevated risk for a fetal chromosome abnormality such as Down syndrome or trisomy 18, when there has been an exposure to a teratogenic agent such as drugs or alcohol, maternal medication, or maternal disease, and when there is a family history of a birth defect or genetic condition for which the parents or their physicians are concerned. Couples may also be seen in the context of infertility or multiple spontaneous abortions. In pediatrics, patients are referred for diagnosis of an inborn error of metabolism, chromosome abnormality, dysmorphism, blindness, deafness, and a wide variety of other conditions that present in infancy and childhood. Finally, adults are referred for testing for adult-onset disorders or disorders with a single-gene etiology present in the family. A great number of patients are now seen in cancer genetics clinics, commonly for presymptomatic testing for *BRCA1* and *2* – genes associated with a high lifetime risk of breast and ovarian cancer. It is obvious that each of these indications for referral could be associated with a high level of anxiety, burden, and/or grief for the family.

In 1974, Dr. F. Clarke Fraser, Canada's first medical geneticist, chaired a committee of the American Society of Human Genetics that was charged with creating a formal definition of genetic counseling. The following definition was subsequently adopted by the Society.

> Genetic counseling is a communication process which deals with the human problems associated with the occurrence, or the risk of occurrence, of a genetic disorder in a family. This process involves an attempt by one or more appropriately trained persons to help the individual or family (1) comprehend the medical facts, including the diagnosis, the probable course of the disorder, and the available management; (2) appreciate the way heredity contributes to the disorder, and the risk of recurrence in specified relatives; (3) understand the options for dealing with the risk of recurrence; (4) choose the course of action which seems appropriate to them in view of their risk and their family goals and act in accordance with that decision; and (5) make the best possible adjustment to the disorder in an affected family member and/or to the risk of recurrence of that disorder [2].

Most in the field of medical genetics agree that this definition still captures the most important elements of the process. Chiefly, first, it highlights the *two-way* nature of the physician–patient interaction, recognizing that diagnosing and treating patients in medical genetics is as much about *listening* to the patients' concerns as about teaching and explaining the recurrence risks, prognosis, and treatment modalities. Second, the definition also highlights the fact that genetic counseling is a *process* of gradual adjustment to new and sometimes devastating information on the family's part and to the changing needs and priorities of the family from the care providers' perspective. Third, Fraser's description includes the important ethical principle of *autonomy*, drawing attention to the fact that with any given diagnosis or list of reproductive or treatment options, patient decisions will be different and that the "right" decision for one patient could be the wrong decision for another. Lastly, the description recognizes that the potential impact of a genetic or possibly genetic diagnosis on a family necessitates a psychotherapeutic component.

Care in medical genetics has evolved to be provided by a multidisciplinary team of health professionals led by physicians, who are often but not always medical geneticists, and which includes genetic counselors, genetics nurses, dieticians, psychologists, and social workers, according to the setting. Given the multidisciplinary nature of care, and the longstanding focus on the psychosocial needs of patients, we posit that medical genetics has been, since its inception, whole person care. In the following pages, we relate a number of examples from clinical practice that illustrate the ways in which medical genetic practice, then and now, can be used as a model for the delivery of whole person care in any specialty.

Medical Genetics in Practice

The broad scope, multiplicity of goals, and dynamic nature of genetic counseling cannot necessarily be captured neatly in a series of steps or stages. However, the process can be loosely described as including a small number of key elements. Similar to Robert Buckman's [3] model and the "SPIKES" series of steps [4] for delivering bad news, the following can be considered as a *Roadmap for Genetic Counseling*.

1. Make a contract – establish mutual goals for the session
2. Assess patients' readiness for results
3. Perform risk assessment, evaluation, and/or diagnosis
4. Give results with sensitivity
5. Care for the patient's emotional reactions – accept and respond appropriately

Steps 1–5 may be repeated as new issues arise.

Although a brief time-limited activity such as breaking bad news is amenable to a protocol that can easily be remembered and implemented under stressful conditions, the *Roadmap for Genetic Counseling* is best understood as representing overlapping elements of the process that may occur at various times and not necessarily in an ordered series of steps. In the spirit of Elizabeth Kubler-Ross' [5] model of the stages of grief, the *Roadmap* provides a helpful "handle" for understanding the elements of the process, as long as it is taken as a model and not as a protocol.

1. Make a contract

In any genetic setting, the most important and first step in a consultation is to clarify the patients' expectations and goals for the session. To borrow a term from the counseling field, this is known as *contracting*. Without taking the time for this step, the assessment and information provided may not fully meet the patient's needs.

Maryse was a 21-year-old woman with cystic fibrosis (CF) who was 10 weeks pregnant. She was referred to Medical Genetics by her obstetrician for genetic counseling regarding the risk to her fetus. CF is a common disease among people of Northern European descent. There is a wide range of severity, but the salient clinical features are repeated respiratory infections and pancreatic insufficiency, and the average life span is 37.4 years [6]. CF is inherited in an autosomal recessive manner. An affected person will necessarily have inherited a faulty copy of the causative gene from each parent.

The genetic counseling student began the session with Maryse by reviewing the histories. She established that the patient's disease was relatively mild and well managed and that this was her first pregnancy. The student then provided a clear and practiced explanation of autosomal recessive inheritance, explaining that the risk to her offspring would be 1 in 2 if her partner is a carrier, or greatly reduced if he is not, and suggested that the next step in the risk assessment would be for her partner to undergo carrier testing (CF has a frequency of about 1/25 in Northern Europeans). She related the options for DNA-based prenatal diagnosis if the partner were found to be a carrier, describing chorionic villus sampling and amniocentesis and their associated risks. The student asked finally if the patient had any questions, and when she replied that she did not, provided the clinic's business card for the patient to make an appointment for her husband's carrier testing, and left the room to review the case with the supervising genetic counselor and medical geneticist. Despite the student's satisfaction that the information she had imparted was accurate and efficiently delivered, she told the supervising staff that she felt that the patient was angry with her and that she was vaguely uncomfortable with how the session had gone.

The genetic counselor returned to the room with the student and asked the patient how she felt about coming to Medical Genetics for a risk assessment. Maryse explained that she was angry. She felt that despite being affected with CF, she was coping well with the condition and was happy with her current quality of life. She felt that there would be no way she could ever terminate an affected pregnancy and felt sure that her boyfriend felt the same way. It would be like saying that her own life had no value and that she herself did not deserve to live. The student and counselor supported Maryse in the position she had taken and said that they would remain available to her in case any other questions arose in the future or her situation changed. They told her they would summarize their discussion in a letter to her obstetrician so that he would similarly understand her point of view. Maryse, in turn, felt *understood*, which had therapeutic benefit in itself. Luckily, the opportunity to provide supportive care to the patient was not lost. If the team had *begun* the consultation with proper contracting, however, the information provided would have been much better tailored to the patient, and the healing role of supportive listener could have been employed much sooner.

2. Assess patients' readiness for results

Let us discuss the initial clinic visit of a 2-year-old boy, Dominic, and his parents. Dominic was referred for genetic evaluation by his pediatrician, who noted him to be behind in his motor milestones and in speech. The parents were aware of the delay and were amenable to exploring the possible etiologies but were not necessarily prepared to receive a genetic diagnosis. Even if Dr. Tremblay, the medical geneticist, were able to recognize a specific condition's phenotype and make a diagnosis immediately, she would be wise to refrain from presenting the diagnosis to the parents until she has had a chance to assess their readiness. While one set of parents might be tired of undergoing multiple tests and appointments in search of a diagnosis and be ready for concrete information, another couple might be wholly unprepared to learn that what they consider to be a mild delay in speech is due to a genetic syndrome and will result in a lifelong and serious altera- tion to their family life. (A further point of semantic confusion is that parents often assume "delayed" children will "catch up" later.) In delivering a genetic diagnosis to parents, the normal expectations of parents for their children – that they will grow up to become independent and responsible citizens, with meaningful employment and life partners, who may have children of their own one day – are instantly shattered and replaced by fear. "What will become of Dominic? How will we educate him? Will I have to quit my job, give up my career to take care of him? What about the other children? We want them to have a normal family life too. Will he ever be able to live independently? Who will take care of him when we are no longer around?" Thoughts then quickly jump to the risks to other family members. "Will our future children be similarly affected? Should we have prenatal testing? What would we do if the results are positive? What about my sister, who is also pregnant? Should I tell her?"

In the case above, Dr. Tremblay noted that Dominic had many of the features of Fragile X syndrome, but she did not immediately share her observations. Fragile X syndrome is a common inherited form of moderate mental retardation due to a trinucleotide repeat expansion in the *FMR-1* gene on the X chromo- some. Its diagnosis in a young boy implies that the boy will have significant intellectual deficiency and that the mother is necessarily a carrier. The mother has a 20% risk for premature ovarian failure, as well as a 50% risk to pass the gene on to each child. The mother's siblings and other family members are also at risk to be carriers and have similarly affected children.

Dr. Tremblay needed to assess the patients' readiness for a diagnosis. She explained to the family that in some children, an underlying genetic cause can be identified that explains the developmental delay but that also has implications for the child's future developmental potential, and can represent a risk for family members. She asked the family how much they were prepared to learn about Dominic and whether they were ready to agree to have him undergo genetic tests (a karyotype and DNA testing for Fragile X syndrome). The parents asked for some time to talk to each other about this, and Dr. Tremblay offered to step out, see another patient and come back. When she returned, the couple stated that they would agree to have Dominic tested and that, while now quite anxious, they would have time to adjust to the idea of a potential genetic diagnosis for Dominic and to prepare themselves emotionally while they waited for the results.

3. Perform risk assessment, evaluation, and/or diagnosis

Confirmatory testing was arranged for Dominic in the form of a karyotype and DNA analysis of the *FMR-1* gene. The results confirmed an expansion in the *FMR-1* gene, and the diagnosis of Fragile X syndrome was made.

4. Give results with sensitivity

Patients will remember the way they are told a diagnosis, forever; they typically remember the exact words used, whether they are told in the hallway or other public area or in a private room, and the poise and comfort level of the person bearing the news. Assuming the patient and physician have established mutual goals for the consultation, the patients were receptive to testing, and the diagnosis has been made, let us jump to the moment of informing the family of the results. Typically included in the information to be discussed are the prognosis, natural history, available treatments and therapies, and options for prenatal diagnosis. Sometimes, the diagnosis is straightforward, and the information to be provided includes some good news along with the bad: there is an available treatment and one can prevent the devastating sequelae of the disease. Other times, this is not possible.

In Dominic's case, the parents came for another appointment with Dr. Tremblay to receive the results, this time without Dominic so that they could have a meaningful discussion without distraction. The parents were prepared for what to them was "the worst" and were edgy and anxious. After brief preliminary greetings, Dr. Tremblay did not launch into a review of the reasons why the couple were there, and the rationale for recommending the testing, or draw out the delivery of the results to an uncomfortable length. She stated clearly yet calmly, "I know you are here to learn the results of Dominic's genetic testing. The results show that Dominic has a condition known as Fragile X syndrome." Dr. Tremblay did not include value-laden phrases such as "I am sorry to inform you" or "unfortunately," as she preferred to leave the interpretation of the news to the parents. She did, however, quietly wait for the reaction of the parents before continuing the discussion.

5. Care for the patient's emotional reactions – accept and respond appropriately

Despite being emotionally prepared for a genetic diagnosis, the parents, like all patients, still needed several long moments to absorb the news. After sighing several times, the mother uttered a simple "Shit" and began to cry. Her husband did not speak but put his arm around his wife's shoulder and gently stroked her back. Dr. Tremblay was comfortable in the silence yet wanted to communicate her understanding of the impact of this news, and empathetically stated, "It is very difficult news to hear, isn't it." This empathetic statement, followed by silence, allowed her to draw the husband out. "We were prepared for this kind of news," he said, "but still – you always hope it's not going to be true. It's still unbelievable." Dr. Tremblay quietly agreed, "Yes, it is. It can take a long time to adjust to news like this." She then asked the couple, "What are some of the thoughts you had as you were preparing yourself these last few weeks for the results?" A discussion ensued, with both parents participating, that allowed Dr. Tremblay to have a clearer idea as to the meaning and impact this diagnosis would have for the family. Notably, she did not *immediately* launch into a factual conversation designed to take away the parents' worry and pain, such as a description of the available therapies and early intervention programs available. There would be time for that. At this moment, nothing one might say could take away the patients' pain at hearing this news. For now, her therapeutic intervention was simply to *be* with the parents, to accept and validate their reactions as normal, and to provide empathetic support. When the parents were ready, Dr. Tremblay briefly listed the likely challenges Dominic would face, and the plan for follow-up, and offered to see them in a month's time to review the prognostic information in more detail. At this next appointment, the couple would be invited to consider the genetic implications of the diagnosis for their future children and their family members, and another circuit of the *Roadmap* would be initiated.

Chances, Choices, and Tools for Prevention

Of course, unlike in Dominic's case, sometimes news of a genetic disorder is accompanied by a clear-cut plan for prevention. One of the great triumphs of the last century was the introduction of newborn screening to detect inborn errors of metabolism. As an example, phenylketonuria (PKU) can be detected in the first weeks of life, and the treatment is a diet low in phenylalanine. As a result, the profound effects of elevated phenylalanine on the neurologic development of an individual who has inherited mutations in the gene for phenylalanine hydroxylase from both parents can be prevented. This is a clear but extreme example of how a necessary component of the diet (phenylalanine) interacts with an underlying genetic endowment (mutations in the gene for phenylalanine hydroxylase) to cause a clear outcome – developmental delay. Another example is galactosemia. A child lacking one of several enzymes involved in the metabolism of lactose can, with dietary restriction of lactose, avoid the life-threatening complications of feeding problems, failure to thrive, hepatocellular damage, bleeding, and sepsis [7].

The situation becomes more complex when one starts to look at adult-onset disease for which disruptions in a single gene have major effects. We would like to consider two disorders that have garnered a fair amount of notoriety: Hereditary breast and ovarian cancer, caused by a mutation in either one of the *BRCA1* or *BRCA2* genes, and Huntington disease due to a trinucleotide repeat expansion in the *HTT* gene. As with all autosomal dominant diseases, the altered genes for both of these diseases can be passed down from a single affected parent to his or her offspring and result in disease, typically in adult life. In the case of patients with *BRCA* mutations, the movement of genetic testing into patient care has been rapid since the discovery of *BRCA1* and *BRCA2* in the last decade of the last century.

It is now clear that mutations in *BRCA1* result in a great lifetime risk for both breast and ovarian cancer. It is also clear that prophylactic removal of breasts and ovaries greatly decreases this risk. In addition, the pathology of the cancers in patients with mutations may be different, and this difference may alter therapeutic options. Genetic test results, thus, need not be devastating; they can also be empowering in that women can take positive steps to avoid the fates of their mothers.

Understanding the choice of taking up testing for *BRCA* mutations requires a physician to understand whole person care. A woman who has lost her mother to breast or ovarian cancer while she herself was a girl or young woman may look at testing in a completely different light from a woman who has lost a sister in adult life. The choices that individuals make may defy science but make great sense when seen from the patient's viewpoint. For example, our clinic has seen examples of young women whose mothers have died at an early age and who are demanding a prophylactic mastectomy. When genetic testing shows that they have not inherited their mother's disease-causing mutation, they may still pressure the team for the mastectomy because they cannot quickly accept – absorb the new reality – that they are at decreased risk. The burden of the disease that they have seen in their family for decades initially trumps the result of the genetic test; it takes time for the results to sink in. The genetics team's contribution to "healing" in this circumstance involved understanding the psychosocial circumstances surrounding the original request for genetic testing, and supporting the patient over the months following the test result as the decreased risk result was integrated into her self-definition.

Let us use the example of the at-risk breast and ovarian cancer patient to illustrate another phenomenon. Patients who present for presymptomatic testing for adult-onset disorders often participate in a mental process known as *preselection* [8]. Patients sometimes hold the erroneous assumption that because they resemble their affected parent, either in physical features or in personality, they will have inherited the disease-causing mutation. Julie was a young woman who came to the cancer genetics clinic to support her sister, Mary, who was undergoing predictive testing for *BRCA1*. Their mother died of breast cancer at age 47, and Mary is "the splitting image" of her mother. Julie had prepared herself to support her sister, and had promised to be there for her every step of the way through the prophylactic surgeries that Mary had already decided she would undergo. Prior to drawing blood for testing, the genetics team asked the sisters what results they are expecting. When they elicited that the sisters had preselected Mary as the positive one, they could intervene to ask, "What will happen if Julie is found to be a carrier, if Julie is not found to be a carrier, or if both of you are carriers?" The genetics team, thus, allowed both sisters to prepare for alternative scenarios and helped to avoid the potential for both sisters to be destabilized, or even devastated by the results.

Reactions to genetic test results evolve over time. As we have seen with our patients who initially cannot integrate a negative *BRCA* gene test result and still request prophylactic mastectomy, denial has many forms. Many patients cannot accept a *positive* diagnosis, particularly of a condition that leads to mental retardation, and request repeat testing, such as expensive karyotyping in a new diagnosis of Down syndrome. Sometimes, shame or perceived stigma prevents individuals from sharing genetic information with their at-risk family members. In these cases, informing individuals of the results of genetic tests must include an understanding and comfort with the very normal denial response, recognizing that it is a normal psychological reaction (at least in the short term) to devastating news. After reassuring the patient as to the standard laboratory methods in place to control for laboratory error and sample mix-up, rather than engaging in a conversation to prove to a patient that the results are indeed correct and forcing them to accept the diagnosis immediately (which would be counterproductive at this time), the geneticist knows that is more effective at this moment to simply empathize with the patient how difficult it is to accept such devastating news. After all, if consent for immediate cardiac surgery is not required, will it really hurt the parents to hold on to the hope that the doctors are wrong for a few more days? Reality will set in soon enough. As for the individual who does not want to share genetic information with his or her relatives, it helps if the genetics team can see the patient in 6 months or a year, as maybe at that time the patient will be less angry and more willing to provide the information to his relatives.

The above examples emphasize the fact that patients often prefer to live for a time in a state of not knowing their genetic status, if it means they can avoid knowing they have inherited the disease-causing mutation, even if it also means they must forego the reassurance that a negative test result would bring. Among the other factors that relate to the receptivity for genetic testing for *BRCA* mutations include community acceptance of testing, the association of breasts with sexuality, and the fear of being refused health and life insurance.

Interestingly, only a small minority of individuals, who know that they are at risk for Huntington disease, choose to have predictive testing to learn whether they have inherited the altered gene from their parent. Those who pursue testing may do so for career or family planning, or for other personal reasons. Presumably, because there is currently no treatment for the disease, most at-risk individuals do not come forward for testing [9]. In many cases, individuals are referred for testing by physicians without discussion of the implication for testing – which is why most Huntington disease clinics have very formal protocols for predictive testing, which include an interview with a psychologist, and an invitation to the patient to bring a support person (who should not be a similarly at-risk family member) as they move through the testing process [10].

The Future of Genetic Testing

Unfortunately, at this time, with the exception of some inborn errors of metabolism, in the presence of genetic mutations, the options for prevention of genetic disease sequelae or for cure are few and far between. This is in marked contrast to the justifiable excitement about breakthroughs in genetics and the great potential they represent for future treatment and prevention. Given the complexity of the application of genetics to single-gene diseases, it is not surprising that it is difficult for genetic practice to live up to its hype in the realm of clinical care. We are not yet at the point where whole genome sequencing and the knowledge of whether one is a carrier for this or that disease susceptibility allele can be translated to direct steps to prevent disease. We do not yet have the evidence that dietary, behavioral, or other environmental factors can make much difference in disease prevention. This being said, such days may not be far off. There are clearly areas where genetic technologies will make a difference. The first area involves the genetics, not of people, but of pathogens. Genetic methodology is essential today to determine both the pathogenicity of organisms and the epidemiology of infectious disease. The day is very close where diagnosis of infectious disease at the bedside will be by means of genetic testing. The second area is that of host resistance to infection. One of the earliest examples of this was the understanding that being a carrier for sickle hemoglobin could lower the risk for malaria. Today, genetic factors underlying host resistance for leprosy, tuberculosis, salmonella, and viral infections are actively being studied in many centers.

Two major buzzwords that permeate the medical literature are genome-wide association studies (GWAS) and pharmacogenomics. The first gives the hope of finding risk factors for common diseases such as schizophrenia, diabetes, inflammatory bowel disease, heart disease, and cancer, to name a few. While GWAS have identified many interesting biological targets, to date these have not translated into many useful clinical applications. GWAS will result in therapeutic options – but not quite yet. With respect to pharmacogenomics, much of the impetus is being driven by economics. There is hope that drugs and other therapeutic agents that are ineffective in the general population may be effective on subgroups that can be identified by genetic testing. While this offers great promise, we are disheartened by the slow acceptance by the medical community of traditional "pharmacogenetic" tests that have been known for years, such as for sensitivity to anesthesia or to chemotherapeutic agents such as 6MP.

Back to the Future

One of the challenges of genetics and its resulting technology is that it functions at the level of the individual, the family, the community, and the society. At the level of the individual, even for the single-gene disorders, it is not possible to predict with certainty such variables as severity and age of onset of disease. For the family, shared risk and the resulting duty to share information conflict with the oft-expressed desire to maintain confidentiality. For the community, shared values relate to the concept of acceptance or rejection of technology. Community acceptance plays a major role in the willingness to undergo genetic testing. Because the frequency of *BRCA* mutations is high in the Ashkenazi Jewish population and because only three mutations in *BRCA1* and *BRCA2* constitute the overwhelming majority of causal mutations, there has been a receptivity to testing in that community. But each culture and society will probably solve these problems in appropriately different ways. For societies, the desire to decrease suffering and the cost of care conflicts with the need to care for the disabled and to respect cultural diversity and individual freedom. Respect for the whole person in genetics as in other areas of medicine will raise important issues and values that need to be clarified and negotiated over time – a long-term project.

In working with patients in prenatal diagnosis, we are often asked by patients following the identification of a major fetal structural anomaly, syndrome, or fetal death, "How can you do this job? How can you deal with patients who are in such terrible situations?" We reply that we are confident in the resilience of the human spirit. We have seen, over and over again, individuals and families adjust and cope with the changed realities and revised expectations of a genetic diagnosis. Harvard-educated sociologist Martha Beck, in her memoire *Expecting Adam* [11], describes rewriting her definition of hopes for her baby, who was diagnosed prenatally to have Down syndrome, and whom she welcomed into her life and raised. Rather than valuing intelligence and workplace success as the most important measure of a person's value to society, Beck came to understand that individuals with disabilities have much to teach us about what it means to love and accept.

As we sit at the crossroads of having the tools to diagnose a great variety of genetic conditions, yet not quite having readily available and effective treatments or cures for many of them, we must rely on the Garrodian model of medicine, and its modern equivalent of whole person care, to be therapeutic. In viewing the patient as the hub in a wheel of a complex social, psychological, and physical environment, we must attend to the impact of a diagnosis and focus our energies on maximizing the patient's adjustment and coping. The healer role can be seen as not necessarily curing the disease but as accompanying the patient along the path to adjustment and to the achievement of a new equilibrium and harmony with his environment. New diagnostic and therapeutic modalities for both single-gene and complex diseases will certainly enter the fray, but with each we will be called upon to help the patient integrate these new options into his life plan and to create meaning where, at first glance, there may be none. It is in facing such challenges together with our patients that we can be truly therapeutic.

References

1. Childs B. The Metabolic and molecular basis of disease. Vol. 1: A logic of disease. 8th ed. New York, NY: McGraw-Hill; 2001.
2. Fraser FC. Genetic counseling. Am J Hum Genet. 1974;26:363–659.
3. Buckman R. How to break bad news. Toronto, ON: University of Toronto Press; 1998.
4. Kaplan M. SPIKES: a framework for breaking bad news to patients with cancer. Clin J Oncol Nurs. 2010;14(4):514–6.
5. Kubler-Ross E. On death and dying. New York, NY: Simon & Schuster; 1970.
6. Cystic Fibrosis Foundation. Patient registry annual data report to the center directors. Bethesda, MD: CFF; 2008. www.cff.org.
7. Elsas LJ II. Galactosemia. In: Pagon RA, Bird TC, Dolan CR, Stephens K, editors. GeneReviews (Internet). Seattle, WA: University of Washington. 4 Feb 1993–2000 (updated 27 Sep 2007).

8. Rolland JS, McDaniel SH. Beliefs and multicultural issues in the new era of genetics. In: Miller S, McDaniel S, Rolland J, Feetham S, editors. Individuals, families, and the new era of genetics: biopsychosocial perspectives. New York, NY: W. W. Norton; 2006.
9. Bernhardt C et al. Decreasing uptake of predictive testing for Huntington's disease in a German centre: 12 years' experience (1993–2004). Eur J Hum Genet. 2009;17(3):295–300.
10. International Huntington Association and the World Federation of Neurology Research Group on Huntington's Chorea. Guidelines for the molecular genetics predictive test in Huntington's disease. J Med Genet. 1994;31(7):555–9.
11. Beck M. Expecting Adam: a true story of birth, rebirth, and everyday magic. New York, NY: Berkley; 1999.

Chapter 15
Whole Person Care on a Busy Medical Ward

Gordon L. Crelinsten

Keywords Evidence-based medicine • Evidence-influenced medicine • Observation skills • Funeral visitation • Condolence letter • Narrative • Jean Dominique Bauby • Role modelling • Teachable moment

By the time medical students and young physicians in training arrive on the medical wards to care for real people, they have a very good understanding of pathology and physiology. They know how biochemical processes can be altered by genes, by microbes, and by the environment to cause and to perpetuate disease. They can list the causes of symptoms such as weakness, dizziness, chest pain, and headache. They know which laboratory tests to order and how to interpret them. They use the imaging techniques that have the best chance of providing the answers to the diagnostic puzzles that confront them.

Once the patient has been deconstructed into problems such as anaemia, weight loss, abnormal liver function tests, or a calcified lung mass on a chest X-ray, the treating team calls into action an array of steps and strategies to deal with each and to reach eventually the correct diagnosis and to formulate an effective treatment plan. The treatment is aimed at eliminating the abnormality either by attacking the cause or by helping the patient accommodate the abnormality to reach a new state of balance.

The challenge on the wards of a busy teaching hospital is to assist and to guide these young people to transition from the care of problems that happen to reside in patients to the care of patients who happen to have problems. This task requires a shift of attention to the container rather than to the contents.

G.L. Crelinsten (✉)
Associate Physician-in-Chief, McGill University Health Centre, Montreal, QC H3G 1A4, Canada
and
Associate Professor, Department of Medicine, McGill University, Montreal, QC H3H 1V4, Canada
e-mail: gordon.crelinsten@muhc.mcgill.ca

T.A. Hutchinson (ed.), *Whole Person Care: A New Paradigm for the 21st Century*,   173
DOI 10.1007/978-1-4419-9440-0_15, © Springer Science+Business Media, LLC 2011

Mrs. Camfield[1] had lived a full life. As an infant, she immigrated to Canada with her parents from Ireland before the Great War; her schooling was interrupted by the necessity to work as a chambermaid to help support her family of five brothers and two sisters when her father died tragically in a streetcar accident. She never was able to finish high school.

She married at twenty, had three children in quick succession and settled into a life of cleaning, cooking, caring and going to church. Her husband started as a truck driver and with hard work and determination built a transportation company which allowed the Camfield's to live well, to educate their children in private schools and to travel extensively.

Over the years, Mrs. Camfield had learned how to control her diabetes, had dealt with the distress of losing a breast to cancer, had mourned her youngest child who died of leukemia and had nursed her husband who finally succumbed to a devastating stroke.

This was the eighty-two year old who was admitted to our ward late one evening with difficulty breathing and the physical signs of severe aortic stenosis. Over time, her aortic valve, the main outlet valve of the heart, had become heavily calcified and its ability to open and to allow adequate blood flow to the body was markedly restricted.

The ward team knew the problem well, knew the tests that needed to be done to characterize the problem fully and clearly and also knew that the only acceptable therapeutic option, once Mrs. Camfield was stabilized, was cardiac surgery to replace her valve, a serious operation made more so by Mrs. Camfield's age and her other medical conditions.

Contemporary medical practice is strongly influenced by the concept of evidence-based medicine. Clinical decision making and the choice of treatment options are based on statistically demonstrated success obtained from large randomized, controlled trials, and the place of intuition, experience, and personal choice based on values or other criteria are regarded as inappropriate. In fact, these trials anonymize the person by ensuring that differences between groups of patients have no effect on the study results. The answers obtained are independent of the patients who helped provide them. The person is a passive conduit in the evaluation of the intervention.

The next morning, Mrs. Camfield had responded to treatment and was able to participate in a discussion about future treatment directions and about the importance of considering a surgical option.

We learned that Mrs. Camfield lived alone in a residence, enjoyed the movies, still went to church every Sunday, and that her oldest granddaughter was to be married in two weeks.

The team started to realize that a decision for surgery, based on available evidence, needed to take into account the needs, beliefs, and plans of Mrs. Camfield. We knew that care for the whole person demands a respect for the subjective in the face of the objective. We knew that the evidence provides direction but that the journey belongs to the patient.

In ward discussions, the subtle distinction of evidence-influenced medicine over evidence-based medicine allows treatment and diagnostic deliberation and debate to recognize that clinical decision making not only involves the rigorously obtained evidence but also takes into account the therapeutic dyad characterized by the experience and interpretation of the physician and the values, character, and choice of the patient.

"What would you do if it were your Mother?" This question is often asked by patients who are overwhelmed with their illness and with the sudden barrage of information thrust upon them. The importance of this question is that it focuses

---

[1]Mrs. Camfield is fictional. Her story is based on years of clinical experience and recollections.

the choices to be made upon an identifiable person with strong emotional connections. The patient expects the physician to filter the options as if they were to be applied to a close loved one, and therefore, not only the best but also the right answer will emerge.

This question personalizes the choice to be made and is another example of conflict between the objective and the subjective. The patient is requesting that the problem be addressed as it relates to the person and not necessarily as a stand-alone issue to be objectively analyzed. The patient has packaged the problem within a person and assumes that the decision will now take the person into account and not just offer a generic solution.

The question needs to be answered by turning it back on to the patient.

"I cannot answer the question as you ask it. I can answer the question for my mother because I know her. I know what burden she is willing to bear for what benefit. I know how she deals with adversity and how her character deals with challenge. I know something of the narrative of her life and of the history of her choices when faced with options. I know her wishes and her goals, and in knowing all of this, I can make a decision close to the one she would make. I do not know you in the same way: only you and those close to you know who you are."

This answer, however, is not sufficient. The patient is asking for guidance but has not provided all of the information. The example of a financial advisor throws some light on the situation. When planning retirement, a prudent person may decide to save and to invest a yearly sum in hopes of establishing a fund to finance a comfortable retirement. Often, the advice of an expert is sought.

The advisor who takes the contribution and says, "Leave it to me, I am the expert, I am trained to do the best thing" may not be the best choice. The careful investor would choose an advisor who says, "What are your goals? Are you a risk taker or a more conservative investor? Are you looking for capital gains or are you concerned about a steady income? Where do you see your investment in 5 years?" Once the advisor knows the client, a plan, using the particular expertise and knowledge of the advisor, can be created that has the best chance of achieving the goals of the client.

"You are not my mother, but if I were to know you as I know my mother, I can help you and guide you to the choice which will best achieve your goals and I will accompany you on that journey."

Mrs. Camfield listened attentively as we described the relative risks and benefits of aortic valve surgery and the potential course of her condition if she chose not to have an operation. The latter would require a palliative approach, treatment to reduce suffering and when the end occurred, no resuscitative efforts.

Mrs. Camfield adjusted the sheets, sat up straight and told us that she understood her choices and her chances. She told us that surgery did not interest her at this time, and her main short term goal was not to cast a cloud over her granddaughter's wedding.

The busy medical ward is not the best environment in which to appreciate the complete significance of disease and suffering. The interaction between medical teams and the patient starts at different points on the illness trajectory and ends before the final stages play out. Most patients seen and cared for have acute exacerbations of chronic problems such as heart failure, renal failure, liver failure, or chronic lung disease.

They are well compensated for a period of time and then for some reason fall off the edge of stability either due to the natural progression of their disease, infection, noncompliance with a medical regimen, dietary indiscretion or due to an acute and sudden uncontrollable complication of the disease process.

To understand whole persons fully in this context requires some knowledge of who they were when stable and who they will become once restabilized. This longitudinal view is a luxury not often provided or available to the young physician who may be grappling with the concept of patient-centred care including the idea that patients have individual preferences and concerns that are situated in social contexts outside of the ward environment.

> In view of Mrs. Camfield's decision not to have surgery, we needed to clarify her understanding of the level of care when her condition inevitably deteriorated. She needed to know that in the event of death no resuscitative efforts would be undertaken. Mrs. Camfield was concerned that her death close to her granddaughter's wedding would not be in anyone's interest and so she requested every effort to keep her alive, and hopefully well, until after the joyous event.

Students chosen to study medicine are all high academic achievers. They cannot be discriminated by their academic rank or by their test scores. They all have letters of reference which laud their abilities, and their personal and biographical letters speak to their proven qualities of leadership, altruism, empathy, attentive listening, and compassion.

Faced with an excess of outstanding candidates, medical schools and postgraduate programs are faced with the difficult task of establishing a process of choice. These young people, all with exceptional academic records, can only be picked according to their personality characteristics that are considered to be essential to the role of physician.

Undergraduate medical school curricula are increasingly being redesigned to include material that emphasizes the healing aspect of medical practice [1]. Students learn that the well-being of patients requires not only scientific understanding of biology and pathology but also an appreciation of the art of connecting with persons [2]. This learning takes place away from the real world of ward medicine. The students are protected from the urgency of the ill and from the responsibility of providing not only answers but also comfort. The former is based on science, while the latter is based on the human connection between two persons seeking a common goal.

On a busy medical ward, the quest for data occupies a large part of the day, and it is difficult to find or to make the time to engage the patient or their families on a personal level, and when asked to do so, the health care teams may put the task at the bottom of an already enormous list.

The appreciation of patients as individuals who stand out because of who they are and not because of what condition they have is a skill as important as the physical examination of the cardiovascular system and requires the development and nurturing of attitudes that are anchored in the traits of personality for which these students were selected in the first place to study medicine.

How can these aspects of medical education and continuous professional development be brought to the bedside and not relegated to the backroom for discussion outside of the mainstream of care and caring?

The knowing of a person begins before verbal or physical interaction. Before we delve into the medical history, the complaints and the related symptoms and before we touch and feel and maneuver body parts, there is a moment in which the doctor and patient enter each other's world. Are there books on the bedside table, pictures of loved ones, of pets, or of places with special meaning, and are there symbols of spiritual connectedness? These clues to the person need to be pointed out and recognized as an important part of the therapeutic encounter. We learn much by looking without speaking and careful observation not only helps to capture information important to physical diagnosis such as pallor, goitre, rheumatoid hands, or evidence of an old stroke but also contributes to characterize the person as different from all others.

> Mrs. Camfield was more than a name and a patient with shortness of breath when we noticed, and pointed out to others, the simple gold cross around her neck, the rosary beads on the bedside table and the picture on the window sill by her bed of a smiling young woman enjoying the St. Patrick's Day Parade.

The emotional component of the practice of medicine is often neglected and not viewed traditionally as an aspect requiring specific attention. A renewed emphasis is emerging on the importance of personal reflection as a means not only to improve practice but also to make it more meaningful [3, 4]. There is a mechanism that allows the principles of reflective practice to be incorporated into the ward routine so that it becomes a recognized part of the ward experience. Protected time is set apart so that the ward teams can share recent experience that evoked emotion or feeling. They describe incidents that made them proud, uncertain, disappointed, sad, happy, and angry. They describe "eureka" moments that brought new insight into old and common problems. They benefit from the experience and from the debriefing provided by peers and near peers who comment without judgement. These "autonomic" rounds legitimize the subjective and personal aspects of caring for the ill and enrich the experience by acknowledging the qualitative elements of doctoring.

> Mrs. Camfield died one week after her granddaughter's wedding. She had the chance to see the wedding video and visited with the couple before they left on their wedding trip to Dublin.
>
> The ward team had the opportunity to share their feelings on the Friday after her death. We noted how easy it was for health professionals to discuss the medical issues and the complications of care but how difficult it was "to give voice to the feelings these events evoked" [5]. We reflected on how our efforts at care allowed our patient her last pleasure and how we felt when she asked us to resuscitate her, not for her benefit, but rather for the happiness of her loved ones. The feelings flowed easily and seemed to give added meaning to the clinical decisions we had made and participated in.

There may be an admonition, "Physicians heal thyself," but this experience pleads, "Physician know thyself."

Even though the actual healing function may reside within the patient, the physician plays an important role not only as a companion but also as a facilitator. Young physicians often do not realize the esteem to which they are held by individual patients and by society. They are also not aware of how this position may help and encourage healing. They may not appreciate how their expertise, as well as their caring, may advance the healing process. We need to learn, and also be able to teach, that the care of the whole person requires an understanding of the physician role "qua" physician and that this role can be integral to the healing process. The physician role requires a knowledge base capable of understanding the biology of disease, and it is this knowledge base that is responsible for the curing function and also mostly responsible for the special social position doctors enjoy. The trick is to use this knowledge base to create a range of options, all scientifically valid, from which the patient can choose.

When death occurs, the personal encounter is completed, but there are learning experiences which endure and can be used to strengthen the concept of physician-hood and further the appreciation of care for persons rather than diseases. The funeral visitation is a solemn event. There is a whispered hum of conversation that hangs in the room. People come and go unnoticed, and attention is fractured into small groups of mourners and comforters. When the doctor enters the room, the hum becomes focused, conversations cease, and the murmur of "That's Jane's doctor," "the doctor is here," "Look, the doctor has just come in," becomes discernable. When doctors experience this for the first time, they come to realize a special-ness inherent in the physician role. The visit not only expresses an honoring of the patient who has died, appreciated and recognized by those who look on, but also forces the humble acceptance of being important in someone else's life.

A doctor's letter of condolence also has special meaning for a family in mourning. The letter signifies a special relationship between the deceased person and the doctor. Encouraged to write letters of condolence, young physicians can be guided to center their attention on the person and not upon the disease. This exercise allows the writer to develop expressive narrative skills in the service of those entrusted to their care. It helps the writer understand who their patient was in life and allows an outlet for this realization [6].

> To the granddaughter of Mrs. Jane Camfield:
>
> Please accept my sincere sympathy at this time of great loss. Your grandmother will live on in the hearts of those who loved her and in the many acts of goodness she performed.
>
> Your grandmother bore her burden with elegant courage and was so happy to see you married. She always had a smile for me. I will miss my visits with her.
>
> I wish and you and yours a future of good health and may you find some comfort in your many memories.

Medicine is a series of patient stories that are told, recorded, and analyzed. These stories need to be heard attentively, appreciated in all of their dimensions, and recorded accurately. There are nuances of verbal and nonverbal expression and striking emotional overtones, which color these stories. A keen attention to patient stories, their content, and the manner in which they are told allows the health professional to practice empathetic listening and to develop a deeper understanding and recognition of the patient as the meaning of the illness begins to become apparent [7]. Efforts to enrich and improve this appreciation of the place of narrative in clinical medicine can be designed and undertaken. Stories written by doctors about doctors, by doctors about patients and vice versa, and stories written by patients who are experiencing or who have experienced illness, can be shared by the ward team, and similarities and differences from their own lives can offer opportunities for rich discussion.

The reality of ward medicine is that many patients cannot verbalize their histories and cannot openly express their feelings. How can caregivers be sensitized to the hidden narrative of these lives and not just rely on the treatment of computer numbers and sophisticated imaging? Can the personhood of these patients be captured and, therefore, serve as an exercise to emphasize whole-patient care?

Jean Dominique Bauby was 42 years old, the father of two and editor-in-chief of Elle magazine in Paris, when he suffered a massive stroke that left him quadriplegic. He was fully alert and conscious but could only move his eyes up and down and blink. All other communication and connection to the world were denied him. This locked-in syndrome is a devastating clinical condition that imprisons the patient in a paralyzed body.

Lying in a bed, Mr. Bauby was fed through a tube, breathed through a tube, urinated through a tube, and was totally dependent on others for his care and well-being. In spite of this condition, Bauby wrote The Diving Bell and The Butterfly by blinking his eyelids in response to the reading of the alphabet while a friend recorded his responses [8]. This laborious test of friendship led to an account of what has been called, "a memoir of life in death" [9].

We learn from the story that even the most diminished patient has the capacity to feel and to sense, not only primitively, but possibly also in a way that is complete with memory, future, and meaning. As the uncommunicative Bauby communicates, "Having turned down the hideous jogging suit provided by the hospital, I am now attired as I was in my student days. Like the bath, my old clothes could easily bring back poignant, painful memories. But I see in the clothes a symbol of continuing life. And proof that I still want to be myself. If I must drool, I may as well drool on cashmere" [8].

When the story is brought to the ward setting and not relegated to the lecture theatre, it can be shared and appreciated in the surroundings of ward reality where often squash games, dinner parties, or recent vacations are discussed over and around the patients who cannot move, cannot talk, and are attached to tubes. The story refocuses the attention on the patient and demands an effort to be conscientious in care and to be sensitive to the whole person, some of whom may be hidden and unnoticed.

Students of medicine receive their fundamental training within formal courses often delivered by lecturers in large rooms. However, students learn as well through unplanned, unscripted encounters and experiences. They see things as they are as well as how they are supposed to be. This implicit side of medical education in which learning outcomes may not be those that were openly intended is called the informal or "hidden" curriculum [10, 11].

The transition from layman to physician is a maturing process as participation in reality becomes more intense. The movement from the classroom to the bedside provides experiences that are outside of the stated educational objectives of the formal medical curriculum. This role change is accompanied by real threats to the idealism that prompted many to seek a future in medicine. Emotional bombardment and overload may lead to emotional neutralization as overcaring may result in inefficiency and self-doubt. There are also striking challenges to ethical integrity that need to be faced. Is consent to treatment really informed? What is the ethical relationship between the physician and the health care industry? What is the role of the family in clinical decision making? Must doctors always tell the truth?

The conscious role modelling [12] of the ward-attending physician is a powerful mechanism to emphasize the experiences and behavior that are required educational objectives for the competent and effective care of whole persons. Clinical knowledge, teaching skill, and personal qualities characterize the role model. If whole-patient care is to be a goal of the clinical experience, then the effective role model has to deliberately, but not artificially, model the skills of sensitivity, empathy, acceptance, and understanding, to name a few. The role model has to be attentive to humanistic problems with the same intensity as to biological problems. The role model has to support the importance of being witness to patient stories and to advocate for their meaning in providing care.

Being a role model is often serendipitous as Paice et al. [13] point out when they paraphrase John Lennon "being a role model is what happens when you are busy doing other things."

These other things include the focused emphasis on the doctor–patient relationship, the genuine interest in the psychosocial aspects of medical practice, the personalization of clinical experience, and the sharing of life stories [14].

The conscious role model is forever vigilant for the teachable moment when a human story can lead to a generalizable lesson.

> Mrs. Camfield asked for a potential limited aggressive treatment option in order not to have her death pale her granddaughter's special day. This event allowed the discussion of how "do not resuscitate orders" are not simply an administrative necessity to insure that care teams are appropriate in their response to a patient's death but are reflections of how patients view meaning at the end of life.

The combination of curing and healing is surely the mandate of contemporary medicine. This requires a balance between understanding what disease does to the body and an appreciation of how illness affects the person. To do both well requires an environment on a busy medical ward that gives equal importance to both aspects of care. It requires teamwork, advocacy, and a commitment to not only attempt to cure biological disease but also to permit and to facilitate the healing of those who are suffering.

References

1. Boudreau JD, Cassel EJ, Fuks A. A healing curriculum. Med Educ. 2007;41:1193–201.
2. Stewart M. Towards a global definition of patient centred care. Br Med J. 2001;22:444–5.
3. Mamede S, Schmidt HG. The structure of reflective practice in medicine. Med Educ. 2004;38:1302–8.
4. Kaufman DM. ABC of learning and teaching in medicine. Br Med J. 2003;326:213–6.
5. Treadway K. The code. New Engl J Med. 2007;357:1273–5.
6. Bedell SE, Cadenhead K, Graboys TB. The doctor's letter of condolence. New Engl J Med. 2001;344:1162–4.
7. Charon R. Narrative medicine: honouring the stories of illness. New York, NY: Oxford University Press; 2006.
8. Bauby JD. The diving bell and the butterfly. Jeremy Leggat, translator. London: Fourth Estate; 1997. p. 25.
9. Schwartz RS. The diving bell and the butterfly, a memoir of life in death. New Engl J Med. 1998;339:856–7.
10. Hafferty FW. Beyond curriculum reform: confronting medicine's hidden curriculum. Acad Med. 1998;73:403–7.
11. Tempp H, Seale C. The hidden curriculum in undergraduate medical education: qualitative study of medical students' perceptions of teaching. Br Med J. 2004;329:770–3.
12. Cruess SR, Cruess RL, Steinert Y. Role modelling – making use of a powerful teaching strategy. Br Med J. 2008;336:718–21.
13. Paice E, Heard S, Moss F. How important are role models in making good doctors? Br Med J. 2002;325:707.
14. Wright SM, Carrese JA. Excellence in role modelling: insight and perspectives from the pros. CMAJ. 2002;167:638–43.

Chapter 16
Teaching Whole Person Care in Medical School

Helen Mc Namara and J. Donald Boudreau

No medical practitioner will ever excel who does not always keep before himself the fact that in every state of man the mind and the body react upon one another and are parts of a whole.

Norman Moore. Lancet, 14 Oct 1893.

Keywords: Teaching • Medical education • Medical school • Medical students • Physicianship • Simulation • Panel • Barriers • Patient–physician relationship • Team relationship • Self-care

Teaching Whole Person Care: Introduction

In an ideal world, whole person care would involve the care for a whole person – physical, psychological, and spiritual needs – by another whole person. This would be a wonderful way to care for each other, but we would probably all come up short. Two limitations become immediately apparent. First, the patients' needs may exceed the skill set of the physician in one or more domains. An individual patient may require, for example, a surgeon and a psychiatrist, as well as a spiritual advisor. Second, it is possible that the profile of needs of a particular patient may be better matched with the unique interests and experiences of one physician over another, even if both have had the same basic skills training. Another consideration is that whole person care is so personal and individual that a "one size fits all" approach to diagnosis and treatment cannot work. In patients with similar medical conditions, we need to consider the context for each individual and what the illness means to them, their families, and their communities at that particular point in time. However, while individual physicians cannot be expected to care for all domains of the

H. Mc Namara (✉)
Unit Chair, Physicianship 3, McGill Medical School, McGill Programs in Whole Person Care, Centre for Medical Education, Faculty of Medicine, McGill University, Montreal, QC, Canada
e-mail: helen.mcnamara@muhc.mcgill.ca

T.A. Hutchinson (ed.), *Whole Person Care: A New Paradigm for the 21st Century*, DOI 10.1007/978-1-4419-9440-0_16, © Springer Science+Business Media, LLC 2011

patient's well-being at all times, they must at least be aware that beyond the most apparent issue of the presenting concerns, there are domains that may either increase the patients' suffering or open a path for the facilitation of healing. The physician must be sufficiently attuned to the patient to find an opening to the latter possibility. In his mentoring and teaching, a founder of palliative care medicine, Dr. Balfour Mount tells the story of a patient he had, a young woman in palliative care, where he spent time learning more about her and found that despite their obvious differences, they shared a love of the music of the Elvis Presley, which turned out to be his "way in" to facilitate her healing through their stronger connection.

Although the teaching of "healing" in whole person care is the focus of this chapter, it may be surprising to the reader to learn that the concept of healing in medicine lacks clear definition. In fact, there have been many attempts to define it in operational terms. In a study based on interviews with experts in the field, it was thought that healing was associated with three main themes: wholeness, narrative, and spirituality [1]. In their definition of healing, Kearney and Mount have also included the concept of wholeness: *Healing is defined as a shift in quality of life away from anguish and suffering, toward an experience of integrity, wholeness, and inner peace* [2]. This shift in quality of life is the overarching goal of whole person care in medicine, and it requires attention to the patient's suffering in all domains: physical, emotional, and spiritual. This means that healing in medicine can only take place in the context of whole person care. Therefore, the teaching of the physician's healer role is synonymous with the practice of whole person care in medicine.

Teaching Whole Person Care: The Medical Education Literature

What does the medical education literature tell us about contemporary strategies aimed at teaching whole person care? Before we embark on this overview, it is important to address a fundamental question: is medical practice (and by extrapolation medical education) composed of two categories of facts, two ways of thinking, or, as it were, two distinct essences? A subsidiary question is: can the teaching of whole person care be equated to the teaching of humanism in medicine? These are weighty questions. They remained a preoccupation as we crafted a blueprint for teaching the healer role.

No doubt the reader will be familiar with the phrase "the art and science of medicine." Generally speaking, the former is linked to the interpersonal aspects of the patient–physician encounter, and it is seen to operate in situations of uncertainty, manifesting itself through excellence in listening skills and that most illusory of personal attributes, "clinical judgment." Science, which is often linked to quantitative research, technology, and the problem-solving aspects of medical practice (e.g., making diagnoses and selecting among treatment options), is believed to operate in a world that is measurable, universal, and predictable and manifests itself through finely honed analytical and reasoning skills. The principle of "nonoverlapping magisteria" has been used to capture this dichotomy [3]. This conception is pervasive in both the professional and lay press. Unfortunately, wide acceptance of this dichotomous state of affairs has had unintended consequences. It may have fostered the idea that the medical mandate has two divergent clinical goals: one goal being the reversal of disorders at the physiochemical level, thus achievement of a cure, while another being the assistance to patients in adapting, in the face of sickness, to a widened gap between what is desired and what is possible. Science is seen to be corralled for efforts at curing, whereas the so-called "art of medicine" is harnessed to the service of healing. It is "the art" that assumes primary responsibility as the handmaid of compassionate caring, albeit in a somewhat supportive role, whereas "the science" presides over the central proposition – fixing the broken body and mind.

Numerous health care programs presenting themselves as humane, accountable, holistic, and/or integrative describe a recalibration of the two ingredients: art and science. Invariably, their promise is that they will control, tame, or channel the latter while simultaneously nurturing the former. The popular and influential "patient-centered method" explicitly acknowledges a duality of clinical purposes by directing clinicians in patient encounters to actively weave back and forth between two strands – between the science, with its pathophysiological perspective of disease, and patients, in all their human complexities [4]. The goal of this method, laudatory as it is, should not be maligned. It may well be anchored in the idea that medicine has no option but to be dichotomous, since human beings are themselves dichotomous. Few would deny the existence of dichotomies in life in general; dualism is inherent to objective reality. A prototype par excellence is particle physics; the reality with which it deals, waves and particles, comprises an irreconcilable duality. That systems of thought and practice are plagued by dualism reflects this fundamental condition of life. Perhaps it is, therefore, entirely appropriate for a clinical method to acknowledge two essences of medicine, adopting a methodology that achieves effective complementarities and simply gets the job done – reverses the gap imposed by disease, where this is possible, and when not in the realm of possibilities, bridges the gap. In the development and deployment of our healing curriculum, the core aspects of which will be presented forthwith, some of us have nevertheless wished to avoid emphasizing dualities, in part, because we have felt that science always seems to prevail and overshadow all other considerations. In response, some of us have argued that an appropriate unifying orientation for medicine's goals might be the well-being of the patient, well-being as understood through a robust and sophisticated appreciation of patients' personal functioning [5], but that is a topic for another chapter.

We have purposely chosen not to characterize our educational goal as that of teaching a healing "art." Notwithstanding Aristotelian definitions of art as "skilled craftsmanship," we feel that there may be downsides to viewing the art of medicine as a species completely different from or, even more invidious, as being somehow at odds with science. The danger is that much of what has traditionally been grouped under "art" (e.g., demonstrating good bedside manner, making therapeutic interpersonal connections, displaying authentic compassion) may be construed as soft or fugacious. These skills may come to be subsumed under opinion and personal preferences and may be considered less accessible to scholarly scrutiny. We want, up front, to immunize our colleagues and students against the notion that teaching whole person care is nothing more or different than "being nice" – in North America, the metaphors of motherhood and apple pie quickly spring to mind. This type of dismissal may resonate with the experience of many readers.

As described earlier in this book, the Whole Person Care Program is founded on the assumption that the primary goal of medicine is healing. Commonality of purpose, as opposed to complementarities of knowledge bases, is the active integrative principle for the range of aptitudes and skills required in clinical work – regardless of whether they are to be discovered in the "art" world or the *weltanschauung* of "scienticism." We have attempted to anchor our teaching program in the beliefs that whole person care can be taught and done so systematically and explicitly. To become a healer implies something additive to heredity, more than the result of family upbringing and extending beyond kindergarten and premedical schooling experiences.

Notwithstanding the presence of epistemological debate, which our introduction delved into in a cursory fashion, it must not only be acknowledged but also be celebrated that there are many textbooks positioning healing as an art. To name but a few: " The Healer's Art" by Cassell, a contributor to this book, and "The Lost Art of Healing: Practicing Compassion in Medicine" by Lown. The literature is also replete with such references. A recent notable example is a commentary published in Lancet in 2008 by the medical anthropologist Kleinman; it is entitled: "Catastrophe and caregiving: the failure of medicine as an art" [6]. We draw attention to a few of the attempts at teaching the art of healing that have met with success. A popular course, designed to help medical students discover things about themselves in the context of learning clinical medicine is called the "The Healer's Art" [7]. Students are prompted to examine their values and emotional intelligence when relating to patients, all the while staying connected to the underlining meaning of the clinical work they do. One of the stated goals of the program is to prevent compassion fatigue and burnout. We too will address the phenomenon of personal alienation later on in this chapter. Another healing-oriented program that emphasizes the relationship between patient and physician, while integrating the best of complementary and alternative medicine with conventional medicine, is the University of Arizona's "Program in Integrative Medicine" [8]. Furthermore, a list of recommended core competencies has been outlined by an educational working group composed of experts in the area [9]. The focus of integrative medicine is the therapeutic relationship with attention also paid to physician self-care and self-awareness. Participants in such programs report that, while exploring their own humanity, they discover emotional wounds and benefit from the opportunity to begin their own healing process, making them more willing to partner with patients in facilitating healing. It stimulates and recalls "the call to service" that draws most individuals to the medical profession in the first place [8].

In yet another program, residents in Family Medicine work with behavioral scientists to identify patient and family strengths and to reflect critically on interactional patterns among themselves, patients, families, and other health care practitioners.

They explain that in the presence of chronic illness both patients and families experience fear, loss of control, and disconnectedness. The teaching of "Healing Relationships" is a curriculum designed to facilitate mutually empowering relationships [10]. The process in this program includes discovering what physicians bring to the work, examining patients' individual, family, cultural, and spiritual contexts; creating sustained partnerships, and empowering patients to take increasing control of their illnesses [10].

The teaching of the healer role has often been conflated with the teaching of humanism. A noncritical acceptance of the art/science, cure/heal, nature/nurture, psyche/soma, and innumerable other dualities may have provided the impetus for a clamor that humanism be provided greater visibility and curricular time in medical education. Regardless of its roots, a brief overview of how humanism can be taught is absolutely germane to our discussion. The range of strategies used to foster humanism has been broad indeed. It has included the study of the humanities (including classic literature), communication skills training (most recently with an emphasis on cultural competency), service learning (which generally refers to volunteer work among disadvantaged populations), and the fostering of self-reflection. In the mid and late twentieth century, the favored entry for humanism in medicine was via the teaching of ethics. This, then, seemed to give way to the targeted teaching of empathy. In the past two decades, the emphasis has been redirected toward tools to foster self-reflection. Reflection has been defined as, *a generic term for those intellectual and affective activities in which individuals engage to explore their experiences to lead to a new understanding and appreciation* [11]. It implies a conscious and deliberate effort to understand and appreciate events deeply and differently. It is assumed that the reflective practitioner will become more attuned to all of the patient's needs. A most highly promising approach to supporting whole person care has been the reaffirmation of professionalism and its related developments such as the creation of a Professionalism Charter and the description of the social contract [12]. These critically important developments are the focus of another chapter in this book.

Narrative medicine has recently entered the world of medical education at multiple levels and with a range of goals and objectives. In a recent review of the literature, three main objectives underlying the introduction of teaching narrative have been identified and it can serve to (1) reveal patients' perspectives, (2) act as a catalyst for self-reflection, and (3) provide emotional support to overworked and harried health care professionals [13]. The combination of creative writing, close reading, and active listening is commonly used to enhance the narrative competence of health care professionals. It is important to add that narrative competence has also been claimed as an approach to therapy, including psychotherapy, and that it has been taught and promoted for patients as well as clinicians.

Although debatable, there are some data to suggest that medical students experience a decline in empathy and a withering of altruism during medical training. For many of the training programs that rely on the humanities, an implicit aim is to mitigate against this loss of idealism. Several reviews have identified the essential features of such programs, one of which suggests that they must (a) provide students with opportunities to gain perspective on the lives of patients, (b) include structured time for reflection, and (c) incorporate focused mentoring [14].

There is a growing understanding of the factors that can hinder our teaching of healing. In a previous study of medical students' apprenticeship experiences at McGill University, Allen and colleagues described a number of perceived barriers to the teaching and learning of whole person care: competing discourses of empathy and efficiency, objectification of patients, power of the medical hierarchy, and the institutionalized practice of "wounding" [15]. They found that second-year medical students were apprehensive about getting to know their patients. Students were led to believe that this was a luxury that would disappear after training due to competing demands on their time. These findings were particularly disturbing as the students in this study were just halfway through their training and already they were anticipating a demise of caring attitudes. This is exactly the opposite of what should be in place as they prepare for the clerkship year – they should be excited at the prospect of being able to put theory into practice and further developing their compassion in the teaching hospitals and clinics. Kleinman has correctly concluded that in some settings it is not only that the concept of whole person care is absent from the curriculum but also that the structure of health care delivery may actually discourage it. He goes on to suggest that a professional education that is solely focused on scientific training may enable the physician as a technical expert but disable him as a caregiver [6]. We must find solutions to this quandary.

There are several corrosive aspects of the learning environment that are largely beyond the control of curriculum planners. For example, reduced admission times and early discharges from hospital can significantly reduce the time medical students spend with individual patients. It presents them with a sort of stroboscopic appreciation of the natural progression of disease and personal trajectories of illness. The untoward effects of a multitude of transient and evanescent social relationships, particularly with patients and also with teachers and peers, have been described in the medical literature [16]. The theoretical framework, described by Hafferty, of the formal, informal, and hidden curriculum can be helpful as we seek solutions. It acts as a powerful reminder that even if interventions intended to promote patient-centered care are placed in the preclinical years, the message may be overshadowed by the strength of the informal and hidden curricula of the clinical years [17]. This may result in what some medical students describe as a frustrating disconnect between what they are taught regarding the importance of whole person care and what they experience in clinical practice. It underlines the critical importance of making sure that physicians, especially those charged with mentorship and teaching, are practicing, modeling, and supporting a whole person care approach to patient care.

Medical school may be an ideal time to set up healthy habits so that the next generation of physicians may end up being happier persons in life and, thus, more prone to adopting whole person care practices in both clinical and educational contexts. Stuber provides some simple concrete suggestions for whole person "self-care," including prioritization of time – learning how to say no and budgeting time properly, keeping friends close and avoiding isolation, using exercise as a tension buster or as an opportunity for nurturing a sense of belonging and community, using relaxation to change thinking and to gain new perspectives, sleeping enough and minimizing disruptions. We could also add proper nutrition and spending time doing things or being with people who make one feel good [18]. A culture change is urgently required and communicating to medical students that being proactive about understanding and meeting their own whole person care needs is a win-win situation for students/peers and faculty. Where medical student stress is reduced, peer support flourishes, faculty mentorship thrives, and the "working–learning–caring environment" is populated with "whole persons" at all levels of care: faculty, student, and patient.

In providing us with the medical students' viewpoint on barriers to self-care, Reis questions the message that in the decision-making process surrounding patient care, it is never appropriate for medical students to consider the implications of their actions for themselves and that such consideration of personal implications is unprofessional [19]. She goes on to suggest that this approach puts professionalism in direct conflict with self-care leading to active discouragement of self-knowledge and self-awareness – in direct opposition to the fundamental requirements for whole person care. Teaching programs in healing and whole person care must actively promote reflective practice and mindfulness while making a clear distinction between altruism (putting the patients' interests ahead of *self-interests*) and the appropriate *self-care* of physicians and medical students. In fact, self-care and altruism must exist simultaneously if we are to care for patients properly while maintaining our own health and well-being in the process. As Reis says, while we should not forget our professionalism when we take off our white coat, it is equally important that medical students are not taught to check their "selves" at the door when they enter the clinic.

In medical school, there is often tension between good patient care (which takes time and graded responsibility) and the pressure to achieve good grades (efficiency and decreased supervision). There is a perception that good patient care may actually harm the medical students' grade and jeopardize their dossier for residency application. If this is the case, then faculty need to rework the evaluation process to reflect our valuing good patient care above all else. Thomas and colleagues found that both distress and well-being (Maslach Burnout Inventory) are correlated with student empathy (Empathy Measure – Interpersonal Reactivity Index), and they suggest that efforts to reduce student distress as part of an overarching goal to promote student well-being could enhance both empathy and professionalism [20]. It is important to teach these concepts and provide the tools by which to achieve them early in undergraduate training and consistently on a regular basis during the postgraduate years and beyond. Some models to accomplish this have been previously proposed [21, 22], one of which is based on the model of a "coping reservoir," a reservoir that has both negative and positive inputs that must be kept in balance to prevent burnout and promote resilience in medical students [21]. Accordingly, there is a clear relationship between resilience and the ability to care such that the two concepts are intertwined and inseparable.

Some have questioned whether healing can be taught, or whether it is, indeed, a received and innate ability [23]. We are of the opinion that as teachers, supervisors, and mentors we can facilitate the learning of healing, much like in our roles as physicians we seek to facilitate the onset of healing in patients. We often use a quote from Yeats in the teaching of healing/whole person care: *Teaching is not the filling of a pail but rather the lighting of a fire.* It is conceivable that our medical students come to us with their healing flame already lit. One may, thus, interpret our educational mission as one of having to gently fan the flame while studiously avoiding the creation of any conditions that will diminish or extinguish it. It is revealing that when we first presented a proposal for teaching whole person care to colleagues at McGill University, we were challenged with: *this stuff can't be taught.* Thankfully, before we could respond, one of the participants at a planning meeting said in a thunderous voice: *Well, we are certainly able to teach the opposite, so let's give this a try.* There is, therefore, tacit acceptance of our ability to minimize or divert attention from whole person care. As the flip side to that coin, we firmly believe that – collectively – we can facilitate the learning of whole person care and perhaps even "unteach" the opposite.

Teaching Whole Person Care: The McGill University Experience

Now that we have presented a few of the issues critical to the pedagogy of whole person care and having introduced some of the salient findings from the medical education literature, we turn our attention to the specifics of the program we have put in place at the Faculty of Medicine, McGill University. The McGill course on the "Physician as Healer" is embedded in the context of a program that revolves around "physicianship" [24]. The term "physicianship" is not in common usage and, thus, deserves to be defined. At our institution, it has acquired three meanings: (a) it encapsulates medicine's core mandate, i.e., healing and the relief of suffering; (b) it refers to the dual roles of physician as healer and physician as professional and posits a set of behavioral attributes necessary for the fulfillment of each; and (c) it refers to a specific curricular component of our medical school's undergraduate program. The Physicianship Component is comprised of a series of courses, including a longitudinal mentorship called "Physician Apprenticeship" and the "Physician as Healer" course. The former course is intended to focus explicitly on the students' transition from layman to physician and to provide a safe environment in which to reflect on the changes that they are undergoing in medical school enculturation. The teachers in that course are called Osler Fellows. The "Physician as Healer" course is organized around a set of six modules and each module addresses a key learning concept related to healing in medicine. The concepts upon which we anchor our teaching are as follows: (1) relief of suffering and promotion of healing, (2) building the patient–physician relationship, (3) patient's perspective and physician's perspective, (4) integrating healing with ethics and professionalism, (5) whole person care in team relationships, and (6) preparing for the high cost of caring (whole person care and medical student wellness). Each concept is associated with specific learning outcomes, and there is a final summative evaluation of learning at the end of the course. The process respects the traditional learning cycle and provides students with an opportunity to provide feedback on both content and process. Although the main part of the course is situated during the third year, enabling it to interface with the clerkship experience, we also conduct a number of introductory whole class interactive sessions in first year. Furthermore, we offer a session reintegrating the healer and professional roles in the fourth year, prior to graduation. The emphasis at this pivotal transition point is to explore where these roles might be conflicting with each other and how to manage this dissonance in clinical practice.

1. Relief of suffering and promotion of healing

Cassell has written extensively on the nature of suffering. He has commented that suffering involves a symptom or process that threatens the patient because of fear the patient has and/or the meaning(s) that are attached to the symptoms [25]. Illness means different things to different patients, and without considering the whole person and their unique experience of the illness, healing is difficult, if not impossible. Furthermore, the same disease in the same patient may mean different things at different times during any illness trajectory. We teach our students that the starting point for the promotion of healing is a clear understanding and appreciation of the patient's suffering, and this, from the patient's rather than the physician's perspective. Healing involves reconciliation of the meaning(s) an individual ascribes to distressing events within his or her perception of personal integrity and "wholeness." This suggests that suffering may be associated with "disrupted wholeness." Whole person care is not limited to only what the physician sees; it must also strive to peer into the suffering patient's arrested, progressing, or otherwise evolving sense of self and wholeness. We expect that in teaching this explicitly, our medical students will learn how to recognize and acknowledge patient suffering and also how to avoid adding to patient suffering, while actively trying to promote patient healing.

This concept is centered on the whole person care of the patient (Fig. 16.1, Module 1), and as such, it is taught by the Osler Fellows in the small group setting with their own group of medical students that they are mentoring throughout the 4-year program.

2. Building the patient–physician relationship

An important distinction is that which exists between a "person" and a "patient." In the Oxford English Dictionary, the patient is defined as *a person who suffers from an injury or disease; a sick person*. However, it is important to remember that the state of "patienthood" resides within a whole person. Physicians must not be concerned solely with the disease as an abstract phenomenon existing apart from the patient. Physicians have the obligation to understand the expression of the disease including its unique manifestations and impacts on the individual patient. How can one become truly patient-centered? We believe that a possible entry is through a focus on patient well-being, with the latter being defined as the patient's ability to

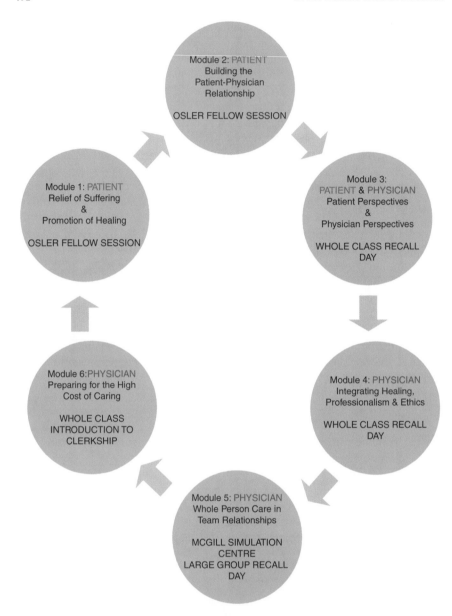

Fig. 16.1 Teaching Whole Person Care: The McGill University experience

pursue his or her achievable goals and functions. The inability to achieve goals and fulfill purposes arises from impairments of function. Functional impairment can occur at any level, from the molecular to the spiritual. Therefore, if the goal is to focus on the patient's well-being, with the primary aim being the restoration of function, to the extent that this is possible, the physician's world automatically continues beyond the patient's physical body into the psychological, social, and spiritual domains [26].

In using the term "patient–physician relationship," we realize that the patient always initiates the relationship. Also, the word relationship is important because many clinical interactions are fleeting in nature, and one may legitimately wonder if they can really qualify as a "relationship." We believe and teach that all encounters with patients, however brief, hold the potential to become healing or wounding. Contrary to what we often hear from physicians, whole person care is not necessarily time-consuming or inefficient. In fact, Donadio describes a relationship-centered care model that allows for compassionate, humanistic health care, regardless of the amount of time spent with the patient, suggesting that the focus and intention brought to the patient interaction (60 s, 3 min or 1 h) becomes the foundation for all future interactions [27]. Our patients tell us repeatedly that time need not be a barrier to a caring patient–physician relationship, relating stories of both extraordinary physician healing and extraordinary physician wounding that took place in a matter of minutes, summarized by a single sentence that they can quote verbatim many years later.

Furthermore, Dobie describes empathy as the capacity to accept, to try to understand, and to connect with another's experience, and she labels this as behavior that is critical to the healing relationship [28]. Another way of describing whole person care could be relationship-centered care where there is the consideration of not just the patient as a whole person but the physician or medical student as whole persons also. Dobie identifies two essential components of relationship centered care: self-awareness and mindful practice. Evidence for this theory is accumulating. A recent paper from the University of Rochester School of Medicine and Dentistry has shown that participation in a mindful communication program was associated with sustained improvements in attitudes relevant to patient-centered care [29].

The patient and physician are united in their mutual goals of the relief of suffering and the promotion of patient healing. Despite the common purpose, there exist power differentials at many points of the health care system. Patients are in a vulnerable state and physicians must never lose sight of that reality. With this in mind, it is important to appreciate that the patient–physician relationship begins even before the patient sees the physician. How did the physician's staff treat the patient in the lead-up process or in the waiting area? We teach students that as much as the patient does not want to be identified by their ill or injured "part," for example, as *the head injury in bed 5*, they also do not want to be cared for by "the medical student" – the caring relationship between two people starts with a name for each one. Our goals in teaching this concept are that our medical students will be able to understand the importance of the patient–physician relationship, appreciate the role of the power differential between patients and physicians, and discuss the attributes required for the creation of a healing patient–physician relationship.

This concept is focused on the building of a "patient-centered" patient–physician relationship (Fig. 16.1, Module 2), and it is also taught by the Osler Fellows in their special individualized small group setting, where they share and discuss their actual clinical experiences in the creation of the patient–physician relationship.

3. Patient's perspective and physician's perspective

We teach our medical students to examine the patient–physician relationship closely by reflectively asking what may be the perspective of the patient entering into this relationship. Also, it is of interest to ask what may be the perspective of the physician and to compare and contrast the two. As patients and physicians, we are clearly working from different positions and the relative importance attributed to information that enters our consciousness will often differ between us. This has been demonstrated with regard to discrepancies between patients and physicians on the relative importance they attribute to different quality-of-life measures. As physicians and medical students, we approach the bedside as unique individuals bringing with us our own culture and beliefs, conscious and unconscious assumptions, needs, emotions, expectations, skills, and our level of presence and/or distractions on that particular day [28]. Our clinical judgment is also influenced by emotions, bias, prejudice, risk aversion, tolerance for uncertainty, and personal knowledge of the patient [30]. Questions that we have found useful to trigger a dialogue on this concept include the following: When does a person become a patient? How does this person become a patient? What does his/her suffering mean in his/her individual context? What barriers might I encounter in relating to this particular patient? How did these barriers arise and how can I overcome them? Why did I have this unexpected reaction to this patient?

In their paper on breaking bad news, Dias and colleagues used patients' experiences to illustrate how physicians practiced whole person care – or not – from the patients' point of view. The patients in this paper described different perspectives on whether cancer patients like to be hugged by their doctors [31]. We use this example to teach students to stop and assess where the patient might be on such issues and to be wary of "one size fits all" approaches to patient care. We expect that our students will be able to understand the importance of both the patient's and the physician's perspective, while appreciating that the physician's self-care may have a significant impact on his/her ability to provide whole person care.

This concept is focused on the recognition of the difference between patient perspectives and physician perspectives in building and maintaining the patient–physician relationship (Fig. 16.1, Module 3). We teach this concept in the context of a Whole Class Recall Day, which involves all clerkship medical students reuniting at the medical school for a day of reflection and learning surrounding these concepts. We present a patient panel and small group sessions in the morning addressing the patients' perspectives, and then we switch to the physician panel and small groups in the afternoon, focusing on the physicians' perspectives, the goal being the exploration of differences and opportunities for increased collaboration, through medical students' questioning and discussion of the issues raised from the perspectives of both patients and physicians.

4. Integrating healing with ethics and professionalism

The role of the "physician healer" is rarely separated from that of the "physician professional." Richard and Sylvia Cruess have argued that physicians function simultaneously in both roles and that each supports the integrity of the other.

This idea is developed further in another chapter of this book. However, while in most situations the healer and professional roles act in the same direction, there are certain situations where there may be conflict, e.g., the "healer" thinks it is best to hug the patient, whereas the "professional" considers that to be a boundary crossing; the "healing" team member covers up for the impaired colleague, while the "professional" is prompted to advocate for removal from patient care and possible disciplinary action. The rules of professionalism exist to protect the integrity of the healer role, and this is a fundamental concept that must be appreciated by physicians. This is also important in our teaching as our clinical experience and stories from patients suggest that medical students may themselves affect the healing process of the patients in whose care they participate. Indeed, they often have a profoundly positive effect. Perhaps this is because they can spend more "quality time" with their patients or because they are still early enough in their training to be able to relate to patients in a more open way.

This concept is focused on the recognition of the challenges and opportunities that may arise in integrating healing, professionalism, and ethics in clinical practice (Fig. 16.1, Module 4). Again, we teach this concept in the context of a Whole Class Recall Day, with all clerkship students reuniting at the medical school for a day of reflection and learning. In this teaching session, we invite the students to explore the contributions they felt they themselves have made to their patient's healing journeys, and they are invited to share their reflections with peers and faculty, including a panel of experts on healing, professionalism, and ethics. We discuss those clinical situations raised by the students where tensions were apparent between the healer role, ethical care, and professionalism, and we examine how best to address these tensions in the integration of these concepts in clinical practice. We are interested in what insights our students can bring to the process based on their personal experiences or observations and whether we can include these in our teaching to the next cohort of physician apprentices in a form of peer to near-peer learning. Our aim for this concept is that medical students will appreciate the importance of integrating the skills of healing with the cognitive bases of bioethics and professionalism.

5. Whole person care in team relationships

It has been suggested that during our training of medical students, whom we wish to be caring and compassionate, it would be reasonable to expect that the teaching and learning environments we provide would be caring and compassionate [32]. However, this is not easy to guarantee. Relating to patients who are suffering on a daily basis may have a negative impact on the well-being of physicians and their relationships with other team members. This is particularly important when these team relationships involve a power differential, such as that experienced by medical students in the clinical setting. When confronted with such situations, students need to be equipped to deal with them in a professional and healing way. It would be ideal if physician-educators could consistently demonstrate the attributes of the healer role in their relationships with team members. It seems self-evident that this would lead to both a positive learning environment for the students and experiential learning of the healer role in the clinical setting. It is patently difficult, and perhaps even absurd, to try to nurture a culture of whole person care of patients in an environment where the learners themselves are being treated as objects rather than whole persons, at times by the very faculty and staff who have been entrusted with their mentorship.

Although it is generally assumed that adverse experiences during training will have a negative impact on medical students, one research team has formally studied the consequences of such experiences [32]. This group found that two thirds of their students had at least one adverse experience, with humiliation the most common reported and having the greatest negative impact. These students reported that it took several hours to several days to get over one of these episodes and the students most commonly avoided that person or department. It is clear that these responses have the potential to negatively impact students' learning. However, although only half of these students sought help, a sixth of the medical students studied admitted that the adverse experiences they encountered made them consider leaving medical school. In relation to this concept, we expect that our medical students will appreciate that they may encounter some negative relationships with team members at some point during their apprenticeship and that they will understand what they can do to protect themselves should they encounter such a situation.

This concept is focused on the whole person care of medical students and physicians in the context of team relationships, and it is taught as part of a Large Group Recall Day at the McGill Simulation Center (Fig. 16.1, Module 5). We teach this concept by creating a safe environment at the Simulation Center using standardized physicians, nurses, and patients to present real-life situations involving negative interactions between medical students and senior team members. The goal of this session is for medical students to understand that negative interactions do occur between team members in the high-pressure area of clinical care and to provide them with tools on how to handle such situations both when they occur and after the fact, in an effort to promote awareness of whole person care for physicians and other team members as an important foundation for the practice of whole person patient care.

6. Preparing for the high cost of caring – whole person care and medical student well-being

Mount suggests that two most important themes in healing are "meaning" and "connection," and he proposes that connection is important in four domains: connection to self, connection to others, connection to nature/the universe, and connection to a higher power [33]. This means that in teaching whole person care, it is critical to understand and teach students how to facilitate patient's meaning-making and to recognize the importance of maintaining or creating new connections at a time when the instinct of the sufferer may be to disconnect. The chapter in this book on "language in medicine" addresses critical aspects of "meaning-making." Furthermore, if we consider the work of Mount in the context of Pearson's advice to medical students regarding the importance of maintaining connections [34], it implies that it is important for us to support students in their attempts to remain connected to themselves throughout medical school, e.g., via mindfulness training. Specific strategies, such as creating or maintaining connectedness to nature, music, or whatever in the universe that provides one with sustenance, have been discussed earlier. Janssen and colleagues suggest that there are three requirements for fostering empathy in medical students: self-awareness, personal well-being, and humanistic development. They also state that to care for others, physicians and medical students must receive care and support for themselves, and this may be best achieved through mentorship, supervision, and peer support, as well as in reflective practice [35]. For this concept, we expect that our medical students will recognize the high cost of caring in the development of the physician as a healer and prepare for, and respond to, this situation in the best way possible.

This concept is focused on the whole person care of medical students (and physicians) in preparation for their entry into the high-pressure world of caring for suffering patients on a daily basis (Fig. 16.1, Module 6). We teach this concept as a Whole Class Interactive Session as the medical students enter clerkship, using experiences – both negative and positive – of the students who have gone before them, with a focus on lessons learned from near-peers such as "what I know now at the end of clerkship that I wish I knew at the beginning" in terms of preparing the medical students for the high cost of caring. This session also relays the positive experiences in clerkship and the benefits that we, as physicians and medical students, are fortunate to experience in the context of our whole person care approach to our patients.

Teaching Whole Person Care: Conclusion

Medical educators are urged to teach that listening to the patient's unique story is "not just one of the most interesting aspects of being a doctor but one of the most necessary to being a good one" [36]. This means that we need to teach our medical students to make the time to listen attentively to the patient – not just with our ears but with all of our other senses also, so that we come away with a "whole narrative," as faithful to the patient's original story as possible, rather than constructing a series of incomprehensible segments within a medical narrative that has subsumed or disregarded the patient's own "real-life" account. In contrast to the way many of us learned to become physicians, we now need to adopt a two-pronged approach by advocating and supporting the whole person care of patients, as well as that of medical students, practicing physicians, and medical teachers. It has been suggested that it is not emotional detachment from patients or oversentimental attachment to patients that makes a good doctor, but rather the words and actions that emerge from an awareness on the part of physicians of "one's inner landscape" [37]. We need to focus on the importance of self-awareness and reflective practice in the creation of healing relationships, whether between patient and physician, medical student and teacher, or between interdisciplinary and peer team members in the relationships that continue to be a fundamental part of patient care. It has also been stated that in the context of patient care, efficiency and cost-cutting may be helpful overall for education and health, but they cannot replace functions such as teaching, learning, and healing, nor can they excuse departures from these central functions [38]. This group further suggests that the functions and structures of management should be redefined to serve the knowledge workers (physicians, nurses, teachers), whose role in health and education is indispensable, rather than burden them with increasing responsibility for management [38]. This is a necessary step in the progression to self-awareness, reflective practice – time to reflect and write – and whole person care for all.

Although we have developed a comprehensive curriculum on healing and whole person care, which is delivered at different stages throughout the 4 years of medical school, we are challenged to combine these efforts at the medical school with active learning approaches and strong patient-centered role modeling by respected attending doctors [39]. One of the ways intended to achieve this at McGill University has been Physician Apprenticeship where each medical student is assigned to a group and a faculty mentor (Osler Fellow) for the duration of medical school. This mentoring relationship often serves as a bridge between didactic teaching and clinical practice, offering a safe space to discuss and address any disconnect. However, one of the next steps must be the explicit teaching of whole person patient care – outlining its benefits for patients, medical students, and physicians – to all faculty members. This could help us harmonize what is taught formally, what is learned informally, and what is practiced on the wards on a daily basis in our caring, teaching, working environment. Dobie suggests that by changing our approach to medical education, we could sustain and develop the wonder and gratitude that medical students bring with them to medical school, rather than see it eroded by medical training [28]. As Malcolm Gladwell once said, *"We learn by example and by direct experience because there are real limits to the adequacy of verbal instruction."* We believe that this is especially true with regard to our teaching of whole person care for patients, medical students, and physicians in medical school.

References

1. Egnew TR. The meaning of healing: transcending suffering. Ann Fam Med. 2005;3:255–62.
2. Mount B, Kearney M. Healing and palliative care: charting our way forward. Palliative Medicine. 2003;17:657–58.
3. Solomon M. Epistemological reflections on the art of medicine and narrative medicine. Perspect Biol Med. 2008;51:406–17.
4. Stewart M, Belle JB, Weston WW, McWhinney IR, McWilliam CL, Freeman TR. Patient-centered medicine. Transforming the clinical method. Abingdon: Radcliffe Medical; 2003.
5. Boudreau JD, Cassell EJ. Abraham Flexner's "mooted question" and the story of integration. Acad Med. 2010;85:378–83.
6. Kleinman A. Catastrophe and caregiving: the failure of medicine as an art. Lancet. 2008;371:22–3.
7. Remen, R. Teaching the heart of medicine: an interview with Rachel Naomi Remen (Internet). San Francisco Medicine. September 2005. http://www.sfms.org.
8. Maizes V, Schneider C, Bell I, Weil A. Integrative medical education: development and implementation of a comprehensive curriculum at the University of Arizona. Acad Med. 2002;77:851–60.

9. Kligler B, Maizes V, Schachter S, Park CM, Gaudet T, Benn R, et al. Core competencies in integrative medicine for medical school curricula: a proposal. Acad Med. 2004;79:521–31.
10. Saba G, Draisin J. Teaching residents to develop healing relationships when caring for the chronically ill. Acad Med. 2000;75:549.
11. Boud D, Keogh R, Walker D, editors. Reflection: Turning Experience into Learning. London: Kogan Page; 1985.
12. Cruess RL, Cruess SR. Teaching medicine as a profession in the service of healing. Acad Med. 1997;72:941–52.
13. Holmgren L, Fuks A, Boudreau D, Sparks T, Kreiswirth M. Terminology and praxis: Clarifying the scope of 'narrative' in medicine. Lit Med. (in press).
14. Stern DT, Cohen JJ, Bruder A, Packer B, Sole A. Teaching humanism. Perspect Biol Med. 2008;51:495–507.
15. Allen D, Wainwright M, Mount B, Hutchinson T. The wounding path to becoming healers: medical students' apprenticeship experiences. Med Teach. 2008;30:260–4.
16. Christakis DA, Feudtner C. Temporary matters: the ethical consequences of transient social relationships in medical training. JAMA. 1997;278:739–43.
17. Hafferty FW. Beyond curriculum reform: confronting medicine' hidden curriculum. Acad Med. 1998;73:403–7.
18. Stuber ML. Medical student and physician well-being [Internet]. http://www.hhpub.com/books/pdf/bam4-c13.pdf.
19. Reis DC. Who am I and why am I here? Professionalism research through the eyes of a medical student. Acad Med. 2008;83:111–2.
20. Thomas MR, Dyrbye LN, Huntington JL, Lawson KL, Novotny PJ, Soan JA, et al. How do distress and well-being relate to medical student empathy? A multicenter study. J Gen Intern Med. 2007;22:177–83.
21. Dunn LB, Iglewicz A, Moutier C. A conceptual model of medical student well-being: promoting resilience and preventing burnout. Acad Psychiatry. 2008;32:44–52.
22. Jensen PM, Trollope-Kumar K, Waters H, Everson J. Building physician resilience. Can Fam Physician. 2008;54:722–9.
23. Bengston WF, Murphy DG. Can healing be taught? Explore. 2008;4:197–200.
24. Boudreau JD, Cruess R, Cruess S. Physicianship – educating for professionalism in the post-Flexnarian era. Perspect Biol Med. 2001;54:89–105.
25. Cassell EJ. The relief of suffering. Arch Intern Med. 1983;143:522–3.
26. Boudreau JD, Cassell EJ, Fuks A. A healing curriculum. Med Educ. 2007;41:1193–201.
27. Donadio G. Improving healthcare delivery with the transformational whole person care model. Holist Nurs Pract. 2005;19:74–7.
28. Dobie S. Reflections on a well-traveled path: self-awareness, mindful practice, and relationship-centered care as foundations for medical education. Acad Med. 2007;82:422–7.
29. Krasner MS, Epstein RM, Beckman H, Suchman AL, Chapman B, Mooney CJ, et al. Association of an educational program in mindful communication with burnout, empathy, and attitudes among primary care physicians. JAMA. 2009;302:1284–93.
30. Epstein RM. Mindful practice. JAMA. 1999;282:833–9.
31. Dias L, Chabner BA, Lynch Jr TJ, Penson RT. Breaking bad news: a patient's perspective. Oncologist. 2003;8:587–96.
32. Wilkinson TJ, Gill DJ, Fitzjohn J, Palmer CL, Mulder RT. The impact on students of adverse experiences during medical school. Med Teach. 2006;28:129–35.
33. Mount BM, Boston PH, Cohen SR. Healing connections: on moving from suffering to a sense of well-being. J Pain Symp Manage. 2007;33:372–88.
34. Pearson J. Teaching the art of healing [Internet]. Minnesota Medicine. April 2009. http://www.minnesotamedicine.com.
35. Janssen AL, Macleod RD, Walker ST. Recognition, reflection, and role models: critical elements in education about care in medicine. Palliat Support Care. 2008;6:389–95.
36. Gunderman RB. Rethinking our basic concepts of health and disease. Acad Med. 1995;70:676–83.

37. DasGupta S. Between stillness and story: lessons of children's illness narratives. Pediatrics. 2007;119:e1384–91.
38. Little M. Health, education and the virtues of efficiency. N Z Dent J. 1995;91:89–93.
39. Branch Jr WT, Kern D, Maidet P, Weissman P, Gracey CF, Mitchell G, et al. The patient-physician relationship. Teaching the human dimensions of care in clinical settings. JAMA. 2001;286:1067–74.

Chapter 17
Whole Person Care, Professionalism, and the Medical Mandate

Richard L. Cruess and Sylvia R. Cruess

The public wants both better medical care and a profession more responsive to its needs. But most of all, people want competent and caring physicians who are committed to the healing of their patients [1].

Keywords Professionalism • Healing • Social contract • Commitment and presence • Altruism • Insight • Trustworthiness

Introduction

The evolution of the practice of medicine, whose history is firmly rooted in the art of healing, is paradoxical. Society has always required and been served by healers since before history was recorded. In Western society, one can trace the roots of the healer to Hellenic Greece with its Aesculapian and Hippocratic traditions. Other cultures have their own traditions, and all appear to be based firmly in a commitment to selfless service to those in need. Prior to the appearance of modern science, curing was rare, but patient satisfaction appeared to be high. From this, one can surmise that whole patient care was being dispensed long before the term was coined. The advent of the scientific revolution in the middle of the nineteenth century, which was essential to the development of the modern medical profession, initially did not appear to significantly alter the relationship between a physician and a patient. Even if Shaw considered the professions to be a "conspiracy against the laity," [2] trust in the medical profession continued to be extremely high until the second half of the twentieth century. Patients were usually cared for by generalists,

R.L. Cruess (✉)
Centre for Medical Education, McGill University, Lady Meredith House,
1110 Pine Avenue West, Montreal, QC H3A 1A3, Canada
e-mail: richard.cruess@mcgill.ca

T.A. Hutchinson (ed.), *Whole Person Care: A New Paradigm for the 21st Century*,
DOI 10.1007/978-1-4419-9440-0_17, © Springer Science+Business Media, LLC 2011

with specialization being present but rare [3]. Scientific medicine, which was becoming much more important to medical practice, was still understandable to the individual citizen who had acquired some education. The latter half of the twentieth century has seen a major change. A combination of specialization and sub-specialization, technological advances that would have been incomprehensible only a few decades earlier, and health care systems whose payment practices encourage the use of procedures and technology have become the new medical reality [4]. The result has been significant changes in the patterns of patient care. This has been accentuated in many jurisdictions by the shortage of primary care physicians who traditionally have assumed a disproportionate share of the responsibility for meeting the fundamental human need for whole person care. In part because of this, trust in the medical profession has diminished at the very time when the medical profession, along with other disciplines practicing the healing arts, has never had a greater ability to alter the course of human disease [5]. As a result, there have been calls for a return to a doctor–patient relationship that can better support the role of the healer. Whole person care describes such a relationship. It is the purpose of this chapter to propose that practicing whole person care is central to meeting the legitimate expectations of both patients and society, something which has not changed throughout the ages. As a consequence, it is a professional responsibility, not only for generalists and primary care physicians, but also for all practitioners.

Professionalism and Medicine's Social Contract

The concept of professionalism has a long history, and the word has been in use for at least 2000 years. Its first appearance in connection with medicine has been ascribed to a Roman physician, Scribonius [6], who defined professionalism as "a commitment to compassion or clemency in the relief of suffering," [7] an essential part of whole person care. He linked it to the act and the tradition of professing inherent in the Hippocratic Oath. This meaning was certainly still operative in the middle ages when the learned professions of medicine, law, and the clergy emerged [4, 8]. They arose in their new form from the guilds and universities of Europe and England (Fig. 17.1) [9]. The professions were given status in society and a considerable degree of autonomy. Medicine, which served a small elite and had minimal curative powers, exerted little impact on the average citizen. In the nineteenth century, science began to transform medicine, making it more effective and, therefore, worth purchasing, at the same time as the industrial revolution provided sufficient wealth so that patients could pay for health care. Society recognized that some form of organization of the delivery of the services of the healer was required and turned to the preexisting concept of the profession to accomplish this [4, 8]. Essentially, public policy in health care was built around the professions, with the medical profession being enthusiastically complicit in this endeavor. In most developed countries, by the middle of the nineteenth century, physicians had come together to form national professional medical associations and had developed

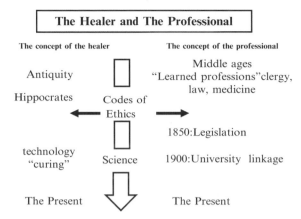

Fig. 17.1 The healer and the professional have different origins and have evolved in parallel but separately. As shown on the *left*, all societies have required the services of healers. The Western tradition of healing began in Hellenic Greece and is the part of the self image of the medical profession. Curing became possible only with the advent of scientific medicine. The modern professions arose in the guilds and universities of medieval Europe and England. They acquired their present form in the middle of the nineteenth century when licensing laws granted a monopoly over practice to allopathic medicine. When science caused medicine to be more knowledge based, the profession moved closer to universities. Codes of ethics have always guided the behavior of both the healer and the professional and science empowers both

codes of ethics governing the behavior of their members. These associations successfully lobbied governments to establish medical licensure, which granted a monopoly over practice to allopathic medicine. At this point, the foundations of the present-day professions were created [4, 10]. Contemporary interpretation of these events indicates that the granting of professional status to medicine served then, and continues to serve, as the basis of a social contract between medicine and society [11, 12]. Under the terms of this contract, medicine is granted a monopoly over the use of its knowledge base, considerable autonomy in practice, prestige and status, the privilege of self-regulation, and financial rewards. In return, physicians and the profession are expected to be altruistic, demonstrate honesty and integrity, assure the competence of practitioners, and be devoted to the public good. While the operational details of both professionalism and the social contract have changed as both medicine and society have evolved, the basic "bargain" has not. Even though individual citizens do not express it, without question whole person care was and remains both a public hope and an important expectation.

Using the term social contract as the basis of analyzing the relationship between medicine and society offers several advantages [12]. In the first place, the term has been in use since the eighteenth century and is still utilized by contemporary philosophers as they discuss the organization of society, including health care services. John Rawls [13] and health care planners such as Daniels [14] are both contractualists and base their discourses on social contract theory. Thus, the broad outline of the historical concept is still widely appreciated and used. Second, it invokes the principle of mutual rights and mutual obligations. Originally, this applied to citizens and those who governed them. In its modern iteration, it is used in a wider sense to illuminate the relationship between those who serve society (such as physicians and other health care workers) and society itself. It highlights the fact that physicians must meet legitimate expectations of the patients and society to maintain their professional status.

The Healer and the Professional

If one is to link whole person care with professionalism, one must understand the relationship of the healer to the professional [9, 15] (Fig. 17.1). Physicians in today's modern and complex society must simultaneously fulfill these two histori-cal roles, which are clearly linked in the public's mind. They share much common ground but are drawn from different traditions and entail different sets of obliga-tions. Neither can they be ignored without altering the relationship of medicine and society. In much of the literature, both roles are subsumed into the term profes-sional, but we believe that separating them helps to clarify their functions, which have always been and remain distinct.

It should be recognized that the terms profession, professional, and professionalism are generic, applying to those occupations responsible for delivering the necessary complex services required by society. Issues concerning health require the services of the healer and as the modern physician emerged, they shouldered a major share of the responsibility for delivering these services [16]. The necessity of adjudicating disputes led to the emergence of the legal profession. Other essential services resulted in the granting of professional status to members of other occupations such as engineering, architecture, etc. While all share many common characteristics, the dominant theme uniting them is expertise used in the service of society.

A schematic representation of the relationship between the role of the healer and that of the professional is shown in Fig. 17.2 [9]. The attributes ascribed to the two roles are derived from the literature. The left side of the Venn diagram lists those attributes unique to the healer, while the right shows those unique to the profes-sional. The area where the two circles overlap includes the attributes shared by both roles. A similar diagram could be created for the legal profession by changing the word "Physician" at the top of the diagram to "Lawyer" and replacing "Healer" above the left-hand circle with "Adjudicator of Disputes." The attributes of the professional would remain unchanged, but the specific attributes of the adjudicator of disputes would be substituted for those of the healer.

It is not the purpose of this chapter to define whole person care. Nevertheless, we propose that the attributes of the healer shown in the diagram represent those necessary qualities that are required for the delivery of whole person care. Among those qualities that are unique to the healer role, caring and compassion, including the ability to listen are a fundamental part of whole person care. When asked what qualities they would like or expect of their physicians, members of the public list

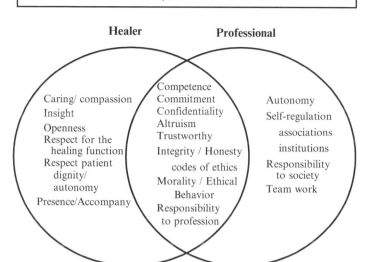

Fig. 17.2 The attributes traditionally associated with and unique to the healer are shown in the *left* hand circle and those with the professional on the *right*. Those shared by both are found in the large area of overlap of the circles. This list of attributes is drawn from the literature on healing and professionalism

these qualities at or near the top [16, 17]. Openness, the willingness to hear, accept, and deal with the views of others without reserve or pretense, is also an essential quality. Respect for the healing function is necessary as it indicates that the physician understands that only the patients have the inherent power to heal themselves. Physicians at best can facilitate this process. Respect for patient autonomy requires that the physician be committed to ensure the subjective well-being and sense of worth in patients, as well as recognizing the patient's absolute right to decide on the nature of their care. Finally, including presence indicates that a physician must be present for a patient without distraction and must fully support and accompany them throughout the course of their care.

There are many attributes that are shared by the healer and the professional and that are also essential to whole person care. Competence must underlie all activities of the physician. Commitment, which serves as an essential foundation of caring and compassion, is a quality that goes back to the time of Hippocrates, as does the obligation to maintain patient confidentiality. The constellation of integrity, honesty, morality, and ethical conduct are necessary to maintain the trust of patients. Without trust, the objective of whole person care, which is healing, is not possible. Finally, altruism requires that the physician place the patient's interests above their own. Clearly, should a patient believe that this is not true, once more healing would not be possible.

The Social Contract and Whole Person Care

In attempting to link the social contract and professionalism with whole person care, it is helpful to refer to the details of the social contract, which is the bridge. Figure 17.3 represents an outline of the expectations of both the public and the medical profession based on an analysis of the literature [11]. It is, thus, a representation of the "bargain" that is the basis of the social contract and hence of medical professionalism. As can be seen, a majority of the societal expectations are fundamental to whole person care. Most actually refer to the healer's role. As outlined above, assured competence is essential. Commitment, presence, and altruism all contribute to timely access and are essential parts of the healer role. The qualities

Patients/ Public Expectations of Medicine	Medicine's Expectations of Patients/Public
• Fulfill the role of the healer	• Trust sufficient to meet patient's
• Assured competence of physicians	needs
• Timely access to competent care	• Autonomy sufficient to exercise
• Altruistic service	judgment
• Morality, Integrity, Honesty	• Role in public policy in health
• Trustworthiness	• Shared responsibility for health
codes of ethics	• Self-regulation
	• Balanced lifestyle
• Accountability: performance,	• Monopoly
productivity, cost-effectiveness	• Rewards – non-financial
• Transparency in decision making &	Respect
administration	
• Respect for patient dignity &	- status
autonomy	- financial
• Source of objective advice on	
health matters	
• Team health care	
• Promotion of the public good	

Fig. 17.3 The expectations of the two major parties involved in medicine's social contract with society

of insight and altruism allow the healer to recognize and preserve the patient's dignity and autonomy, which are so necessary to whole person care. Also, trustworthiness is essential to help a person heal.

Conclusions

In this chapter, we propose that whole person care is the professional responsibility of all physicians. This is based upon the belief that all societies have and will remain in need of the services of the healer. While linking the concepts of profession and social contract to health care is relatively recent, we believe that a social contract has always existed between healers and the societies they served. In modern times, professionalism has been the means that society has chosen to organize the services of the healer. Healers have always had status in society and often substantial rewards on the understanding that they would meet societal needs and expectations. These needs and expectations hinge on what is required to effect healing, and the whole person care concept represents a powerful means of assuring that the physician will be the healers that societies have always required.

References

1. Sullivan WM. Introduction. In: Cruess RL, Cruess SR, Steinert Y, editors. Teaching medical professionalism. New York: Cambridge University Press; 2009. p. 1–7.
2. Shaw GB. Introduction. In: The doctor's dilemma. Harmondsworth: Penguin Books; 1946. p. 75.
3. Stevens R. Medical practice in modern England. The impact of specialization and state medicine. New Haven: Yale University Press; 1996.
4. Starr P. The social transformation of American medicine. New York: Basic Books; 1982.
5. Schlesinger M. A loss of faith: the sources of reduced political legitimacy for the American medical profession. Milbank Q. 2002;80:185–235.
6. Hamilton JS. Scribonius Largus on the medical profession. Bull Hist Med. 1986;60:209–16.
7. DeRosa P. Professionalism and virtues. Clin Orthop Relat Res. 2006;44:28–33.
8. Krause E. Death of the guilds: professions, states and the advance of capitalism, 1930 to the present. New Haven: Yale University Press; 1996.
9. Cruess SR, Cruess RL. The cognitive base of professionalism. In: Cruess RL, Cruess SR, Steinert Y, editors. Teaching medical professionalism. New York: Cambridge University Press; 2009. p. 7–31.
10. Cruess RL, Cruess SR. Teaching medicine as a profession in the service of healing. Acad Med. 1997;72:941–52.
11. Sullivan W. Work and integrity: the crisis and promise of professionalism in North America. 2nd ed. San Francisco: Jossey-Bass; 2005.
12. Cruess RL, Cruess SR. Expectations and obligations: professionalism and medicine's social contract with society. Perspect Biol Med. 2008;51:579–98.
13. Rawls J. Justice as fairness: a restatement. Cambridge: Harvard University Press; 2003.
14. Daniels N. Just health care. Cambridge: Cambridge University Press; 2008.
15. Freidson E. Professional dominance: the social structure of medical care. Chicago: Aldine; 1970.
16. Neufeld VR, Maudsley RF, Pickering RJ, et al. Educating future physicians for Ontario. Acad Med. 1998;73:1133–48.
17. Coulter A. What do patients and the public want from primary care? BMJ. 2005;331:1199–201.

Chapter 18
Whole Person Care: Conclusions

Tom A. Hutchinson

Keywords Burned out • Cicely Saunders • Therapeutic relationship • Hierarchy • Vulnerability • Mortality • Chronic disease • End-stage kidney disease • Chronic kidney failure • Dichotomy • Algorithm • Surgeon • Synergistic • Placebo • Longings • Expectations

Is whole person care a clear solution to problems plaguing twenty-first century medicine, including the paradox that we have more security, health, and material comfort, and live longer than humans at any other time in history, and at the same time appear to be more unhappy, anxious, and dissatisfied than ever before? We believe that mindful whole person care is a solution to the problem of unhappy patients who increasingly complain about the care they are receiving and to healthcare workers who are increasingly stressed out and burned out on the job [1], despite greater technological ability to solve medical problems than has ever been available to mankind. The solution that we are suggesting is not window dressing or simply better manners, but a change in the patient–healthcare worker relationship that takes lessons from the palliative care movement and applies them in a much wider context. But make no mistake, whole person care is not palliative care by another name, but a new paradigm for practicing medicine that is relevant to all parts and specialties of medical practice.

When Cicely Saunders set up St Christopher's Hospice as the first modern palliative care hospice, she attempted to set up a comprehensive system of care that dealt with the needs of dying patients [2]. The success of the palliative care movement that she started [3] and the appreciation of patients and families suggest that she went a long way to achieving that goal. Of course, not all of anybody's needs can actually be met by any person or institution, so there had to be something else going on. The something else we believe was a profound change in how healthcare workers viewed

T.A. Hutchinson (✉)
Professor, Faculty of Medicine, Director, Programs in Whole Person Care, McGill University, 546 Pine Avenue West, Montreal, QC H2W 1S6, Canada
e-mail: tom.hutchinson@mcgill.ca

and related to themselves and the persons for whom they were providing care [4, 5]. She initiated a therapeutic relationship based on the following: the need for and the unavoidable hierarchy associated with professional expertise and evidence-based practice, absolutely equal standing and value as persons, and a mutual presence made more mindful and open by the acute awareness of shared human vulnerability and inevitable mortality. It is this therapeutic relationship that is the new paradigm that whole person care aims to bring to the rest of medicine.

An obvious question is whether whole person care is necessary. We can understand that this may be necessary and important for dying patients who have an irreversible disease process, but with the advances in medical technology that can solve more and more problems, surely the proportion of people who are sick for any significant period of time is bound to decrease, and we will find quicker and more efficient technologic ways to deliver whatever care is necessary with the minimum of human interaction. In fact, what has happened globally is that serious chronic disease is on the rise [6], and advanced technology sometimes creates more chronically ill people with overwhelming human needs, who remain sick for longer and who tax the resources of society. How could this be?

A good example is end-stage kidney disease, a severe chronic illness that requires regular dialysis treatment, a rigorous dietary and fluid regimen, multiple medications, and frequent doctor's visits and checkups to detect and treat complications for the duration of the patient's life or until they receive a kidney transplant, which requires its own intensive follow-up and care. In Canada, in 1981, there were 5,500 patients alive with chronic kidney failure [7]. In 2006, there were 34,000 [8], and the number is still rising. Bad diet? Too little exercise? Toxic environment? Perhaps partly, but the primary reason is that people who used to die now live with chronic renal failure. This is a success story [9] that has been repeated in other fields [10], which partly explains why we probably have a higher proportion of our population in the North America ill with serious chronic illness now than at any point in our history. And the problem is likely to increase. We have a greater need for whole person care than at any point in the past, and the need is likely to increase.

Let us look for a moment at the needs of patients with end-stage renal disease. These patients need human help and support dealing with the multiple challenges of end-stage renal disease and its treatment while at the same time ensuring that they receive the treatment that they need to remain as physically healthy as possible. It is a difficult balance to maintain. Sometimes, the demands of the treatment itself are so time consuming and require so much of the available medical resources that patients complain that they are not treated as whole persons receiving a service but as items on an assembly line whose views are disregarded by an arrogant medical team [11]. This is not whole person care encompassing curing and healing but further wounding in the service of life prolongation. And yet, it may still be worth it for patients who would otherwise die. But surely more is possible and desirable for patients with this and other chronic diseases that are now so prevalent. We may not get a magic bullet to make all disease go away, but we do have a huge and largely unrecognized resource – the nontechnologic internal resources of the patients who are ill and the people who care for them. Whole person care aims to combine this resource and its potential for healing with the resources of biotechnology and its potential for life prolongation and cure to maximize the duration and quality of life of people in our communities.

The image that we use to represent whole person care is the caduceus metaphor [12] shown in Fig. 18.1, with the white snake representing the Hippocratic curing side of medicine and the black snake representing the Asklepian healing side. As mentioned previously (Chap. 4) and is evident from Table 18.1, where we elucidate more extensively the specific features of the Hippocratic and Asklepian sides of medicine, we do believe that this is a very real dichotomy. We do not believe that

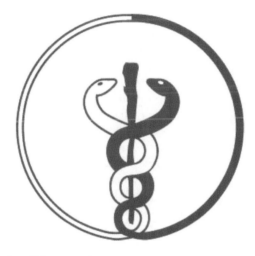

Fig. 18.1 The metaphor of the two snakes

Table 18.1 The metaphor of the two snakes and the full medical dichotomy

	White snake (Hippocratic)	Black snake (Asklepian)
Patient		
Problem	Symptoms or dysfunction	Suffering
Possibility	Being cured	Healing
Action	Holding on	Letting go
Goal	Survival	Growth
Self-image	At the effect of disease	Responsible for coping with illness
Doctor		
Focus	Disease	Person with illness
Communication	Content	Relationship
	Digital	Analog
	Conscious	Unconscious
Power	Power differential	Power sharing
Presence	Competent technician	Wounded healer
Epistemology	Scientific	Artistic
Management	Standardized	Individualized
Effect	Real	"Placebo"

the dichotomy can be (or needs to be) resolved. It would, in our view, be impossible to create an algorithm or design a machine to logically integrate these two contrasting strands of medicine, which is why we need real people to practice good medicine – whole persons who can encompass the dichotomy inherent in medical practice [13] to provide the best help to the whole person who is the patient presenting for care.

A question that might reasonably be asked is whether it is possible, or even necessary, for one person to encompass both sides of the medical dichotomy. Our answer is unequivocally yes. Even novice healthcare workers can begin to do this once they realize the healing potential of whole person care. In fact, we find that many medical students are already familiar with the Asklepian aspect of medicine when they enter medical school. It is sometimes a desire to help in this way that got them into medical school in the first place. Some of them keep this side alive as they learn more about the Hippocratic side. In others, the Hippocratic side replaces the Asklepian side, until there is almost nothing left but a memory. But you may say perhaps that is inevitable and cannot somebody else do the Asklepian side, the family for instance. Here is an instructive story from the New York Times [14]: "When my mother found out she had myelodysplastic syndrome, the terrible blood cancer that eventually took her life, she oscillated between numb despair and acute panic. When she was panicked, nothing those who loved her did or said could calm her down, let alone console her. And yet we soon learned that if we could reach Stephen Nimer, her principal physician at the Memorial Sloan–Kettering Cancer Center, by telephone, or if, better still, Dr. Nimer could make time to see my mother, however briefly, her awful distress would abate – at least for a while. Observing my mother's exchanges with Dr. Nimer, I could not help wondering why what he said consoled her. For he never played down the lethality of her disease, nor did he hold out false hope. Doubtless, Dr. Nimer's long experience with gravely ill people, the hard-won human skills he acquired over decades of practice, played a central role. But it was my sense at the time, and it is my sense now, more than three years after my mother's death, that the comfort my mother derived from speaking with him was also due to her own conception – her very traditional conception – of their relationship. She was a person who had no time for so-called alternative medicine, nor did she believe that her will would somehow be strong enough to counter the scientific realities. And yet, when all was said and done, I think that my mother's relationship with her principal doctors can only be fully understood – and was only fully effective – because it was in some ways as shamanistic as the relations our ancestors knew before the advent of modern scientific medicine."

So, patients sometimes (we would say virtually always) need the Asklepian attitudes and skills from their physician, which is exactly our experience. And in a strange paradox, the person they often want it from most is the person perceived to be highest on the technological/hierarchical medical ladder. We have found, for example, that a surgeon who really listens or says a kind word can have an impact far greater than a palliative care physician (like me for instance) who has spent hours talking with the patient. It might seem unfair, but it begins to give some idea not just of the importance and power of the Asklepian side but also of the power of the two sides to potentiate each other.

There are synergistic cross-links at every point in the table. The example above might be seen as the cross-link between the competent technician (Hippocratic) and the wounded healer (Asklepian). We are suggesting that the higher that you are perceived by the patient on the competent technician scale, the more difference your willingness to put yourself in the wounded healer role will make. There are analogous connections at every point in the table. Physicians who are clear about the scientific evidence and standardized guidelines for treating a specific problem (Hippocratic) can more safely and creatively use art (Asklepian) to individualize treatment for a specific patient. As dialysis patients sometimes express it "teach us how to cheat safely." A physician who communicates content in clear digital language (Hippocratic) avoiding obvious errors and mistakes will likely be someone with whom the patient will feel safer developing a trusting therapeutic relationship (Asklepian).

For patients themselves, the same dichotomy and synergy is operative. Relief of suffering through healing that comes with beginning acceptance and reconnection with significant others (Asklepian), which we frequently see in patients with terminal illness, makes symptoms such as pain much easier to control with medications (Hippocratic). Patients who are holding on to their old identity of not being sick may find it difficult to be adherent with a complicated regimen (Hippocratic). It is difficult to follow a demanding regimen of treatment for a disease that you have not fully accepted is real, but this may change dramatically when you begin to let go of your old identity and accept that you really are sick and need treatment (Asklepian). And this cross-linkage and synergy may extend down to a biologic and cellular level.

At the bottom of the table, we use the terms "real" on the Hippocratic side and "placebo" on the Asklepian side, and we have already commented (Chap. 4) on how this unfairly devalues the Asklepian side. But what about connections between the two sides at this level? First, it appears obvious that biologic changes in disease, as for instance when we successfully treat a pneumonia with antibiotics, will bring with it multiple beneficial effects on the patient's well-being that are not limited to the symptoms directly related to the pneumonia (such as dyspnea or fever). The patient may feel relieved, grateful, newly optimistic, and so on. This effect is one of the reasons that curative medicine is so justifiably gratifying.

But what about a cross-link in the opposite direction? Can a "placebo" effect lead to "real" measureable biologic change? This is an historically problematic possibility [15] perhaps because in the past dramatic changes in reported cases [15, p. 31–33] have been linked to deception of the patient [16]. But can a completely honest and respectful relationship with the patient, which is the key to promoting healing, also have effects on the Hippocratic (curing) side of the medical dichotomy? A patient like Marc Levasseur makes me wonder about it. Marc was a man in his 50s with a glioblastoma that had spread to both sides of his brain. I was called to see him because his oncologist felt with the advance of his tumor on MRI scan and attendant increase in symptoms of weakness, difficulty walking and some slurring of speech his prognosis was limited (probably months). He could not return home and needed palliative care help with symptoms, placement and facing end of life.

Marc was a delightful warm bear of a man who fully accepted that he was dying, felt very loving toward the world since he had accepted his illness, and wanted to give back some of the wisdom he had gained since his illness. He was already doing this on the ward where he helped and interacted with staff and other patients but wanted an audience, preferably medical or nursing students, to whom he could give the message that they should use their hearts as well as their heads when they became doctors and nurses.

Over the ensuing week, two things happened. First, Marc began to become weaker, and one evening he fell when going to the bathroom. He was found by a nurse sitting on the floor in a pool of urine and unable to get up. He said that she treated him roughly and disrespected his dignity. This upset him deeply and on the morning following the episode he was not his usual self. He appeared disturbed and said that he had given up on his previous plans to give back to the world. We had a conversation. In the course of our talk, he came to see that the nurse's disdain said something about her but nothing about him. It was one of those intense conversations in which I called on the best in him (not always in gentle terms) and he responded. His mood improved and he again wanted to reach out to the world.

The second thing that happened was that I shared my frustration at not being able to find a suitable audience for Marc with a colleague who told me that she was looking for a palliative care patient for a television interview. When I asked Marc if he would be interested he was like a man called to arms. He gave me a look that expressed surprise and deep gratitude that I had followed through. He was excited in the weeks leading up to the interview and appeared to be getting daily stronger. Just before the interview, Marc had an MRI scan and went to see his oncologist.

Marc's brain tumor had unexpectedly regressed on the MRI, which fitted with his improvement in function. His oncologist expressed surprise but said he no longer felt Marc was dying. Marc attributed his improvement to our interactions and the anticipation of the TV program.[1] His oncologist attributed the change to the Temodal he had received. And I really do not know, although it does make me wonder. And perhaps wonderment is an appropriate response to our current state of ignorance about and hopes for the mind–body connection. We are aware of results in animals showing that atherosclerosis can be dramatically decreased in rabbits on a high cholesterol diet by personal care and attention from their minders [17], and data showing that gene expression for response to stress can be turned on and off by mothering behavior in mice [18]. Recent research in patients with lung cancer showed that the addition of palliative care to regular treatment

---

[1] Marc did the interview, which went well, but he was disappointed with the resultant TV program, which severely curtailed his contribution. This improved after a conversation with my colleague who helped him understand better the context of the program. He continued to do relatively well and was discharged from the hospital to a long-term care residence. At the time of writing (2 years later), he continued to have serious problems with his health but was splitting his time between the residence and the apartment of his new girl friend. He was very happy that his story as told here would be included in a book for doctors and health care professionals. He specifically requested that his real name be used because he felt his story was part of his legacy.

significantly (and surprisingly) prolonged survival [19]. We have much more to learn about the biologic effects of the so-called placebo response, but the effects are probably powerful and real.

However, we are not presenting these possible biologic effects of Asklepian medicine on disease, or indeed the other cross-links and synergies in the table, as the primary justification for whole person care. This elucidation of whole person care only begins to point out some of the benefits of something that cannot be fully captured in our dichotomous table. And we do not believe that studying the table will supply sufficient motivation and energy for whole person care. That will require a deeper source of energy that will grow rather than diminish the more we use it, an energy that will supply what our patients need and nurture us in the process.

Virginia Satir suggested that we have many layers, only the topmost of which shows on the surface. And at the deepest level, providing energy for all the rest, are our longings. These are our deep and unmet desires for things such as love, connection, peace, wholeness. We all have them, but they have generally become concretized, diverted, and finally hidden under layers of expectations, perceptions, feelings, and coping mechanisms [20]. An old mentor of mine, Alvan Feinstein, said that to be successful (in research) you need fire in the belly and ice in the head. We believe that whole person care answers a deep longing in both patients and healthcare workers to treat and be treated as whole persons. This longing is the fire in the belly that clinicians need to remain in touch with in their work. Sometimes, the effects look like ordinary patient care, although patients will notice the difference, and sometimes the effects are extraordinary. Consider the following story about William Osler [21]:

> One remembers a young brother with severe whooping-cough and bronchitis, unable to eat and wholly unresponsive to the blandishments of parents and devoted nurses alike. Clinically it was not an abstruse case, but weapons were few and recovery seemed unlikely. The Regius, about to present for degrees and hard pressed for time, arrived already wearing his doctor's robes (gowns). To a small child this was the advent of a doctor, if doctor in fact it was, from quite a different planet. It was more probably Father Christmas.
>
> After a very brief examination this unusual visitor sat down, peeled a peach, sugared it and cut it in pieces. He then presented it bit by bit with a fork to the entranced patient, telling him to eat it up, and that he would not be sick but would find it did him good as it was a most special fruit. Such proved to be the case. As he hurried off Osler, most uncharacteristically, patted my father on the back and said with deep concern "I'm sorry Ernest but I don't think I shall see the boy again, there's very little chance when they're as bad as that." Happily events turned out otherwise, and for the next forty days this constantly busy man came to see the child, and for each of these forty days he put on his doctor's robes in the hall before going in to the sick room.

Perhaps at a remove of over 100 years, we can forgive Osler for appearing to use some magical deceit and ask ourselves the more relevant question of where in the world did Osler find the imagination, energy, and time to do all that for this one patient? Do we all have to do that all of the time? Of course not, but we can find some of that energy for ourselves and practice a depth and breadth of medicine that we only dreamed about when we started medical school. For myself, I find this a very individual process that is not aided and often hampered by institutional constraints, financial imperatives, measures of efficiency and even quality, career advancement and even, with notable exceptions, other physicians. But there are exceptions among physicians, and my hope is to see these exceptions become more numerous and begin to coalesce into communities of support and practice as we are now beginning to see at McGill. We will in time, I hope, become a profession aimed at managing not only a satisfactory social contract with the public and self-regulating measurable standards of practice [22] but also a mutually energizing association of fellow learners supporting each other in practicing the best medicine of which each of us is capable – whole person care.

References

1. Spickard Jr A, Gabbe SG, Christensen JF. Mid-career burnout in generalist and specialist physicians. JAMA. 2002;288(12):1447–50.
2. Clark D. Part 2, The expansive years (1968-1985). In: Cicely Saunders – founder of the Hospice movement. Selected letters 1959-1999. New York, NY: Oxford University Press; 2002. p. 127–33.
3. Clark D. Cicely Saunders – founder of the Hospice movement. Selected letters 1959-1999. New York, NY: Oxford University Press; 2002. p. V–VII (Mount B, Foreword).
4. Saunders C. A therapeutic community: St. Cristopher's Hospice. In: Schoenberg B, Carr AC, Peretz D, Kutschereds AH, editors. Psychosocial aspects of terminal care. New York, NY: Columbia University Press; 1972. p. 275–89.
5. Kearney M. Mortally wounded. New York, NY: Simon & Schuster; 1997. p. 13–4 (Saunders C, Foreword).
6. Yach D, Hawkes C, Gould CL, Hofman KJ. The global burden of chronic diseases: overcoming impediments to prevention and control. JAMA. 2004;291:2616–22.
7. Canadian Organ Replacement Register. 1999 Report. Vol. 1, Dialysis and renal transplantation (includes data 1981–1997). Ottawa, ON: Canadian Institute for Health Information; 1999 Jun. p. 1–5 (Section 1, Information from the facility profile questionnaire, 1997).
8. Canadian Institute for Health Information. 2008 Annual report – treatment of end-stage organ failure in Canada, 1997 to 2006. Ottawa, ON: Canadian Institute for Health Information; 2008. p. 11 (Section 2, Renal replacement therapy for end-stage renal disease).
9. Hutchinson TA. The price and challenges of extraordinary success: treating end-stage renal failure in the next millenium. CMAJ. 1999;160(11):1589–90.
10. National Cancer Institute. U.S. National Institutes of Health. Estimated U.S. Cancer Prevalence [Internet]. Rockville, MD. 2010. http://cancercontrol.cancer.gov/ocs/prevalence/prevalence.html#survivor.
11. Allen D, Wainwright M, Hutchinson T. 'Non-compliance' as illness management: hemodialysis patients' descriptions of adversarial patient-clinician interactions. Soc Sci Med. In press.
12. Kearney M. Introduction. In: A place of healing: working with suffering in living and dying. Oxford, UK: Oxford University Press; 2000. p. XIX–XXII.
13. Hutchinson TA, Hutchinson N, Arnaert A. Whole person care: encompassing the two faces of medicine. CMAJ. 2009;180(8):845–6.
14. Rieff D. The way we live now. Miracle workers? [Internet]. New York Times. 17 Feb 2008. http://www.nytimes.com/2008/02/17/magazine/17wwln-lede-t.html?_r=&ei=51241&en=12388136d24f.
15. Harrington A. Chapter 1, The power of suggestion. In: The cure within: a history of mind-body medicine. New York, NY: W.W. Norton & Company; c2008. p. 31–66.
16. Robinson W. A misguided miracle: the use of placebos in clinical practice. Ethics Behav. 1998;8(1):93–5.

17. Nerem RM, Levesque MJ, Cornhill JF. Social environment as a factor in diet-induced atherosclerosis. Science. 1980;208:1475–6.
18. Weaver ICG, Cervoni N, Champagne FA, D'Alessio AC, Sharma S, Seckl JR, et al. Epigenetic programming by maternal behavior. Nat Neurosci. 2004;7(8):847–54.
19. Temel J, Greer JA, Muzikansky A, Gallagher ER, Admane S, Jackson VA, et al. Early palliative care for patients with metastatic non–small-cell lung cancer. N Engl J Med. 2010;363:733–42.
20. Satir V, Banmen J, Gerber J, Gomori M. Chapter 7, The transformation process. In: The Satir Model. Family therapy and beyond. Palo Alto, CA: Science and Behaviour Books; c1991. p. 147–73.
21. Bliss M. Chapter 10, Sir William. In: William Osler: a life in medicine. Toronto, ON: University of Toronto Press; c1999. p. 369–401.
22. Medical Professionalism Project. Medical professionalism in the new millennium: a physicians' charter. Lancet. 2002;359:520–2.

Appendix: The Nature of Persons and Clinical Medicine

Eric J. Cassell

Keywords Relationships • Clinical knowledge • Love • Sexual • Sexuality • Esthetic dimension • Narrative • Illness • Reasoning • Emotiveness • Emotive • Unitary • Inner life • Fear • Trust • Anxiety

Eudora Welty said, "Relationship is a pervading and changing mystery…brutal or lovely, the mystery waits for people, whatever extreme they run to" (*Writing and Analyzing a Story*, Eudora Welty 2002). Nowhere is that mystery more important than in clinical medicine where relationships abound, waiting to provide information and aids or barriers to the attentive clinician. How odd is this? A person can go to see a physician who is a stranger and within minutes the physician has a finger in the patient's rectum. And the person (now a patient) says thank you. What made that otherwise inexplicable event possible? We know it was the doctor–patient relationship, but the name does not explain it. What happened was guided by a complex set of rules and entitlements that applied to both the patient and the physician. We might guess that the doctor learned those rules and entitlements (not called such) during the long years of training. For all we know, this exact situation has never happened to the doctor (or the patient) before, yet we expect the physician's behavior to be as described. Why did the patient undress, much less bend over to expose the reluctant anus to the finger's penetration, something almost universally abhorrent? Perhaps the patient contains the same rules and entitlements (or their mirror image). This suggests that role behavior (for they were playing the parts required by their respective roles) resides in both of them. The degree to which our daily behaviors are rule guided is startling, since we generally believe our behaviors are spontaneous and responsive to our chosen purposes.

E.J. Cassell (✉)
Emeritus Professor of Public Health, Weill Medical College of Cornell University, New York, NY 10021
and
Adjunct Professor of Medicine, Faculty of Medicine, McGill University, PO Box 96, Shawnee on Delaware, PA 18356, USA
e-mail: eric@ericcassell.com

T.A. Hutchinson (ed.), *Whole Person Care: A New Paradigm for the 21st Century*, DOI 10.1007/978-1-4419-9440-0, © Springer Science+Business Media, LLC 2011

We all know these rules, at least tacitly (or they would not work), which makes it possible for clinicians to take a history from a patient and use daily living as a test of function. Knowledge of the rules of daily living is a crucial part of our *clinical knowledge.*

Knowledge of persons then is knowledge of people in the complicated web of relationships in which life is conducted. In every facet of life, the person is functioning in a largely rule guided manner. Spend some time observing people in their daily lives, but stop and dwell on the different situations for sufficient time to see how similarly persons in each situation behave. If you look closely at each individual in these situations, however, the careful observation will also reveal how differently each acts and how different is each from the others. This is each person's own perception; as an individual acting individualistically. I have spelled it out in such detail to make clear how much most, usually without awareness, already know of clinical utility and how much there is to be known.

All persons have a capacity to love to a greater or lesser extent. Even when we are in love or are sure of our loving and being loved, it is a wonderment. On the contrary, except for the most unfortunate, love – flowing in both directions – is a fact of infancy and young childhood. From that young experience, we get the basic characteristic of the feeling of love; it is a merging – a connection – between two people. Of course, under even the best of circumstances the merging of loving persons (or at least the feeling of merging) is of relatively short duration, but their belief in their love may be enduring.

When people are sick, especially very sick, their ability to connect to others – particularly caregivers – is greater than at other times. This is the source of the sometimes very strong attachment of the very sick to their clinicians. Here is one of the situations when the fact and the manner of the attachment of sick persons to their caregivers are reminiscent of the attachment of these persons to their mothers in infancy. Not surprisingly, many persons who care for the sick also seem to have more than the usual ability to form connections. With these strong connections goes the ability to be more aware of the feelings of the other person. In general, the loving attachment seems to be a conduit to the feelings, thoughts, and even the body of the merged persons. We know so little of this because it is so difficult to study and because it shares in the disbelief in such things in daily life.

All persons are sexual to one degree or another. Physicians in general were often not good at taking a sexual history from patients because they were often embarrassed by the subject. When the HIV/AIDS epidemic came along, a sexual history became very important and clinicians learned that it was not difficult; you just had to know how. Very sick patients usually lose sexual desire and do not have sexual thoughts until they start to recover. It is one of the functions, like reading the newspaper, lost in serious illness but a good sign of recovery when it returns. On the contrary, patients who are chronically ill, even if dying, may experience sexual thoughts and sexual desire. For that reason, questions about sexuality should be part of taking a history even in a dying patient. Sexuality is not simply about physical desire and orgasm even in healthy persons; intimacy and the feeling of connection is an integral part of the experience and may be vitally important to a patient even in the absence of normal erectile or vaginal function. Because people may be embarrassed to ask for help in these circumstances, clinicians should remain aware of the possibility. Clinicians show their recognition of these and other intimate problems by asking simple and unembarrassed questions.

All persons have a past, present, and a future. The past as remembered is a lived series of events, and when they are spontaneously recounted it is in terms of the things that matter personally: events, relationships, primarily, but sometimes circumstances such as sickness. Persons generally see the present and themselves in the present as an unremarkable extension of that past – the past merely unrolling to the present. In questioning people about the past, it may be portrayed as a series of discrete events that represent what is important to the questioner or it may be sought and described as a narrative, a story about the person in which events are embedded in the more general story and tied to other events, such as holidays or anniversaries. In doing this, the narrative prepares the person for its extension into the future as the future is continuing to unroll. It is not surprising that illness in the past and experiences with caregivers, medications, and hospitals will condition a person's reactions to present illness, caregivers, and hospitals. It is interesting that the family's past is often considered by persons as part of their past and it also conditions present illness.

The future is always uncertain, and it cannot be otherwise. People tend to have enduring ideas about what the future will bring and how they will make it happen. The future is the canvas where the optimists and the pessimists paint different pictures. Everybody indulges in hoping and their hopes are part of their construction of the future. Hope seems to be constructed of both desire and expectations and is a process of thought arising in part from personality and the contributions of others – particularly physicians. The desire to remain one's self, no matter how bleak the expected future, is more important than the wish to merely remain alive. Maintaining or restoring hope is an important function of physicians. It allows patients to regain purpose, motivation, expectations, and goals even in the face of death.

A person is more than a spatial object, something you can see and touch. A person is also a temporal object like a piece of music that extends through time. As such, *persons have an esthetic dimension* where one can judge whether the seeing or knowing about the person through time presents a harmonious aspect to consideration. This understanding of the esthetics of a life over time fits nicely with the use of the narrative to describe a person over time. One part of the story of a life or a part of a lived life fits with the preceding and the following parts of the narrative. This is like reading a book where its parts hang together or conversely the parts of the life are in discord or unbalanced, or like looking at a picture and seeing that one element "goes" nicely in relation to the other parts of the picture or, conversely, is jarring. There can be no objective measurement of this idea of "fit," but it is not usually idiosyncratic and there will mostly be agreement among observers. Reflect on what you know of the lives of different people and you will see that in some, life is lived in a harmonious fashion, while in others the parts – lasting days, weeks, months, or years – are discordant, out of balance, or do not fit together. It is almost as if parts of the life were lived by different persons. The belief that the life as lived should be concordant allows us to say that what happened to someone does not seem to fit their life as lived.

Illness may represent an unpleasant shift in the narrative, a disruption of the preceding story, a bump in the pattern – sometimes of major dimensions. Little can be done about this because it is in the impersonal nature of sickness. The process of care, however, can be carried out with active thought given to fitting into the esthetic balance of the person's story and thereby reducing the ugliness of the illness and its care. This requires that clinicians acquire an esthetic viewpoint of their patient's life, and this requires conscious effort. Most of us have practice in taking an esthetic perspective because that is what allows us to know about the coherency and accordance of characters in movies or fiction. This is innate because all persons have an esthetic sense, a sense of order, harmony, and beauty (as they know it).

Persons are thinking all the time. Your mind is almost certainly and almost constantly occupied by a stream of thought varying from moment to moment as your focus, interests, occupations, and preoccupations shift. Content of the stream of thought, which is mostly like silent speech, also arises from memory as the information from the world evokes ideas and associations that have been stored in both distant and recent memory. These thoughts are *personal.* Mine are mine and yours are yours, and as far as we know or have thus far discovered (despite clues to the contrary), yours do not become mine, nor does mine become yours. The mental life is not a machine; it is personal so that as all this activity goes on material is provided for further thought and that thought influences the focus of the subsequent mental activity that may change what is of interest and further change the direction of thought, and so on. As I suggested, the train of thought is also a commentary on activities so that as the person is occupied, for example, with illness or symptoms, the train of thought will offer a meaning to explain the symptoms. Sometimes, the focus of thought becomes captured by one subject – for example, a fear, so that all aspects of thought are in the service of what can become monomania. Actually, what is thrown up by all this mental activity are ideas in the form of words and their meanings, and it is the meaning that we dwell on when thoughts become concrete. So, the sick person interprets everything in terms of sickness and its manifestations; fearful person sees only further support for fear, and so on.

For example, shortness of breath previously interpreted as meaning that the stairs are steep becomes evidence suggesting heart disease, fatigue become evidence of escalating weakness; gradually, a case may be built that further supports both the idea that the person is sick and a pessimistic picture of the future. It matters little (in the short run) whether the individual *actually is* sick; what matters is the evidence arising from the inevitable flow of thought. The clinician can have a major impact on the content and direction of the stream of thought.

Also continuous and in part feeding the stream of thought and fed by it is the *unending assessment of its world by and the assignment of meaning to events –* mostly out of awareness. Sensation – the major senses and the minor – are joined to perception, and mood, which are also constantly in play. Each of these is a distinct mode of appraisal and together or separately they provide constant (but personalized) intelligence about the world – both inner and outer – that may or may not become part of the flow of thought. The output of the mind's continuous activity of appraisal is a flow of meaning. Meaning has an impact in virtually every dimension of the person from the molecular to the spiritual. That is to say that meanings not merely are ideas in a dictionary but also contain body sensations, feelings, and spiritual expressions. Meaning are both social – the meanings of words and many other things – held in common in social groups, but also personal – supported by a private glossary. That is to say that the word apple is the common meaning applied to the round, firm, fleshy fruit of the rosaceous tree that comes in many varieties, and which also makes sense in the phrase, "She's the apple of my eye." But apple also has personal meanings to you – taste, the feel in your mouth, etc. – which may be different than that to me, and so on. Similarly, you know that certain clinical facts mean that the patient has pneumonia, an infection of the alveoli, but pneumonia has some special meanings to you because of the cases you have seen.

Persons understand their world as they believe it to be primarily by two kinds of thought, reasoning and emotiveness. Reasoning is based on what are accepted as facts and is able to follow ideas to their ends, take them apart, combine them to form new ideas, and generally go beyond the information given. Truth is generally thought to come from correct reasoning, but logical thought only produces truth if the ideas on which it is based are true. Reason is a method of thinking that can be used to understand and follow any set of ideas whatever their subject is. If the ideas are faulty – internally incoherent, or such as that cannot be logically connected with other ideas, then the reasoning will be faulty.

Emotive thought also operates on content from perception and memory producing specific instantaneous evaluations that are felt as emotions. Emotions are feelings, affections such as pain, pleasure, love, amusement, amazement, anger, sadness, dejection, joy, etc. Much less is known about emotion and emotiveness than about ideas and reasoning because from antiquity emotions (which were called the passions) were thought to contaminate thinking and interfere with reasoning. This is incorrect; they are a central and essential element of the mental life. Certainly, the emotions that sick patients have about their sickness are as much a part of the sickness as are the symptoms. Sometimes, when patients tell us about something we ask, "How do you feel about that?" That is really a request for their emotional reactions, but the phrase has come to mean both thinking and feeling. There is certainly no thinking about sickness that is free of emotion if you are the one who is sick.

Emotion is as primitive as the existence of animals. Motion, the sine qua non of animality from paramecium to man, requires at least two feelings to explain why the animal goes here rather than there: desire and fear. Just as there is a flow of thought where ideas seem to be central, there is a stream of thought where mood is the content. The list of human emotions is well over a hundred in number. Emotion may be experienced in three distinct ways: First, as transitory where one brief experience of emotion may follow another as the emotional reactions to thoughts and experiences. Or one emotion may endure. For example, anger may last for hours past its inciting event. Finally, an emotion such as anger may become the dominant mood. Then, we might not say that the person is angry but that the person is an angry person. The dominant mood could as well be joy, despair, sadness, or love. It seems to be the case that the emotiveness of sick persons is blunted, just as their cognition is impaired and executive control diminished. While there is experimental evidence of the impairments of cognition and executive control, the evidence for the impact of sickness on emotiveness is anecdotal. Patients may report, for example, that although they know that they should feel love for a family member visiting and they say the words, they do not feel the emotion.

People generally seem to consider themselves unitary beings. If you ask them that if they are more than one "I," they usually don't think so. "Who are you?" "I am me." "Are you more than one me?" "No, just me." "Okay, if you are just one, who writes your dreams?" "I do." "So, why don't you understand them?" "I don't know."

It appears to be the case, however, that below the surface of consciousness there are other entities that in certain circumstances (for example, in hypnotic states) can openly voice opinions that are not necessarily the same as those expressed in ordinary everyday conscious states. This has been known for at least 150 years, demonstrated in the famous French neurology clinics of Jean Martin Charcot and Pierre Janet. The importance of highlighting ordinary everyday consciousness is that in the everyday setting, persons are strongly influenced by rules of everyday life. The rules are not merely precepts that apply in daily society but also beliefs, acceptable behaviors, and conventional modes of dress, patterns of speech, and other guidelines for living in the world of dailiness. These *other, inner, voices* are not ruled by dailiness. On the contrary, they are shy and hesitant. They are easily dismissed, and they are overridden by doubt. Doubt is the everyday mind's pronouncement that these inner thoughts and ideas should not be heeded and are perhaps nonsense. Actually, however, when doubt arises it means the inner voice is suggesting something that would be denied as impossible in the everyday world. By the time you have finished reading this section, many of you will experience this aspect of doubt for yourselves. The reason to point up this phenomenon is to make it clear that the inner life of the mind is more likely to be complex than simplistic. It is also evident that the experiences of sick persons, their reactions to their illnesses and care, and their behaviors may in part be responses to events, feelings, and experiences of early or later childhood, which are lost to conscious recall. Some offer their past experiences back to early childhood as an explanation for what they think now, or what is happening now. Memory of the past is quite clear for some and variable for others. The accuracy of these early memories may, however, be open to question. It has been said that unhappy or negative memories are shorter-lived than happy ones, but traumatic memories back to childhood may be selectively remembered in considerable detail. There can be no doubt, on the contrary, that there can be selective rejection of information from awareness. This means that although past memories may be quite clear, what reaches awareness may not be the whole memory. It is also the case that the past can be rewritten to serve the purposes of the present.

It cannot be disputed that events in childhood back to infancy may form the basis for an adult pattern of behavior and that these events, even though they have this impact, may not come to awareness. Events in this sense are restricted not only to brute facts but also to the person's emotional response to recall of early relationship with parents, siblings, caretakers, or others. These memories may not be merely forgotten in the sense that with a little jog from another person or a subsidiary recollection they will again come to mind, but may be actively repressed. Even actively repressed early memories or their emotional content – memories that are not and cannot be brought to consciousness – may have an impact on behaviors, including speech and bodily responses to stimuli (including sexual stimuli), which seem to come out of the blue or seem completely unexplainable. All of this may be particularly important in illness in which things happen, for example, complete dependency, which are in themselves reminiscent of childhood. When that happens, the door may be opened for the effect of childhood events and their emotional content, remembered, dissociated (incomprehensible and, therefore, shoved aside before even being remembered), or repressed (remembered, but hidden from consciousness), to have an impact on the course of the illness.

Fear is an emotion as universal as desire in animals. Generally, fear is described as an aversive emotional response to a specific stimulus – persons know what, in the situation, they are afraid of. Sometimes, the fear is momentary, perhaps in response to an impending needlestick. Other times, the fear is a pervasive emotion that invades everything, the fear of the hospital for example. Fear of surgery is another example. Sometimes, fears seem to be less specific such as about dying, unfamiliar situations, loss of control, or dependency. When that is the case, it is often possible to track down what the patient is afraid of about hospitals or surgery: loss of control or dependency. If the exact details of the fear can be elicited, it can often be laid to rest. It has become common, especially in specialized surgical settings such as cardiac surgery units, for the patient to be told in exquisite detail about what is going to happen. Well-prepared patients are less afraid, have less postoperative pain and other complications, and generally do better.

Fear is an emotion that can have bad consequences from the molecular to the spiritual, and the effort to resolve it is worth whatever time it takes. The most effective antidote to fear is information; however, to be useful, the information should be focused around the particular concerns of the patient, at a level the patient can understand. Too much information, or undesired information, can lead to more fear. Information is transmitted in the context of a therapeutic relationship, and for the information to be accepted and to do its job the relationship must be trusting. Trust is not blind trust. That is why it is so important to be truthful and honest. If you say something will not hurt, that has to be true. It is much better to be honest about a painful procedure explaining in detail what you (or others) will do about the pain. Simple reassurances are rarely helpful, and the words "Don't worry" are probably as useless as anything in medicine.

People in strange and threatening settings, such as, for some, hospitals or other medical situations, can be expected to be frightened. If they deny fear or if fear is unapparent, it should be actively, but gently, sought and once understood, specific reassurance can be offered. Sometimes, people have fears that seem understandable, but on further questioning the fear is not what it first appeared to be. The fear of death is very common, but often – perhaps most often – the real fears are not death but the fear of separation from others or from the group, or fear about the dying process.

The importance of finding the true source of fear is that effective amelioration becomes possible.

Anxiety, like fear, is a normal response to certain kinds of threatening situations. Anxiety is, however, more complex than fear. It is important to distinguish the kind of anxiety that can occur in anybody as distinct from the psychological anxiety disorders such as generalized anxiety disorder, post-traumatic stress disorder, panic disorder, and social anxiety disorder. Whereas fear has an identifiable object, anxiety is vaguer, and it is less easy to identify what is at the root of the anxiety. For example, persons may have distinct fears of death or of dying, but they may also become anxious where they believe death threatens. When anxiety is present, it is experienced as variable feelings of dread, tenseness or jumpiness, restlessness, and irritability. There may be an anticipation of bad things or general apprehension. Restlessness, trouble concentrating, anticipating the worst, and waiting for the ax to drop are characteristic, as are nightmares and bad dreams. The anxious person's world threatens, but what is actually the source of the threat is not obvious. Physical manifestations are almost universal and can, at times, be quite extreme: heart palpitations, shortness of breath, and chest pains that may seem like a heart attack to the person. Fatigue, nausea, stomach aches, headaches, diarrhea, or other physical symptoms may make the anxious person sure that he or she is physically ill. Physiological manifestations are common such as elevated blood pressure, increased heart rate, sweating, pallor, and dilated pupils. However, anxiety can make itself known by mild feelings of unease, irritability, and apprehension without obvious physical symptoms or go all the way to a full-blown panic attack where the person is sure that death is imminent.

Why all of this is present may often be completely unknown to the person. Sometimes in a patient who is sick, threatened by serious possible consequences, or in a threatening (to the person) environment, the source seems obvious to an observer. But it is not obvious to the patient even as the cause is pursued. There are a number of reasons for the obscurity of the causes of anxiety in individuals. One is that the source is so scary to the person that it is repressed. That is, the person not only does not know the source of the anxiety but also cannot know because the idea is intolerable.

Here is a simple but illustrative example, a mother is anxious each time her child is on a trip – not fearful, anxious – but she does not know why. Everybody says that it is obvious that she is afraid something is going to happen to the child, and she agrees that it must be that, but the anxiety persists. A physician asks whether she is afraid of a car crash in which the child will be killed. As she listens to the words, she is almost overwhelmed with horror at the thought, but agrees. The anxiety stops and now she is sometimes fearful when the child is away, but does her best to insure that the child will travel safely and not be involved in an accident. The idea of a car crash was repressed because the thought of her child's death was impossible to bear, so she repressed it. It may have been that a trusting relationship with the physician provided the safety that allowed her to confront and accept the fear, and not be so overwhelmed by it. This is an uncomplicated example, but many are not so simple. Even in this instance, conflict is present between the apparent need to repress the danger to the child and the need to protect the child from the danger. Different voices, more than one self and myriad memories, some conscious, some forgotten, and some repressed, suggest a mental life below awareness that might be marked by more than one meaning and more than one emotion for the same events and relationships. Where there is more than one meaning, conflicting memories for the same event, and more than one way of responding to similar stimuli, there is the potential for conflict. Where action to mitigate threat is thought to be necessary but conflict exists whose nature is not available to consciousness, anxiety follows. This is because persons cannot defend against a threat whose real nature is not known to them. The source of the conflict that is always present in anxiety may be as simple as in the instance noted above where a fear is repressed but situations in which the fear is evoked continue to occur.

The conflict may be more complex. For example, a person may seem to be very anxious in response to the threat of death, but it is really not death itself, but conflict about it that is evocative. A very sick person has come to terms with his impending death, but his wife is extremely upset at the idea of his death and he feels that his acceptance of death is a betrayal of his intense love and loyalty. He is afraid of what will happen to his wife when he dies, but he is tired of fighting an illness when the inevitability of death seems to offer surcease. As a consequence of this conflict of which he is unaware, he becomes anxious, and his anxiety is wrongly interpreted by observers as evidence of his fear of death.

Anxiety is sometimes aroused in situations where different selves in the same person come into conflict. An older woman found herself anxious in situations where she kept asking herself, "which me am I supposed to be, the compliant, hard working, but resentful me, or the hardworking but interested and creative me." Without being aware of such a conflict, anxiety is evoked, which resolves when the conflict is made clear. Anxiety is extremely common, especially in the medical setting. There are effective antianxiety drugs, but they do not expose, clarify, or generate understanding of the conflict that always exists. It may not require sophisticated psychotherapy to uncover and resolve the conflict. This is preferred to medication and certainly better than allowing someone to endure chronic anxiety.

For some clinicians, what I have described as the conflict always found where there is anxiety would be described as ambivalence, in serious illness wanting to live but not wanting to suffer, wanting to be cared for but feeling guilty about it. The person is of two minds, ambivalent, conflicted, and these feelings are commonly sources of anxiety. There may be partial awareness of these feelings of conflict, or even perhaps clarity about them, but the tension that creates the anxiety is not being able to have both desired outcomes even when they are known.

Every person has a body. The body can do some things and not others. People become habituated to their body's enormous range of abilities and incapacities. They generally know exactly what every part can do of which they are or can be conscious. These capacities become accepted as a part of their person ("me"). This physical view of persons has been partly hidden by the cultural importance of and attention to individuality developed over the past number of centuries in Western European and American societies. Individuals presented as though there were no bodies. People also generally know when parts are not working properly and these impairments of function – if they come on quickly enough to be noticed and are lasting and important enough – become symptoms as they are joined to other incapacities. On the contrary, if impairments of function emerge only slowly, are easily accommodated, or are deemed unimportant, even quite impressive impairments will soon be adapted to or dismissed. This is why careful questioning is so important as a part of the evaluation of a patient. This is particularly so because of the importance of impairments of social, psychological, and spiritual function that is part of the understanding of sickness described in this chapter.

Things happen to bodies – they can be injured or get sick. Bodies sometimes bleed, smell bad, make embarrassing sounds, have embarrassing functions, make inopportune demands, create strong desires, sometimes look bad, and become old and slow, and sometimes ugly (These facts are frequently denied or hidden in everyday life.). Persons grow up with profound ignorance about how the body works, even though most people learn about it in school. Certain functions such as that of the bowels and urinary system are even less well known because of everyday stigmata about them. Sexual organs are also poorly understood, although, in general, sex education has advanced greatly in recent years. Modesty keeps people from really knowing about their sexual function.

Unfortunately, clinicians can have considerable knowledge about diverse diseases but be quite ignorant about the body's everyday functions. This limits their ability to ask questions in the hunt for impairments. It also reduces their ability to make things function better.

Everybody dies. Human beings, alone among the animals, know about the inevitability of their death. This knowledge has effects at virtually all ages, is often the hidden listener in the clinician's communications with patients, and has its place in the process of care at many of its stages. Dying, as we have come to know, may not be the passive event of somebody becoming dead, but a human function that may go well or ill depending on clinicians' actions (including their words).

Index

A

Altruism, 63
Anxiety, 225–244. *See also* Death anxiety
Anxious resistant attachment pattern, 50
Asklepian healing, 211
Attachment theory and health
    anxious avoidant attachment, 50
    anxious resistant attachment pattern, 50
    borderline personality, 50
    careseeking and caregiving, 48–49
    secure attachment, 49–50
Attitude, 67, 104
Awareness, 64, 65, 85. *See also* Clinician
    self-awareness
Ayurvedic medicine (AM), 137

B

Borderline personality, 50, 52
Brain tumor, 214
Breast cancer, 28
Burnout (BO), 116–117

C

Caregiving
    breast cancer, 102
    depression, 104
    lung disease, 103
    lymphoma, 103
    medical practice and treatment, 102
Chronic disease, 210
Chronic kidney disease, 27
Chronic kidney failure, 210
Clinician self-awareness
    contemplative awareness, 121
    dual awareness, 120
    mindful self-awareness, 120
    practice, 123

    preparing the mind, 120
    self-empathy, 120
    self-knowledge, 119–120
Compassion, 150
    altruism, 63
    definition, 62
    HCP-patient sufferings comparison,
        63–64
    interconnectedness, 63
    mindfulness, 64
    self-compassion (*see* Self-compassion)
    self-reflection, 64
Compassion fatigue, 112
Complementary therapies (CT)
    ayurvedic medicine, 137
    health-promoting diet, 138–139
    integrative medicine
        hospital-based healthcare teams, 143
        interdisciplinary professional
            relationships, 142
        mixed method approach, 143
    medical treatment and patient
        emotions and beliefs, 135
        exclusion and inclusion criteria, 136
        healing, 134
        placebo effect, 136
        RCT, 134
        reductionist methods, 134, 136
    physical exercise, 139
    spiritual growth, 141–142
    stress management, 139–140
    symptom management, 140–141
    traditional Chinese medicine, 137

D

Death anxiety
    atherosclerosis, 100
    attitude and behavior, 104

Death anxiety (*Continued*)
  caregiving
      breast cancer, 102
      depression, 104
      lung disease, 103
      lymphoma, 103
      medical practice and treatment, 102
  distal defense, 99
  health-related behavior, 99
  human awareness, 105
  human emotions, 97
  humility and self-compassion, 106
  medical culture, 106
  meditation, 105
  mortality salience, 98
  proximal defense, 98
  religious faith, 101
  self-esteem, 100
  systemic lupus erythematosus, 6
  terror management function, 98
  unconscious death thought, 101
Dementia, 84, 89
Detached concern, 60–61
Dichotomies
  analog communication
      digital language, 40
      nonverbal manifestation, 40
      prosody, 40
  components, 37–38
  congruent physician-patient relationship,
      38–42
  curing and healing, 35
  diagnostic process, 32–33
  disease recognition and validation, 32
  double-blind randomized clinical trials, 35
  evidence-based medicine, 35–36
  externalization effect, alcoholism, 32
  face perception, 36–37
  first-rate intelligence test, 31
  Hippocratic *vs.* Asklepian
      clinical trials, 35
      communication, 40–41
      epistemology, 40, 41
  humanity, 32
  left/right cortical dichotomy, 36–37
  placating and blaming, 38–39
  Satir's communication stances, 38
  superreasonable stance communication, 40
  two therapeutic relationships, 33–35
  wave-like properties, 31
Doctor–patient relationship, 102. *See also*
      Words
Down syndrome/trisomy 18, 162

E
Empathic engagement, 112, 113
Empathy
  definition, 60
  detached concern, 60–61
  emotional attunement/resonance, 60, 62
  exquisite, 113
  HCP–patient interactions, 61
  limitations, 59
  mirror neurons, 61
  "not my job" phenomenon, 61–62
  overidentification, 62
  sympathy, 60
  trivialization risk, 61
End-stage kidney disease, 210
Ethology, 48–49
Evidence-based medicine, 174
Evidence-influenced medicine, 174
Exercise, 129
Exquisite empathy, 113

F
Fear, 225–227

G
Genetic counseling, 162–163
Genetic testing, 169–170
Genome-wide association studies
      (GWAS), 170
Glioblastoma, 213

H
Healing, 151, 184
  abusive relationship, 25
  alcoholism
      alcoholics anonymous, 24–25
      familial effects, 23
      healthcare workers, 26–27
      integrity and wholeness, 26
      terminal stage, 26
  Asklepian, 211
  breast cancer, 28–29
  Buddhism, 26
  chronic kidney disease, 27
  compassionate caregiving, 55–56
  complementary therapies, 134
  devastating problem, 25
  diagnostic categories, 23
  dilemma, 27
  dimensions, 24

healer-patient archetype, 29
healing factor, 29
kidney failure, dialysis, 26, 27
medicine, 26
mindfulness, 69, 77, 78
moment-to-moment basis, 25, 27
palliative care, 28
patients suffering, 29
professionalism, 204–205
psychosocial transition, 25
quality of life, 24, 25
quality of life dimension, 24, 25
self-care, 118–119
teaching in medical school, 184
walking placebo, 86–87
words, 85–104 (*see also* Words)
wounding and suffering, 25–26
Healthy diet, 129
Hippocratic curing, 211
Human vulnerability, 210
Humorism, vii
Huntington disease, 167

I
Intention, 67
Interconnectedness, 63
Intrinsic values, 153

L
Language
clinical setting, 83
diagnosis, 89–90
elderspeak, 88–89
military metaphor, 90–91
therapy failure, 92–93
words, 93–112 (*see also* Words)
Left/right cortical dichotomy, 36–37
Listen, 84

M
McGill Simulation Center, 196
Medical dichotomy, 211
Medical education, 153–154
Medical education, health care
       professionals
compassion (*see* Compassion)
empathy (*see* Empathy)
goal, 59
positive/negative connotation, 59–60
self-esteem (*see* Self-esteem)

Medical encounters
mindful, 72–74
mindless, 75–76
Medical genetics
contracting, 164
cystic fibrosis (CF), 164
Down syndrome/trisomy 18, 162
patient care, 166–167
patient readiness assessment, 165–166
risk assessment, 166
roadmap, 163
whole person care, 163
Medical ward
condolence letter, 178
continuous professional development, 177
emotional connection, 175
evidence-based medicine, 174
evidence-influenced medicine, 174
formal medical curriculum, 180
funeral visitation, 178
imaging technique, 173
informal/hidden curriculum, 179
Jean Dominique Bauby, 179
medical team-patient interaction, 175
narrative skill, 178
observation skills, 177
patient-centred care, 176
patient treatment, 173
role modelling, 180
teachable moment, 180
undergraduate medical school
       curricula, 176
Metaphor, 90–91
Military metaphor, 90–91
Mindful meditation, 142
Mindfulness, 64–67, 129
definition, 69
health care professionals training, 70–71
health care setting, 79–80
medical encounters
       mindful, 72–74
       mindless, 75–76
meditation, 120
mindful patients, 71–72
mindful practitioners, 69–70
multidisciplinary teams, 74–75
participatory medicine
       clinical encounter, 78, 79
       patient care and coping strategies,
               78–79
       physician-patient relationship,
               77–78
       rehabilitation, 78

physicians burnout *vs.* patient outcomes, 76
self-compassion, 70
twenty-first century
    barriers, 80–81
    mindful health care delivery, 77
Mindfulness-based stress reduction (MBSR), 72
Mortality, 210
Mortality salience (MS), 98
Myelodysplastic syndrome, 212

N
Narrative, 94
Nature of persons and clinical medicine
    adult pattern of behavior, 224–225
    anxiety, 225–226
    clinical knowledge, 219
    death, 227
    doctor-patient relationship, 219
    emotions, 223–224
    esthetic dimension, 221
    fear, 225
    hypnotic state, 224
    inner life, 224
    love, 220
    personal thought, 222
    physiological manifestation, 226
    reasoning and emotiveness, 223
    sensation, 222
    serious illness, 227
    sexual person, 220
    sickness, 221
    trusting relationship, 226
Neff Self-Compassion Scale, 74
Negative affective priming, 87
Nocebo effect, 86–87

O
Overidentification, 80

P
Palliative care, v. *See also* Whole person care
Participatory medicine
    clinical encounter, 78, 79
    patient care and coping strategies, 78–79
    physician-patient relationship, 77–78
    rehabilitation, 78
Patient-healthcare worker relationship, 209
Patient panel, 194
Patient-physician relationship, 191–193
Personal values, 153
Personhood, 152–153
Pharmacogenomics, 170

Phenylketonuria (PKU), 167
Physicianship, 190
Placebo effect, 85–87
Prayers, 151–152
Prevention
    Asklepian mode, 130
    cost-benefit ratio, 128
    diet, 131
    disease-focused measure, 127
    Hippocratic mode, 130
    meaning and connection, 129
    primary, 127
    quality of life, 131
    randomized trials, 131
    secondary, 128
    whole-body, 129
    whole person, 129
Prevention paradox, 127
Professionalism, and medical mandate
    doctor-patient relationship, 202
    healing, 204–205
    patient satisfaction, 201
    scientific medicine, 202
    social contract
        altruism, 206–207
        codes of ethics, 202–203
        commitment and presence, 206
        insight quality, 206–207
        medicine-society relationship, 203
        public-medical profession
            expectation, 206
        public policy, 202
        relief of suffering, 202
        trustworthiness, 206
    societal needs and expectation, 207

Q
Quality of life (QOL), viii, xi
    healing journey, 24, 25
    and spirituality, 158
    whole person prevention, 129, 131

R
Randomized controlled trial (RCT), 134, 136
Relief of suffering, 213
Religious belief, 154
Revolution in genetics
    BRCA mutation, 170
    chances, choices and tools for prevention
        breast or ovarian cancer, 168
        Huntington disease, 167, 169
        phenylketonuria, 167
        preselection process, 168

diagnostic and therapeutic
modality, 171
Garrodian model, 161–162
genetic counseling, 162–163
genetic testing, 169–170
homeostasis, 161
medical genetics
contracting, 164
cystic fibrosis, 164
Down syndrome/trisomy 18, 162
patient care, 166–167
patient readiness assessment,
165–166
risk assessment, 166
roadmap, 163
whole person care, 163
pharmacogenomics, 170
Ryff-Well-Being Scale, 74

S
Science-based healthcare, vii–viii
Secure attachment, 49–50
Self-care
burnout, 116–117
clinician self-awareness
contemplative awareness, 121
dual awareness, 120
mindful self-awareness, 120
practice, 123
preparing the mind, 120
self-empathy, 120
self-knowledge, 119–120
compassion fatigue, 112
discussion, 109
end-of-life care, 115–116
exquisite empathy, 113
healing connections and meaning-based
coping, 118–119
hospice medicine, 110–112
quality of lives, 109–110
rainmaker, 117–118
self-awareness-based model
organizational benefits, 122
proposed model, 121–122
soul and role, 118
wounded healer
psychodynamics, 114–115
recovery from trauma, 113
Self-compassion, 70
inner and outer dialogue, 65–66
kindness and understanding, 65
mindfulness, 66
vs. pity, 65
vs. self-esteem, 64–65

Self-esteem, 64–65, 100
Separation–attachment theory
attachment solution
anxious avoidant attachment, 50
anxious resistant attachment
pattern, 50
borderline personality, 50
careseeking and caregiving, 48–49
secure attachment, 49–50
compassionate caregiving and
implications
allostatic load, 55
healing, 55–56
stress response system, 55
cybernetic theory, 48
object relations theory
abandonment and engulfment, 52
aloneness, 52
ego relations, 50–51
fusion concept, 52
illusion, 51–52
mother–child interaction, 51
transitional phenomena, 51
separation challenges, illness
competent and compassionate, 47
Horton's view, 45–46
illness narratives, 46
limbic system, 47
paralimbic circuit, 47
physical illness crisis, 47
spiritual imperative
attachment security and insecurity, 54
attachment style, 54
healing, 53
internal working model, 54
linguistic analysis, 53–54
Silence, 88
Sleep, 129
Social contract, 216
altruism, 206–207
codes of ethics, 202–203
commitment and presence, 206
insight quality, 206–207
medicine-society relationship, 203
public-medical profession expectation, 206
public policy, 202
relief of suffering, 202
trustworthiness, 206
Sociolinguistics, 83
Soul and role, 118
Spiritual belief, 155
Spiritual dimensions
death, 156–157
healing, 151
medical education, 153–154

needs and concerns
  death, 155
  illness, 156
  religious belief, 154
  spiritual belief, 155
  suffering, 154
neglect in medicine, 149–150
obstacles in medical practice, 150
personhood, 152–153
prayer, 151–152
quality of life, 158
Spirituality, viii
Stress management, 129
Suffering, ix–xi
  bodies, 9
  integrity of the person, 10–11
  medicine goals
    body function, 16–17
    diagnosis, 20–21
    disorder, 17
    dying patient-family communication,
      18–19
    pathophysiology, 19–20
    person's well-being, 15–16
    sickness, 16–17
  pain, 10
  self-conflict, 11
  whole person
    accepted, valued and admired, 13
    in action, 12
    biological, physical, psychological,
      and spiritual, 13–14
    embodied and purposeful, 12
    empirical self, 14–15
    ever-present relationships, 13
    medicine, 11–12
    sickness, 12
    volitional, habitual and instinctual,
      12–13
Sympathy, 60

T
Talk, 87–106. See also Language
Teaching in medical school
  comprehensive curriculum, 198
  healing, 184
  McGill University experience
    cost of caring, 196–197
    ethics and professionalism, 194–195
    patient and physician perspective, 194
    patient-physician relationship, 191–193
    physician apprenticeship, 190
    physicianship, 190

relief of suffering, 191
team relationship, 195–196
medical education literature
  art of medicine, 185
  barrier, 188
  healing relationship, 187
  medical students, 186
  nonoverlapping magisteria principle,
    184–185
  patient-centered care, 188
  patient-centered method, 185
  reflection, 187
  self-care and altruism, 189
  whole person care program, 186
  working-learning-caring environment,
    189
mentoring relationship, 198
self-awareness and reflective practice, 197
skills training, 183
Therapeutic relationship, 210
Traditional Chinese medicine (TCM), 137, 143

W
Well-being, 129–131
Whole person care, xi
  admission criteria, 7–8
  disseminated germinal testicular cancer,
    101–202
  obstetrician and labor relationship, 6–7
  systemic lupus erythematosus
    clinical interactions, 3–4
    curing and healing, 4–5
    death anxiety, 6
    dialysis, 202
    dimensions, 3
    friendly interview, 3
    self-monitoring, 3
    transition state, 202
Words
  caregivers, 84
  clinical encounter, 83
  diagnosis, 89–90
  fighting against disease, 91–92
  geriatric baby talk, 88–89
  healing, 84–86
  interlocutor, 84
  patient shared concerns, 84–85
  silence, 88
  soft talk, 87–88
  verbal interactions, 83
Wounded healer
  psychodynamics, 114–115
  recovery from trauma, 113

Printed by Printforce, the Netherlands